Complications
Abortion's Impact on Women

By

Angela Lanfranchi

Ian Gentles

Elizabeth Ring-Cassidy

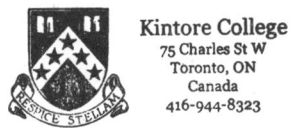

Kintore College
75 Charles St W
Toronto, ON
Canada
416-944-8323

The deVeber Institute for Bioethics and Social Research

Copyright 2013 by Angela Lanfranchi, Ian Gentles and Elizabeth Ring-Cassidy

All rights reserved. No part of this book may be reproduced, transmitted in any form or by any means, electronic, mechanical, photocopying, recording, or otherwise, or stored in a retrieval system, without written permission from the publisher, except by a reviewer who may quote brief passages in a review.

First published in 2013 by

The deVeber Institute for Bioethics and Social Research

415 Oakdale Road, Suite 215

Toronto M3N 1W7

Ontario, Canada

www.deveber.org   Email: bioethics@deveber.org   Phone: 416-256-0555

Cataloging data available from Library and Archives Canada.

ISBN 978-0-920453-36-0

Printed in Canada

Complications: Abortion's Impact on Women

Table of Contents

Preface and Acknowledgements   i

Introduction   1

I The Big Picture

    Abstract   5

1. Spiritual and psychological healing after abortion   9
2. Maternal and infant mortality: A global perspective   17
3. So many missing girls: Abortion and sex selection   45
4. Has abortion reduced the crime rate?   57
5. Informed consent: A woman's right   75

II The Medical Impact

    Abstract   89

6. Immediate physical complications of abortion: An overview   95
7. Biology and epidemiology confirm the abortion-breast cancer link   109
8. Prenatal testing and abortion for fetal anomaly   143
9. Physical complications: Infection and infertility   167
10. Physical complications: Injury, miscarriage, placenta previa   183

11. Physical complications: Autoimmune diseases	195
12. Physical complications: Maternal mortality from abortion	201
13. Medical or drug-induced abortion: How safe?	211
14. Multi-fetal pregnancy reduction (MFPR)	221
15. Premature or preterm births after abortion	235
16. Pain during and after abortion	247

III The Psychological and Social Impact

Abstract	253
17. Psychological outcomes: Abortion and family formation	257
18. Depression, suicide, substance abuse: Contested research	271
19. Intimate partner violence and abortion	285

IV Women's Voices

Abstract	301
20. Who are the experts? What 101 women told us	303
21. Women's voices: Narratives of the abortion experience	319
Conclusion: Abortion's impact on women	357
References	367
Glossary of terms	411
Index	421
About the Authors and the deVeber Institute's Contact Information	433

Preface and Acknowledgements

This book has been nearly ten years in the making. It arises out of a concern that the steadily growing body of information about the harmful complications of abortion for women and their subsequent children should become widely known. These complications are physical, psychological, social, and spiritual. In order to present direct evidence of the malaise brought on by abortion in contemporary society, we have included in our study the results of interviews of over 100 women who have undergone that experience. Words cannot express our gratitude to the women who shared with us the stories of their abortions.

Complications could not have been finished without the help of many people. We are deeply grateful to Deborah Zeni, MD, Will Johnston, MD, Rene Leiva, MD, Paul Ranalli, MD, David Reardon, PhD, Priscilla Coleman, PhD, Daniel Bader PhD, and Barbara McAdorey for their valuable contributions. Brent Rooney answered many questions about preterm births. We thank the Edward Jackman Foundation, as well as many private donors who financed the publication costs. Special thanks to Martha Crean and Lorraine McCallum who have worked tirelessly to perfect the book. Kathy Matusiak supplied indispensable administrative assistance. Jean Echlin, Mary Pon, Angelina Steenstra, Denise Mountenay and Patricia Dolente interviewed women about their abortions. We thank Bambi Rutledge for her continued support. A host of volunteers and summer student interns did an immense amount of research, writing, checking of references and other tasks. They include Petra Gombos, Nadia Tanel, Duc Mai, Raphael Ma, Elaine Drake, Elaine Zettel, Jennifer Zettel, Madeleine Gubbels, Katie Hanlon, Catherine Farrell, Peter O'Hagan, Regine Leung, Genevieve Bonomi, Shannon Brown, Barbara Farlow, Amy MacInnis, Safina Allidina, Thien-An Nguyen, Mary Webb, Adam Giancola, and Lorraine Smith-MacDonald. Brian Hurley, LLB, provided information about women who laid charges against their abortion providers. Paul Broughton and Aimée Rochard provided invaluable editorial support.

Finally, we gratefully acknowledge the commitment and labour of our Board of Directors, Advisors and Associates who ensured the Institute's completion of this work.

Introduction

For all three authors the driving force behind this book is the concern about the ill effects—largely unknown, and for the most part unpublicized—of induced abortion on women. *After several years of intensive research we are more than ever persuaded of the urgency of communicating this information to medical professionals, counsellors, and to women who are contemplating having an abortion.*

What we have written is based on rigorous research: more than 650 papers, mostly in medical and psychological journals, as well as a number of books and official publications. *Some of the findings are startling, and even counter intuitive.* Some of them contradict the statements of official bodies that have been charged with the responsibility of providing accurate information to women. Our chapter on breast cancer, for example, provides solid documentation, both biological and epidemiological, that challenges the National Cancer Institute's official position on the link between induced abortion, and the subsequent risk of breast cancer. We also provide solid documentation, from several countries, that challenges the statement of the American Psychological Association that induced abortion has no adverse psychological effects upon women.

It has also been assumed in many quarters that women's reproductive health cannot make real strides forward in countries where abortion is not available on request. Our investigation of women's health in countries that do not permit abortion on request, compared with those that do, does not bear out this assumption.

On the other hand, it is evident that the majority of women undergo induced abortion without experiencing any adverse consequences, physical or psychological. Yet there is disturbing evidence that the emotional impact of an abortion can lie dormant for decades, manifesting itself late in a woman's life. The last section of Chapter 20 contains a number of stories collected by palliative nurse Jean Echlin from women on their deathbeds who were haunted by abortions long past.

The wide practice of abortion has been attended by some unexpected and unfortunate consequences. In China, India and other countries ultrasound imaging has been used for 40 years or more to detect the sex of the child before birth, and to discard those who are unwanted. In the overwhelming majority of cases this has meant the elimination of female children and a consequently much higher ratio of males to females. There is evidence that sex-selective abortion is also occurring in North America.

Two economists have argued that the legalization of abortion in the US had the beneficent effect of reducing the crime rate. However, the same correlation was not found elsewhere, and other economists have suggested different reasons for the US decline in crime since the 1980s. In any case, the legalization of abortion has been accompanied by deleterious social consequences that have more than cancelled out any supposed beneficent effect on the crime rate.

In recent years informed consent has become an increasingly important issue in relation to abortion. In spite of the insistence of various official bodies that abortion has no negative consequences for women, several US states have passed "Right-to-know" laws, which have created difficulties for abortion providers who have failed to inform their clients of the risks surrounding abortion. In addition, *US courts have accepted the validity of the sworn testimony of thousands of women as to the negative impact abortion has had upon them.*

As we are coming to know, the physical consequences of surgical abortion are more widespread and serious than previously thought. The complication rate for chemically-induced abortions is much higher.

We are convinced that the biological and epidemiological evidence for a link between induced abortion and the later development of breast cancer is so overwhelming as to be irrefutable. We invite readers to review the evidence cited in Chapter 7 and judge for themselves.

Prenatal testing to detect genetic defects and anomalies in the fetus has become increasingly common. Unfortunately, the practice has not been accompanied by any increase in the support to parents, or to their children with genetic disorders. Still less is testing being used to prevent or treat illness and disability to help unborn children.

Concerning infertility, or subfecundity, there is limited but strong evidence that induced abortion is linked to an increase in both. Induced abortion also carries the risk of perforating the uterus and rendering the cervix incompetent. These complications can also result in infertility.

A recent paper in an influential American journal of obstetrics and gynecology has advanced the astonishing claim that abortion is safer for women than childbirth. This conclusion flies in the face of recent, massive studies in four countries showing that women who have abortions experience a sharply higher death rate than women who give birth.

Two recent systematic reviews have made it settled science that women who have *one or more abortions significantly increase their risk of later giving birth to a preterm or low birth weight child*. These children suffer from significantly higher rates of several disabilities, notably cerebral palsy, intellectual impairments and autism. The social cost of the increased rate of premature births due to abortion is immense.

On the psychological and social fronts, abortion has been found to have unfortunate consequences for the family. This is the subject of Chapter 16. The debate also continues to rage over abortion's impact on women's mental health. A recent meta-analysis published in the *British Journal of Psychiatry* concluded that women who had one or more abortions suffered an 81 per cent greater risk of mental health problems than women who did not. The author and her conclusions were subject to bitter criticism, but the editors upheld the validity of the paper, and their decision to publish it. Again, we invite readers to review the evidence presented in Chapter 17 and judge for themselves.

Another issue is *not* the subject of debate: the relationship between induced abortion and intimate partner violence. *Studies from across the world establish a strong correlation between induced abortion and intimate partner violence.* Plainly put, women who seek abortion are more likely to suffer physical abuse than those who do not. Why this should be so is the subject of Chapter 18.

We end this book by listening to what women themselves have to tell us about their abortion experience. Their stories are riveting and full of surprises. A common theme among stories told by 101 women to researchers from the de Veber Institute is regret at having the abortion and firm resolve never to have another. These stories, as well as many more from other sources, expose the illusion that abortion is a free choice and a liberating experience for women. In short, the narrative evidence from many women calls into the question the oft-repeated assertions by various experts, that abortion has minimal psychological effect upon women.

As we have indicated, the findings contained in this book will surprise, shock, and even provoke incredulity. Yet they are all based on extensive research in the scientific literature. Every important statement in this book is supported by a footnote reference, as well as an entry in the bibliography. Anyone with access to the internet will not find it difficult to follow up these references and check them for themselves. The authors will also be happy to answer any comments and enquiries that you the reader may have.

Angela Lanfranchi, Ian Gentles and Elizabeth Ring-Cassidy

Section I: The Big Picture

Abstract

Chapter 1, Spiritual and psychological healing after abortion, outlines the strides that have been made in recent years in bringing psychological and spiritual healing to women after induced abortion. For many women, the grief they experience is devastating.

It may manifest itself in symptoms of depression, anxiety, anger, coldness, suicidal thoughts, and resort to non-medical drugs. Grief can sometimes be suppressed for many years before it resurfaces.

Acknowledging grief is the first step in healing. But because abortion carries a social stigma, those who grieve often experience what is known as disenfranchised grief, in that they are not permitted to pour out their feelings to family or close friends. There are now many organizations, individuals and online resources that offer women assistance after an abortion. In addition, many books and self-help manuals have been written to help women along their path to healing and to furnish awareness to those providing support during the healing process.

Forgiveness too is an essential part of healing after abortion. It allows a woman to restore her relationship with herself, with the people around her, and for many women, with God. Forgiveness can also allow her to begin a new relationship with the child she has lost. Fortunately, the taboo against publicly acknowledging the distress caused by abortion is beginning to weaken. The reality of that distress, to which thousands of women have testified, is more and more recognized. These developments can only benefit the healing process.

Chapter 2 scrutinizes the widely-held assumption that maternal health can only improve where induced abortion is freely and legally available. There are at least four countries where abortion has been completely banned in the past two to three decades: Poland, Chile, El Salvador

Chapter 1:

Spiritual and psychological healing after abortion

Chapter 2:

Maternal and infant mortality: A global perspective

Chapter 2:

Maternal and infant mortality: A global perspective

and Nicaragua. These countries have not experienced any deterioration in maternal or infant health. In fact, the two largest—Poland and Chile—boast dramatic improvements. So have countries where abortion has long been unavailable, such as Ireland, Egypt and Uganda.

By contrast, the record of countries where abortion is freely available, such as the US, the UK, Russia, Hungary, Guyana and South Africa, have a notably worse record than nearby countries where abortion is illegal. These findings may be counter intuitive, and contradict the assumption that banning abortion will only drive women into the hands of illegal abortionists.

Why is this so? The reality seems to be that countries that do not allow abortion are much more likely to make sustained efforts to improve the quality of care for pregnant women and mothers. They offer better emergency obstetric care, transportation to emergency obstetric care, delivery by trained birth attendants, education for women, and better post-natal care for mothers and infants. The most dramatic strides forward have been in Chile and Poland. Maternal mortality in Chile plunged from 93 to 2 per 100,000 between 1960 and 2007. Childhood mortality from cerebral palsy in Poland declined from 20.4 to 2.4 per 100,000 live births between 1986 and 2006. In short, countries that do *not* offer abortion on request have a much better record of promoting maternal and infant health than countries that do.

Chapter 3:

So many missing girls: Abortion and sex selection

Chapter 3 explores a relatively new phenomenon: sex-selective abortion. Since the 1970s, ultra-sound imaging and amniocentesis have made it possible to detect the sex of the child before birth. The unexpected consequence of these new technologies has been the selection of babies of the unwanted, or "wrong" sex for abortion. This has led to skewed sex ratios in a number of countries, most notably China and India. Estimates of the numbers of female babies destroyed through sex-selective abortion in the past two to three decades are 160 million or higher. In China, the traditional preference for male children was exacerbated by the one-child policy, under which parents who had more than one child faced severe penalties, including forced abortion.

India too has cultural reasons for favouring sons to daughters, and since the 1990s the gap between male and female births has continued to widen. The same is true of other Asian countries such as Vietnam, Nepal and Korea. Only South Korea, by taking strong measures, has managed to rebalance its skewed sex ratios. Some Asian immigrants to the US and Canada have been found to practise a strong son preference, and a number resort to sex-selective abortion. It is sobering to reflect that beginning in the 1970s it was "western governments [that] actively promoted abortion and sex selection in the developing world, encouraging the liberalisation of abortion laws and subsidising sales of ultrasounds as a form of population control."[1]

Chapter 3:

So many missing girls: Abortion and sex selection

The rise of sex-selective abortion has produced an ethical dilemma for supporters of the unfettered right to procreative freedom. Is free choice the good that trumps all others, even when it leads to the deaths of hundreds of millions of female children before birth?

Another consideration is that sex-selective abortion, by causing a shortage of marriageable women, has had extremely negative social consequences, one of the most vicious being human trafficking.

Chapter 4 analyzes the assertion made by two American economists that legalizing abortion in the late 1960s and early 1970s caused a significant decline in the crime rate twenty years later. Their argument was that by eliminating unwanted children, abortion eliminated many people who, if born, would have become criminals from the late 1990s to now. This argument has been challenged on three grounds:

Chapter 4:

Has abortion reduced the crime rate?

1. The drop in the US crime rate can just as persuasively be linked to the decline in the cocaine/crack epidemic during the same period.

---

1   Pilkington E. Sex selection and the rise of Generation XY: A new book explores western involvement in what has become a scourge of the developing world: sex selection of babies. The Guardian. June 17, 2011.

Chapter 4:

Has abortion reduced the crime rate?

2. The United Kingdom, which also legalized abortion at about the same time, has seen crime rates rise rather than fall.

3. The great increase in the number of abortions in the US since legalization has been accompanied by a very large rise in the number of children born to single mothers. Single parenthood is associated with higher levels of child poverty, which has not been shown to have done anything to improve the crime rate.

Since the 1950s it has become a well-established principle in law that a physician is obliged to provide patients with information on the risks of a proposed medical procedure before embarking on it. This is known as the principle of informed consent, which is the subject of Chapter 5. The application of informed consent to abortion cases has been controversial.

Chapter 5:

Informed consent: A woman's right

Several states in the US have passed "Right-to-know" laws, requiring physicians to inform their patients about the risks connected with induced abortion, and about the alternatives. It has nevertheless proved difficult to bring suits against physicians or abortion providers for failure to inform women of the risks of the procedure. Courts have routinely ruled that, in the absence of physical injury, failure to inform a patient of possible psychological harm is not sufficient ground for a lawsuit.

Recently, however, "Right-to-know" laws in several American states have begun to create difficulties for abortion providers. Three cases in three different states have seen women win damages from their abortion providers for failing to inform them of the increased risk of developing breast cancer after abortion.

Chapter 1

Spiritual and psychological healing after abortion

> "I don't feel scared any more…I do believe that I can be forgiven. Isn't that great? A miracle at last!"

KEY POINTS

- Many women and families grieve deeply after an abortion, as with other pregnancy losses.

- Grief, which is not openly acknowledged, publicly mourned, or socially supported can become disenfranchised and complicated.

- Healing has many dimensions—physical, social, psychological, and spiritual.

- Each person heals in her own way and on a unique timeline.

- There are many resources and supports available to those seeking healing after abortion.

- Forgiveness is an essential step in healing after abortion.

- Many people find it helpful to memorialize and name the child.

INTRODUCTION

In this book we explore current research and personal stories about the impact of abortion on women and families. While there are similarities that can be statistically analyzed, each woman's experience of abortion is unique. Her reaction to her pregnancy, the reaction of those around her, her sense of herself and her purpose in life, her social situation, support offered to her or criticism, or conflict, judgment and coercion to abort will all influence whether she continues her pregnancy, or has an abortion.[1] These same factors influence her response after the abortion. Many women experience grief for the lost child. This grief may manifest itself in symptoms of depression, anxiety, anger, coldness, a resort to non-medical drugs, and suicidal thoughts. Abortion can be traumatic and feelings of grief can be suppressed for many years before resurfacing. However, some women can experience healing after abortion. In this chapter we explore that phenomenon of healing. We recognize too that not only women, but also fathers, siblings, grandparents, extended family and friends may grieve after an abortion.

Healing occurs on many levels. Physical healing is generally short term. Immediate complications that should be reported to a physician include excessive bleeding, fever and infection. Long-term complications arising from abortion have also been identified, and are discussed in Section II. Psychological and spiritual healing is often more complex and is related to the way that abortion has affected a particular woman. The decision to abort may involve friends, the father, and the woman's family, which means that healing of these relationships may be a necessary component of overall healing from an abortion. Because abortion involves a death, women often seek religious consolation and spiritual healing. A re-examination of moral and religious beliefs also occurs because abortion results from deliberate human action. There is no specific timeline for healing, which can occur at different times and in different ways throughout a woman's life.

HEALING AFTER PREGNANCY LOSS

Grief after abortion is like grief after other pregnancy losses. Unlike the loss of an older child or adult, loss during pregnancy is the loss of a child

---

1   Cozzarelli C, Sumer N and Major B. Mental models of attachment and coping with abortion. Journal of Personality and Social Psychology 1998 February; 74(2): 453-67.

that the parents, family and friends have not seen or touched. The grief felt, however, is very real. The Perinatal Bereavement Services of Ontario explains:

> When a pregnancy ends with miscarriage, ectopic pregnancy, medical termination, stillbirth or neonatal death, the parents may experience anger, hopelessness, lowered self esteem and other feelings. It is healthy and helpful to allow the parents to feel, name and express their emotions. Holding in feelings may cause delayed grief reactions. The shared grief felt by parents, families and friends will be expressed in different ways. No two people grieve alike.[2]

Those grieving the loss of a pregnancy may find support among family, friends and professionals. Some take part in individual or group therapy, and online support is available. Support is also offered during subsequent pregnancies as women continue to heal from previous losses during later pregnancies.

HEALING AFTER INDUCED ABORTION

Healing after induced abortion has both similarities to healing after miscarriage or stillbirth, and unique aspects. It is normal to grieve after an abortion, and to grieve the lost child. This grief is personal and each person experiences it differently and will take a different path to healing and finding peace.

Grief after abortion, however, is often disenfranchised, because the loss is not openly acknowledged, publicly mourned, or socially supported.[3] Because abortion carries a social stigma, those who grieve from it perceive little or no support from friends and family for their feelings of loss. They feel equally unable to express their desire to grieve to those who supported their choice, for fear (if not the actual experience) of being told there is nothing to grieve.[4] The prevailing view of abortion as a psychologically benign procedure[5] and the fierce political controversy surrounding it mean

---

2   Pregnancy and Infant Loss Awareness Network (PAIL Network). Pregnancy and infant loss: about us. PAIL Network 2012. www.pailnetwork.ca .
3   Speckhard A and Rue V. Complicated mourning: dynamics of impacted post abortion. Pre- and Peri-natal Psychology Journal 1993; 8(1): 5-32.
4   Ibid., p. 16.
5   This is the current position of the American Psychological Association (APA).

that the grief of those who have suffered abortion is often unacknowledged or dismissed. This disenfranchisement of grief can further complicate it.[6] Complicated grief occurs when the painful emotions of sorrow, numbness, guilt and anger following a loss are long lasting and do not resolve in acceptance of the loss. Instead they continue to debilitate and interfere with the life of the grieving person.[7] Openly acknowledging the loss that occurs with abortion and the grief accompanying that loss is the first step in healing.

In certain situations, the risk of complicated grief may be particularly high. In one study of women who aborted after learning of an adverse prenatal diagnosis, 25 per cent became critically affected after the loss, while 13.7 per cent continued to experience complicated grief fourteen months after the abortion. Kersting recommended developing specific interventions and programs to prevent that grief.[8] Increasingly, the medical and counselling communities are identifying women's need for assistance after abortion as more research shows the psychological risks, and as women seek help for themselves.

HEALING—A JOURNEY

An important part of grieving after abortion is for a woman to tell the story of her pregnancy and abortion. It can require great courage and strength for a woman to do this, and allow herself to feel the pain of grief. She may seek assistance when she is ready to tell her story, or she may need first to listen to others' stories and be assisted with other symptoms that she is experiencing, before being ready to share her own story. There are many organizations, individuals and online resources that offer assistance after an abortion. These services are available on both a short and long-term basis. It should be stressed that women who experience thoughts of suicide should immediately seek professional help. Psychotherapy can be helpful especially for women who are experiencing complicated grief or for those struggling with destructive behaviours, or severe anxiety or depression. Through individual counselling or group discussion women find support to explore their emotions, build support networks around them, and find

---

6   Speckhard and Rue. See n. 3, p. 16.
7   Mayo Clinic. Complicated grief. December 2012. http://www.mayoclinic.com/health/complicated-grief/DS01023.
8   Kersting A, Kroker K, Steinhard J, Ludorff K, Wesselmann U, Ohrmann P, Arolt V and Suslow T. Complicated grief after traumatic loss: a 14-month follow up study. European Archives of Psychiatry and Clinical Neuroscience 2007 December; 257(8): 437-43.

forgiveness and peace. For some, the anonymity of visiting websites that offer online support is preferable, and this can also be a simple and convenient way to take the first step towards healing. Women may rely on a variety of forms of assistance at different stages of their healing journey. By telling the story of her abortion and beginning to explore her emotions about that event, a woman embarks on a journey that helps her to find peace, and decrease the suffering she may still be experiencing.

Abortion Recovery International (ARIN) is an international affiliate organization that connects abortion recovery centres, programs and services. Its affiliates must provide services that are "personal, confidential, non-judgmental and open to all."[9] ARIN encourages individuals and families to seek out care that is confidential, does not pressure them to tell their story, provides a prompt response to inquiries, has no political component, is respectful and professional, and avoids "quick fixes." They provide referral to counselling services in both the United States and Canada.

Some other major organizations that offer healing after abortion include:

- Lumina, which offers group therapy, retreats, referrals to professional therapists for one-on-one therapy, and a network of people who have experienced abortion.

- Rachel's Vineyard, which offers weekend retreats and weekly support groups, in addition to training for mental health professionals.

- Ramah International, which promotes Christian post-abortion ministry and offers resources that can be used by recovery groups.

- Project Rachel, which provides post-abortion outreach through the Catholic Church, making local referrals to trained therapists, clergy, retreats and support groups.

Pregnancy resource centres and crisis pregnancy centres often host abortion support groups. These centres can be found locally or through Optionline.[10]

---

9   Abortion Recovery International (ARIN). About us: principles of care. Abortion Recovery International: Restoring Lives and Relationships after Abortion. 2013. http://www.abortionrecovery.org/aboutus/principlesofcare/tabid/247/Default.aspx.
10   www.optionline.org, or 1-800-712-HELP.

Online support is available through many websites, including Abortion Changes You (abortionchangesyou.org), which guides the reader through pathways to healing.

In addition, many books and self-help manuals have been written on this topic, designed to help the reader along her path to healing and to provide awareness to those providing support during the healing process.

Whether they receive support through group therapy or one-on-one therapy, online resources or print materials, women who have had abortions are encouraged to continue seeking healing using a variety of means until their symptoms lessen, their depression or anxiety eases up, their self-destructive behaviours end, and their relationships are restored.

FORGIVENESS

Forgiveness is considered an essential part of healing after abortion. Many women have unresolved feelings of shame and guilt arising from the volitional nature of abortion. It can be painful to revisit and re-evaluate the decisions that they and the people around them made that led to the abortion. Both pro-abortion and anti-abortion women report that the act of forgiveness is a very important step in the healing process.[11]

Christian Counselling

Christian counsellors assure women of God's mercy and forgiveness towards those who genuinely desire it. The woman must not only accept external forgiveness, but in turn forgive herself, as well as the other people involved in the abortion.[12]

Project Rachel, the Catholic Church's approach to healing after abortion, recommends that those who counsel women after abortion:

> affirm her courage in seeking healing, acknowledging how difficult it can be to talk about decisions that evoke guilt and shame, and how difficult it is to reveal the painful emotional and behavioral

---

11 Hess RF. Healing after abortion: a search for forgiveness. Journal of Christian Nursing 2009; 26(3): 154-8.

12 Wilson BK and Haynie L. Experiences of women who seek recovery assistance following an elective abortion: a grounded theory approach. DNS dissertation, Louisiana State University Health Sciences Center School of Nursing, 2004.

consequences of having made poor choices.[13]

Project Rachel lists other steps towards healing after abortion, which can include, in no particular order: recounting one's story, dissipating anger, forgiving others, understanding abortion and accepting it as the death of her child, grieving for the lost child, remembering or considering the child's sex, naming the child, beginning a new relationship with the child, surrendering her child to God, memorializing the child, assurance of God's mercy, and self-forgiveness.[14]

Japanese Buddhist "Mizuko"

Japanese Buddhist tradition includes the mizuko kuyo ritual for post-pregnancy loss, which requires a full apology from the parents to make amends to an aborted child. Mizuko means water child, referring to a baby that was conceived and lived in the womb but was not born alive. "In contrast to the child in darkness because of an ordinary miscarriage or by natural death after being born, the child here discussed is in its present location because its parents took active steps to prevent it from being born alive in our world. If the parents merely carry out ordinary memorial rites but fail to make a full apology to their child, their mizuko will never be able to accept their act."[15]

Forgiveness allows a woman to restore her relationship with herself, the people around her, and her God. It can also allow her to begin a new relationship with the child she has lost, and continue the grieving process.

MEMORIALIZING THE CHILD

In restoring their relationship with the child, women often find healing by writing a letter to their child, and naming him or her. Some choose to remember their aborted child in a more public way. In the United States there is a National Memorial for the Unborn where families can share their grief with others who have suffered a similar loss and name plaques are

---

13   United States Conference of Catholic Bishops (USCCB), Committee on Clergy, Consecrated Life, and Vocations. *Project Rachel Ministry: a post-abortion resource manual for priests and Project Rachel leaders.* Washington, DC: USCCB, 2009: p. 14.
14   Project Rachel Ministry. See n. 13, pp. 15-20.
15   Wilson JT. Mourning the unborn dead: American usage of Japanese Buddhist post-abortion rituals. PhD Dissertation [Unpublished], University of North Carolina at Chapel Hill, 2007. http://udini.proquest.com/view/mourning-the-unborn-dead-american-goid:304844080/.

mounted to memorialize aborted babies.[16] In Japan and Taiwan there are mourning rooms in temples and programs to help parents grieve and atone for abortions.[17] Memorializing the child can help women and families to find peace after the loss from abortion.

Pregnancy loss, particularly if caused by a medical or surgical abortion, can be a very difficult experience. It is unique for each individual; hence, grieving and healing occur in different ways and on different timelines for each person. Healing and peace is attainable, and with appropriate assistance women are able to restore their relationships with themselves, their child, God and the people around them. Today there are more counsellors and programs available than ever before, and every day women are journeying towards healing after abortion. The remainder of this book reports the latest medical, psychological and sociological evidence about the effects of abortion, as well as the stories of many women who have experienced abortion first hand. The topic is controversial, and discussion of the research presented in the following chapters is often avoided, especially in North America. But the voices of women who have had abortions cannot be silenced. Attempting to deny their narratives will only hinder the healing process for these women and their families. While we document much bias in recent research, we do not promote any specific political or religious approach. Our aim is to share the stories accurately, to summarize research findings honestly, and to offer clarity and real hope to those who are suffering. Their emotional and spiritual agony is often acute, but so is the peace that can be found when it is recognized and women are helped on their journey towards healing.

---

16   National Memorial for the Unborn. 2010. http://www.memorialfortheunborn.org/tabid/55/default.aspx.
17   Thorn V. Project Rachel: Faith in action, a ministry of compassion and caring. In *Post-abortion aftermath*, ed. Mannion M, Kansas City, MO: Sheed and Ward, 1994: 144-63.

Chapter 2

Maternal and infant mortality: A global perspective

KEY POINTS

- Based on official statistics, four countries that have banned abortion in the past two decades (Poland, Chile, El Salvador, Nicaragua) have experienced dramatic improvements in maternal and infant health.

- Countries where legal abortion has long been unavailable (Ireland, Egypt, Uganda) have done significantly better at maintaining or improving maternal and infant health than neighbouring countries where abortion is legal on request.

- The record of the US, the UK, Russia and Hungary, where abortion is legal, has been generally worse than nearby countries where there is restricted access to abortion.

- The keys to reducing maternal mortality include:
    - Skilled attendance at birth
    - Improved education for women
    - Emergency obstetric care (including caesarean sections)
    - Transportation for emergency obstetric care
    - Community outreach
    - Improved referral systems

Introduction

Maternal mortality is generally defined as "the death of a woman while pregnant or within 42 days of termination of pregnancy, regardless of the site or duration of pregnancy, from any cause related to or aggravated by the pregnancy or its management."[1] World-wide maternal mortality has declined significantly over the past three decades, from an estimated 526,300 deaths in 1980 to 342,900 in 2008. Expressed as a maternal mortality ratio (MMR), maternal deaths shrank from 320 to 251 per 100,000 live births.[2] The leading causes of maternal mortality are hemorrhage (bleeding) and hypertension (high blood pressure).[3]

Unsafe abortion is defined as "a procedure for terminating an unintended pregnancy carried out either by persons lacking the necessary skills or in an environment that does not conform to minimal medical standards, or both."[4] Unsafe abortion has been labelled as a significant contributor to maternal mortality worldwide. The World Health Organization (WHO) estimates that every year between 60,000 and 75,000 maternal deaths are caused by unsafe abortion, or about thirteen per cent of all maternal deaths worldwide. They further estimate that five million additional women require medical care as a result of unsafe abortions.[5]

If these estimates are reliable, it might seem that legalized abortion would go a long way towards reducing the health burden of unsafe abortion, thereby reducing maternal mortality in general.[6]

---

1 World Health Organization (WHO). Maternal mortality ratio (per 100 000 live births). Health Statistics and Health Information Systems. http://www.who.int/healthinfo/statistics/indmaternalmortality/en/index.html.
2 Hogan MC, Lopez AD, Lozano R, et al. *Building momentum: global progress toward reducing maternal and child mortality.* Seattle, Washington: Institute for Health Metrics and Evaluation, 2010: 1-84, p. 7.
3 Khan KS, Wojdyla D, Say L, Gulmezoglu AM and Paul FA. WHO analysis of causes of maternal death: a systematic review. The Lancet 2006 April; 367(9516): p. 1072.
4 Department of Reproductive Health and Research, World Health Organization (WHO). *Unsafe abortion: global and regional estimates of incidence of unsafe abortion and associated mortality in 2008,* 6th ed, Geneva: WHO , 2007: p. 1.
5 Ibid., p. 14.
6 Singh S. Hospital admissions resulting from unsafe abortion: estimates from 13 developing countries. The Lancet 2006 November; 368(9550): 1887-92; Johnston HB, Gallo MF and Benson J. Reducing the costs to health systems of unsafe abortions: a comparison of four strategies. Journal of Family Planning and Reproductive Health Care 2007; 33(4): 250-7.

However, the relationship between legality and safety is not that clear. Ninety-eight per cent of what WHO defines as "unsafe abortions" occur in developing countries, since industrialized countries tend to have more permissive abortion laws.[7] One study attempts to link high MMR to countries with restrictive laws—nevertheless, the author also notes that "countries in any of the six categories that have a high mortality ratio due to unsafe abortion are likely to be those with the least effective and accessible health care services, making complications and deaths from unsafe abortion more likely."[8] In other words, the countries that have the most deaths from abortion also tend to be the countries that have worse health care in general, higher levels of maternal mortality and mortality in general, and lower incomes than countries with low levels of abortion-related death.

What is surprising is that for many countries, the link between legal abortion and improved maternal mortality, even MMR related to abortion, is the reverse of what its advocates claim. Countries that have legalized abortion such as South Africa and Guyana have not seen the predicted maternal health benefits. By contrast, several countries that have disallowed abortion, such as Chile, El Salvador, Nicaragua, Egypt, and Uganda, have seen significant reductions in maternal mortality. The major factors involved are improvements in general maternal care, especially in emergency obstetric care (EmOC), the attendance of skilled health workers at birth, and advancements in women's status and education. Provision of safe, legal abortion has not been a factor in these countries' success.

Moreover, research on abortion that refers to high levels of unsafe abortions and subsequent deaths contains various limitations that undermine its conclusions. Estimates of abortion incidence and complications due to them can be very difficult to arrive at for some developing countries owing to a lack of recorded data, and so researchers end up having to make assumptions and extrapolations from what data they are able to collect. In addition, distinguishing complications due to spontaneous abortions from those due to induced abortions is extremely difficult, and some researchers make dubious assumptions, which in turn affect their numbers.[9]

---

7   Dabash R and Rhoudi-Fahimi F. *Abortion in the Middle East and North Africa.* Washington, DC: Population Reference Bureau, 2008: p. 1.
8   Berer M. Global perspectives—national laws and unsafe abortion: the parameters of change. Reproductive Health Matters 2004 November; 12(24 Supplement): 1-8, p. 4.
9   Prada E, Mirembe F, Ahmed FH, Nalwadda R and Kiggundu C. Abortion and postabortion care in Uganda: a report from health care professionals and health facilities. Guttmacher Institute, 2005; p. 10; Berer 2004. See n. 8, 1-8.

As we shall see, there is abundant evidence that legalized abortion is not a requirement for improving women's health. Several countries have already adopted effective means of reducing maternal deaths and advancing maternal health, without including abortion in the mix. Given the countless documented problems with the abortion procedure even where it is legal and supposedly "safe", and given the evidence presented below that maternal health initiatives work best without an abortion component, the conclusion is inescapable: the case for including abortion in maternal health initiatives is unproven.

SOUTH AMERICA—THE CASE OF CHILE

Chile has become a focus for studies on maternal health. Compared to other countries in the Americas, it has one of the lowest rates of maternal mortality.[10] Abortion has also been completely illegal in Chile since 1989.[11] In the last half century, Chile has experienced a major decrease in maternal health mortality, indicating that legalized abortion is not necessary to achieve a low maternal mortality ratio. Similar findings have been observed in two Central American countries that have made abortion illegal: El Salvador and Nicaragua.[12]

Chile is a country that has undergone significant changes to its health care services following a reform in the 1980s. The government transformed the ways in which health services were organized and were made accessible to the public. Notably, in the 1980s free delivery was made universal in Chile.[13] Koch found that the maternal mortality ratio was reduced by two main factors: increased education for women and better health care in

---

10 Ruiz-Rodríguez M, Wirtz VJ and Nigenda G. Organizational elements of health service related to a reduction in maternal mortality: The cases of Chile and Colombia. Health Policy 2009 November; 90(2-3): 149-55.
11 Population Division of the United Nations Secretariat. Abortion policies: a global review—Chile. United Nations Population Division Department of Economic and Social Affairs, 2002. Online edition: http://www.un.org/esa/population/publications/abortion/index.htm.
12 Leiva R. Illegal abortion and safety: the case of El Salvador (Letter in response to "Transparency in the delivery of lawful abortion services" by Rebecca J. Cook). CMAJ 2009, February 3. Accessed 25 July, 2012: http://www.cmaj.ca/content/180/3/272/reply#cmaj_el_53631?sid=e3298cf7-d9ea-4e90-9711-ec808ccf37ae; Mendieta W, Bohemer L and Cabrera RJ. Nicaragua and abortions (Letter). Washington Times. December 20, 2007.
13 Population Division of the United Nations Secretariat. Abortion policies: a global review. United Nations Population Division Department of Economic and Social Affairs, 2002.

general.[14]

Chile furnishes an excellent case study of the experience of maternal and abortion mortality *after* the complete banning of induced abortion.[15] It is also instructive to compare Chile with other South American countries that allow abortion on request, such as Guyana.[16]

Chile and Guyana: A Statistical Comparison

In a similar span of time, Guyana and Chile have adopted very different abortion laws, providing two interesting case studies. Induced abortion was legal in Chile from 1931 to 1988, but only to save the life of the mother. In 1989, it was made illegal in all cases.[17] In Guyana, abortion was completely prohibited by the Criminal Law Act up until 1995 when it was made legal on request.[18]

A recent paper in *The Lancet* provides estimates of MMRs between 1980 and 2008 for 181 countries, and plots their trends.[19] Chile had 70 maternal deaths per 100,000 live births in 1980, falling to 21 deaths per 100,000 live births in 2008, a drop of 70 per cent.[20] Guyana, by contrast, had an MMR of 216 per 100,000 live births, in 1980, falling to 143 per 100,000 live births in 2008, a decline of only 32 per cent.[21] Thus, with a complete ban on abortion, Chile has been able to achieve a much lower MMR than Guyana, which continues to experience serious maternal health problems.

Chile can also be analyzed as a singular case of maternal and abortion mortality before and after the complete banning of abortion.[22] A recent study assessed time series of both maternal and abortion mortality ratios

---

14   Koch E, Thorp J, Bravo M, Gatica S, Romero CX, Aguilera H and Ahlers I. Women's education level, maternal health facilities, abortion legislation and maternal deaths: a natural experiment in Chile from 1957 to 2007. PLoS ONE 2012 May; 7(5): e36613; Schuberg K. Abortion ban does not mean more maternal deaths, Chilean study finds. *CNS News*. 25 July 2012. http://cnsnews.com/news/article/abortion-ban-does-not-mean-more-maternal-deaths-chilean-study-finds.
15   Leiva. See n. 12.
16   Koch et al. See n. 14.
17   Ibid.
18   Ibid.
19   Hogan MC, Foreman KJ, Naghavi M, et al. Maternal mortality for 181 countries 1980-2008: a systematic analysis of progress toward Millennium Development Goal 5. The Lancet 2010 April; 375(9726): 1609-23.
20   Ibid.
21   Ibid., p. 1615.
22   Koch et al. See n. 14.

from 1960 to 2007.[23] MMRs were highest in 1961, at which point 34 per cent of maternal deaths were due to abortion. Over the entire period, however, MMRs decreased by 94 per cent (from 294 to 18 per 100,000 live births), and abortion mortality ratios decreased by 98 per cent (from 93 to less than two per 100,000 live births). Far from interrupting these decreases in maternal mortality, the complete banning of abortion in 1989 seems only to have accelerated them.[24]

After 1989, the MMR fell by over half, from 41 to eighteen per 100,000 live births. The abortion mortality ratio fell from 16.5 to 1.7 per 100,000 live births—a drop of almost 90 per cent. Therefore, it is clear that the complete ban on abortion in Chile has been accompanied by even more rapid improvements in maternal health and mortality than before the ban.

Chile has achieved striking success in improving maternal health. Furthermore, very little of what maternal mortality remains is due to abortion.[25] Out of the 44 maternal deaths in Chile in 2007, four were attributed to abortion. Of these four, two were due to ectopic pregnancy complications and two were unspecified.[26] Thus, abortion has had little impact on improving maternal mortality levels.

Discussion of Chile's Success

Why has a relatively poor country like Chile achieved such a dramatic success in improving maternal health and reducing maternal mortality from induced abortion? Education is a critical factor. In a recent study researchers observed "…a direct association between women's education levels and declining MMRs (maternal mortality ratios)."[27] This finding was reaffirmed by a preliminary study by Koch on the impact of abortion legalization on maternal mortality. Increased education for women seems to have the greatest impact on maternal mortality reduction, with decreasing MMRs corresponding to women's increased years of education. Education was also associated with a decreasing fertility rate, and in improving quality of health care facilities.[28]

Other factors, such as improved care before delivery, delivery by trained

---

23 Leiva. See n. 12.
24 Ibid.
25 Koch et al. See n. 14.
26 Ibid.
27 Gonzalez R, Requejo JH, Nien JK, Merialdi M, Bustreo F and Betran AP. Tackling health inequities in Chile: maternal, newborn, infant, and child mortality between 1990 and 2004. American Journal of Public Health 2009; 99(7): 1220-6, p. 1225.
28 Leiva. See n. 12.

birth attendants and emergency obstetric care, all play an important role in overall maternal health.[29] In the words of Ruiz-Rodriguez and colleagues, "…there is clear evidence that—when adjusting for country income level—provision of, and access to, maternal health care services, particularly emergency obstetric care, are associated with a reduction in maternal mortality."[30] Ruiz-Rodriguez and colleagues also found that the quality of maternal care was directly influenced by the amount of training received by birth attendants and maternal care providers. In Chile, midwives must complete a four-year university degree and by 2009, a health professional was present at over 90 per cent of births in the country.[31]

In addition to proper training for health providers, it is essential that these providers be available throughout the country, not just in urban clinics. By 1992, in Chile, "…the midwife was one of the professional health cadres that was most closely correlated with the geographic distribution of the population."[32] Therefore geographic accessibility to services and having well-trained birth attendants are crucial factors in maintaining excellent maternal health in Chile. The example of Chile suggests that other poor countries are capable of similar improvements. Gonzalez and colleagues note that "the observed decreasing mortality trends suggest that increasing access to health care services among populations most in need can translate into significant reductions in maternal and child mortality."[33]

EL SALVADOR AND NICARAGUA

In 1997, a new penal code was enacted in El Salvador that removed all grounds for induced abortion. Before the criminalization of abortion the MMR was 155 per 100,000 live births. By 2006 it was 71 per 100,000 live births, a drop of more than 50 per cent.[34]

A 2006 study carried out by the Ministry of Health in El Salvador determined that out of 2,468 maternal deaths only six were connected to abortion, two of which were due to ectopic pregnancies. In other words, almost no maternal deaths were related to abortion. They were caused by simple complications that could have been easily prevented by providing

---

29   Ibid.
30   Ruiz-Rodríguez et al. See n. 10, p. 150.
31   Ibid., p. 150.
32   Ibid., p. 152.
33   Gonzalez et al. 2009. See n. 27, p. 1224.
34   Mendieta et al. See n. 12.

education and resources for the pregnant women in question.[35]

The experience of Nicaragua has been similar. In November 2006, the government of Nicaragua passed an absolute ban on abortion. Within a year, maternal mortality decreased by 23 per cent.[36] The majority of maternal deaths were caused by treatable conditions, such as post-birth hemorrhaging.[37] The experiences of El Salvador and Nicaragua provide additional evidence that countries that ban abortion outright do not experience major increases in maternal mortality.

THE ACHIEVEMENTS OF EGYPT

Egypt provides another notable success story in the battle against maternal mortality. In a 1992-93 study, the country's maternal mortality ratio was calculated at 174 for every 100,000 live births. Through a series of initiatives during the 1990s, the Egyptian government worked to improve maternal health care and women's well-being. By 2000, the MMR had plunged by 52 per cent, to 84 per 100,000 live births.[38] There was also a reduction in deaths due to induced abortion, from the already low total of 13 (representing two per cent of maternal deaths) in 1992-93 to six (one per cent), a decline of over 50 per cent, mirroring the overall decline in the country's maternal mortality ratio.[39]

Several factors contributed to this decline. Crucially important was skilled attendance at birth. In addition, "the network of adequate essential obstetric care and primary health care facilities has been improved, and long distance to a hospital and lack of transportation are now less of a barrier to care."[40] These interventions had already begun in the mid 1980s in Egypt. By the 1990s, the major avoidable factor causing maternal deaths was substandard care.[41]

Since 2000, the MMR in Egypt has declined even further, to 43 per

---

35 Ibid.
36 Ibid.
37 Ibid.
38 Campbell O, Gipson R, Issa EH, et al. National maternal mortality ratio in Egypt halved between 1992-93 and 2000. Bulletin of the World Health Organization 2005; 83(6): 462-71, p. 462.
39 Khadr Z. Monitoring socioeconomic inequity in maternal health indicators in Egypt: 1995-2005. International Journal for Equity in Health 2009 November; 8(38): p. 38.
40 Campbell et al. See n. 38, p. 469.
41 Khadr. See n. 39.

100,000 live births in 2008.[42] Again, maternal health service provision was crucial to this reduction. There was skilled delivery at 71 per cent of births in 2005.[43] A real improvement in women's socioeconomic status and education during the past twenty years has also been noted: "illiteracy among women aged fifteen and older declined thirteen percentage points; [the] gross enrolment ratio for basic and secondary education increased from 79 per cent in 1996 to 88 per cent in 2004; and enrolment in secondary education increased from 44.1 per cent in 1996 to 70.1 per cent in 2006."[44]

Abortion Law in Egypt

Abortion is illegal in Egypt except to preserve the life of the mother. Maternal mortality due to abortion is low, and declined even faster than the general decline in MMR, from two per cent of maternal deaths to one per cent. However, there is evidence that abortion still accounts for a significant number of medical complications. A 1998 study revealed that nineteen per cent of all obstetric and gynecological admissions to health facilities were due to abortion, and that the abortion case fatality rate for these institutions was 0.43 per cent. However, when the spontaneous abortions (35 per cent) are deducted, only 12.3 per cent of obstetric and gynecological admissions were for complications arising from induced abortion. Furthermore, most of these complications were not severe, requiring less than a day's stay in hospital.

Another study relating to abortion found that 21.9 per cent of the women interviewed required medical assistance for their last abortion.[45] However, the study made no differentiation between spontaneous and induced abortions, so it is impossible to determine the effects of induced abortion from these findings.

To summarize, Egypt has succeeded in significantly reducing maternal mortality from abortion while maintaining a highly restrictive abortion law. The country's success stems from its advances in emergency obstetric care, attendance of skilled personnel during birth, and general improvements in women's education and well being over the past thirty years. Despite recent turmoil, Egypt is a stellar example of a poor country that has progressively bettered its women's health while remaining steadfast in its refusal to sanction abortion.

---

42   Hogan, Lopez, Lozano, et al. See n. 2, p. 61.
43   Khadr. See n. 39.
44   Ibid.
45   Yassin KM. Incidence and socioeconomic determinants of abortion in rural Upper Egypt. Public Health 2000; 114(4): 269-72, p. 270.

A Bright Light Against a Bleak Background: Uganda and the Soroti District

Uganda is one of the poorest countries in the world. This poverty is reflected in its health system that, in spite of improvements over the past fifteen years, is still woefully inadequate.[46] Only 40 per cent of births in Uganda are performed in a health facility, and postpartum care—critically important for maternal and child health—is negligible.[47]

Maternal mortality is difficult to estimate because of the lack of solid data, but by all accounts it is grim. Yet surprisingly, there are some indications that it may be improving. A 2010 report estimates that Uganda's maternal mortality ratio has decreased from 604 per 100,000 live births in 2000 to 352 in 2008.[48] The Uganda Demographic and Health Survey for 2006 also documented an apparent decrease, from 527 maternal deaths per 100,000 in the decade prior to 1995 to 435 for the ten-year period prior to 2006.[49] These findings are not conclusive, however.[50]

Abortion in Uganda

Abortion in Uganda is illegal except to preserve the life or health of the mother.[51] Although abortion is thought to be widely practiced underground in Uganda, we will see that these estimates of abortion's prevalence can be called into question.[52] Nevertheless, complications from abortion account for a substantial proportion of obstetric admissions to hospitals and health centres.[53]

---

46   Orinda V, Kakande H, Kabarangira J, Nanda G and Mbonye AK. A sector-wide approach to emergency obstetric care in Uganda. International Journal of Gynecology and Obstetrics 2005; 91: 285-91.
47   Uganda Bureau of Statistics (UBOS) and Macro International Inc. Uganda demographic and health survey 2006. Calverton, Maryland, USA: UBOS and Macro International Inc., 2007; p. xxiv.
48   Hogan, Foreman, Naghavi, et al. See n. 19, p. 1618.
49   Uganda Bureau of Statistics (UBOS) and Macro International Inc. See n. 47, pp. 281-2.
50   Ibid., p. xxviii.
51   Population Division of the United Nations Secretariat. Abortion policies: a global review—Uganda. United Nations Population Division Department of Economic and Social Affairs, 2002.
52   They estimate about 297,000 induced abortions occur yearly, but this estimate is open to question. Singh S, Prada E, Mirembe F and Kiggundu C. The incidence of induced abortion in Uganda. IFPP 2005 December; 31(4): 183-91.
53   Okong P, Byamugisha J, Mirembe F, Byaruhanga R and Bergstrom S. Audit of severe maternal morbidity in Uganda—implications for quality of obstetric care. Acta Obstetricia et Gynecologica Scandinavica 2006; 85(7): 797-804; Mbonye AK, Mutabazi MG, Asimwe JB, Sentumbwe O, Kabarangira J, Nanda G and Orinda V. Declining maternal mortality ratio in Uganda: priority interventions to achieve the Millennium Development Goal. International Journal of Gynaecology and Obstetrics 2007 July; 98(3): pp. 287-8.

A study and report by Singh and colleagues estimated that in Uganda, 84,758 women per year experience complications from abortion.[54] Of these, anywhere from 23 to 50 per cent are due to spontaneous abortion.[55] A comprehensive study by Mbonye and colleagues found that abortion accounted for eleven per cent of direct obstetric deaths.[56]

It is impossible to say whether this represents a decrease in Uganda's rate of deaths due to abortion, given the smallness of the 1992-1993 study that Singh and colleagues cited.[57] Nevertheless, the findings of Mbonye and colleagues definitely challenge the assumption of high rates of death due to abortion, even while confirming high rates of complications due to abortion. This may mean either that women presenting with complications after abortion are not as ill as women presenting with, say, hemorrhage, or else that Ugandan hospitals are better able to provide care for post-abortal women so that they do not die as frequently. Either way, in Mbonye's study, abortion had the lowest case fatality rate of all the direct obstetric complications (0.6, in contrast to a case fatality rate for all obstetric complications of 2.2). We shall now examine one region within the country that has seen a large reduction in maternal mortality.

A Success Story: The District of Soroti

In the midst of a generally bleak maternal health picture, Uganda does have a notable success story.[58] In 2001, the World Health Organization, in partnership with the local government, launched its "Making Pregnancy Safer" (MPS) initiative in Soroti, a very poor district with a maternal

---

54   Singh et al. See n. 52, p.185.
55   Prada et al. See n. 9, p. 35; Jewkes RK, Fawcus S, Rees H, Lombard CJ and Katzenellenbogen J. Methodological issues in the South African incomplete abortion study. Studies in Family Planning 1997 September; 28(3): 231-2; Mbonye AK. Abortion in Uganda: magnitude and implications. African Journal of Reproductive Health 2000 October; 4(2): 104-8; Kaye DK, Mirembe M, Bantebya G, Johansson A and Ekstrom AM. Domestic violence as a risk factor for unwanted pregnancy and induced abortion in Mulago Hospital, Kampala, Uganda. Tropical Medicine and International Health 2006 January; 11(1): 90-101; Moodley J and Akinsooto VS. Unsafe abortions in a developing country: has liberalisation of laws on abortions made a difference? African Journal of Reproductive Health 2003 August; 7(2): 34-8.
56   Mbonye et al. See n. 53, p. 288.
57   Singh et al. See n. 52, p. 189.
58   Uganda's MMR went down from 600 per 100 000 live births in 1990 to 310 per 100 000 live births in 2010. Maternal Mortality Estimation Inter-Agency Group. *Trends in maternal mortality: 1990 to 2010: WHO, UNICEF, UNFPA and the World Bank estimate*. World Health Organization, 2012; p. 45.

mortality rate much higher than the rest of the country.

The MPS initiative worked to implement an Emergency Obstetric Care (EmOC) referral system, placing ambulances at strategic locations to help with accessibility. In addition, it initiated extensive education efforts in the community, educating people to recognize warning signs of obstetric complications and the importance of EmOC care. This focus on EmOC and the implementation of the necessary referral system, "led to dramatic outcomes. Within five years the MMR had plunged by more than 75 per cent."[59] All this was accomplished on a budget of US $200,000.

The major lessons learned from such a success are twofold: the importance of Emergency Obstetrical Care and the involvement of the community. The Soroti district had a catch-phrase as the motto of its program: "for each mother, there must be a baby to go back with and for each baby, there must be a mother to go back home with."[60]

This success story is pertinent to the debate on abortion. There are some who assume that the legalization of induced abortion is a necessity for improving women's health.[61] But the Soroti success story calls into question this assumption. There, the gains in maternal health were accomplished without legalizing abortion. Admittedly, the lack of any breakdown of the causes of maternal deaths makes it impossible to be completely certain that abortion deaths decreased along with other maternal deaths. What should be emphasized, however, is that there is no reason to assume that freely available abortion is an independent cause of improved maternal health.

Data from South America and Egypt have already shown that impressive gains in reducing maternal deaths from abortion have been achieved through improvements in the health system, without any legalization of abortion. Other factors that will improve maternal health in Uganda are an attack on poverty and malaria—which take a heavy toll, particularly on mothers—as well as better treatment of women suffering

---

59 World Health Organization (WHO). *MPS: making pregnancy safer—implementing the MPS initiative in Soroti district, Uganda*. World Health Organization, 2010; p. 24.
60 World Health Organization (WHO). Bulletin of the World Health Organization: maternal health care wins district vote in Uganda. WHO. 24 July 2012. http://www.who.int/bulletin/volumes/84/11/06-031106/en/index.html.
61 Gorrette N, Nabukera S and Salihu HM. The abortion paradox in Uganda: fertility regulator or cause of maternal mortality. Journal of Obstetrics and Gynaecology 2005 November; 25(8): 776-8.

from complications after childbirth.[62] None of these measures requires the legalization of abortion.

SOUTH AFRICA AND THE LEGALIZATION OF ABORTION

Overview of South Africa

In 1994, South Africa held its first fully democratic elections. One of the new regime's early priorities was improving maternal and child health, resulting in the construction of more than 1300 primary health-care clinics, and the removal of user fees for many maternal and child health services.[63] There has been an increase in deliveries in the presence of a skilled attendant; most women receive at least one antenatal visit by a health professional, and they have their babies at a health facility.[64] Despite these improvements in the health system, maternal and child mortality not only remain high in South Africa, but have continued to grow. According to a recent report, the MMR was 250 per 100,000 live births in 1990, 330 in 2000, 360 in 2005 and 300 in 2010. The country is classified as making "no progress" in terms of moving towards improving maternal health.[65] As a result, South Africa presents a situation in which there is "the paradox of a supportive policy and funding environment, high rates of use of maternal and child health services, and yet poor and in many cases worsening health outcomes."[66]

Abortion Law in South Africa

Abortion law in South Africa has undergone two alterations.[67] Up to 1975, abortion was illegal except in the case of danger to the life of the mother. The Abortion and Sterilization Act of 1975 extended legal abortion to cover fetal abnormality, rape and incest, and the physical or mental health of the

---

62 Government of Uganda: UNGASS country progress report January 2008-December 2009. United Nations Development Programme, 2010; p. 45; Mbonye et al. See n. 53, p. 289; Lalonde AB, Okong P, Mugasa A and Perron L. The FIGO save the mothers initiative: the Uganda-Canada collaboration. International Journal of Gynaecology and Obstetrics 2003 February; 80(2): 204-12, p. 210.
63 Chopra M, Daviaud E, Pattinson R, Fonn S and Lawn JE. Saving the lives of South Africa's mothers, babies, and children: can the health system deliver? The Lancet 2009 August; 374 (9692): 835-46.
64 Ibid., p. 836.
65 Maternal Mortality Estimation Inter-Agency Group. See n. 58, 44.
66 Chopra et al. See n. 63, p. 836.
67 Population Division of the United Nations Secretariat. Abortion policies: a global review—South Africa. United Nations Population Division Department of Economic and Social Affairs, 2002.

mother. In 1996, following intense debate, the South African parliament passed the Choice on Termination of Pregnancy Act, which permits abortion on request up to twelve weeks. From thirteen to twenty weeks, abortion is permitted for the reasons allowed under the 1975 Act, and also if "the continued pregnancy would significantly affect the social or economic circumstances of the woman." After week twenty, abortion is permitted if two medical practitioners "are of the opinion that the continued pregnancy would endanger the woman's life, would result in severe malformation of the foetus or would pose a risk of injury to the foetus." All abortions must be performed in government-designated facilities, although up to the twelfth week a midwife can perform the abortion. No spousal or parental consent is required, even for minors.

The 1996 Act gives South Africa the most permissive abortion law in Africa, and one of the most permissive in the world.[68] The numbers of legal abortions have risen, but there is evidence that illegal abortion continues as well. In one study, the authors found that of 151 women interviewed upon being admitted to hospital with incomplete abortions, nearly a third (46) had had their abortion outside designated facilities.[69] Ignorance of the law, unawareness of where to obtain a legal abortion, fear of staff rudeness, fear of discovery, and long waiting lists were the main reasons for taking the illegal route.[70]

Maternal Mortality and Abortion in South Africa

According to a widespread belief, the legalization of abortion reduces the prevalence of unsafe abortion and thereby improves maternal health, while restricting access to abortion does the opposite.[71] Studies looking specifically at South Africa have drawn similar conclusions.[72] However, there are contradictions and surprises among the data, which cast doubt

---

68   Buchmann E, Kunene B and Pattinson R. Legalized pregnancy termination and septic abortion mortality in South Africa. International Journal of Gynaecology and Obstetrics 2008 May; 101(2): 191-2.
69   Jewkes RK, Gumede T, Westaway MS, Dickson K, Brown H and Rees H. Why are women still aborting outside designated facilities in metropolitan South Africa? BJOG 2005 September; 112(9): 1236-42, p.1240.
70   Ibid.
71   Berer. 2004. See n. 8, p. 4.
72   Berer M. 2004. See n. 8.; Jewkes R, Rees H, Dickson K, Brown H and Levin J. The impact of age on the epidemiology of incomplete abortions in South Africa after legislative change. BJOG 2005 March; 112(3): 355-359; Mbele AM, Snyman L and Pattinson RC. Impact of the choice on termination of pregnancy act on maternal morbidity and mortality in the west of Pretoria. South African Medical Journal (SAMJ) 2006 November; 96(11): 1196-8.

on these conclusions and point to a different reality.

The decline in maternal deaths in South Africa from 1994 seems to have plateaued.[73] There were 120 deaths due to abortion in the triennium 1999-2001, or an average of 40 per year, accounting for 4.9 per cent of maternal deaths. In 2002-2004, there were 114 deaths, or an average of 38 per year, accounting for 3.5 per cent of maternal deaths (a decrease of 1.4 per cent). This gave a maternal mortality ratio for those years of 5.03 per 100,000 live births. However, in the triennium 2005-2007, there were 136 deaths due to abortion, or about 45 deaths per year, accounting for 3.4 per cent of maternal deaths and a *higher* MMR of 5.23. An extensive study by Fawcus and colleagues analyzed data on maternal deaths in the Cape Peninsula from 1953 until 2003. They found that there was "a sharp decline in the MMR starting in the 1950s and reaching its lowest level of 31.2 in the triennium 1987-1989. Since then, the MMR has risen again and markedly so since the late 1990s to 112/100,000 deliveries in 2002."[74]

Evidently, legalized abortion has not led to clear improvements in maternal health. The reason for the discrepancy between conventional wisdom and the experience of South Africa is that the significance of other factors in improving maternal health are often downplayed while the importance of legalized abortion is overemphasized. As well, many studies, including those influential in effecting the legalization of abortion in South Africa, contain notable methodological flaws that undermine the strength of their arguments.

IMPROVED MATERNAL HEALTH: OTHER FACTORS

The causal relationship between legalized abortion and improved maternal health is not as strong as it is often perceived to be. Evidence indicates that overall improvements in health care and education are more significant to improving maternal health than legalized abortion. A 2009 study by Piane notes the importance of intrapartum (meaning during the birth process) care for maternal health, arguing that "interventions such as prenatal care, postpartum care, family planning and safe abortion are justified after near

---

73   Jewkes, Rees, Dickson, et al. 2005. See n. 72, p. 358.
74   Fawcus SR, van Coeverden de Groot HA and Isaacs S. A 50-year audit of maternal mortality in the Peninsula Maternal and Neonatal Service, Cape Town (1953-2002). BJOG 2005 September; 112(9): 1257-63, p. 1260.

birth interventions are already in place."[75] These basic medical interventions that can significantly reduce maternal mortality are often lacking in poor countries, resulting in a higher MMR. Similarly, a study by Berer, while arguing for a general correlation between permissive abortion laws and decreased maternal death due to abortion, makes the following revealing admission: "countries in any of the six categories that have a high mortality ratio due to unsafe abortion are likely to be those with the least effective and accessible health care services, making complications and deaths from unsafe abortion more likely."[76] The possibility that this might be a link as strong as, or stronger than, restrictive laws, does not seem to occur to her, but the evidence from South Africa suggests that it may well be the case.

Restrictive Laws or Failures in Care?

The Fourth Report on Confidential Enquiries into Maternal Deaths in South Africa found that 54.4 per cent (74 of 136) of deaths due to abortion in the triennium 2005-2007 were "clearly avoidable within the health system."[77] This means that over half of the deaths could be attributed to failures in care, not necessarily to a prevalence of unsafe abortion.[78] Brown and colleagues noted that patients admitted to hospital for gynaecological related sepsis—a major cause of maternal death—were often cases caused by late recognition of sepsis and inadequate antibiotic usage as prescribed by health professionals. Consequently, health-care providers "are failing to accurately assess the clinical severity of the women's condition and treat them appropriately."[79] A study by Mbele and colleagues suggests that improvements in maternal mortality at Kalafong Hospital were due to improved care of critically ill women after abortion upon the introduction of a strict protocol to manage women after abortion and that "women with abortions were presenting earlier and the complications were

---

75   Piane GM. Evidence-based practices to reduce maternal mortality: a systematic review. Journal of Public Health 2009 March; 31(1): 26-31, p. 27.
76   Berer. 2004. See n. 8, p. 4.
77   National Committee on Confidential Enquiries into Maternal Deaths (NCCEMD). *Saving mothers 2005-2007: fourth report on confidential enquiries into maternal deaths in South Africa: expanded executive summary.* Pretoria: South Africa: National Department of Health, March 2008, p. 3. http://www.doh.gov.za/docs/reports/2007/savingmothers.pdf.
78   Notably, specifics are not given and there is ambiguity as to whether "avoidable" means that the abortions could have been done safely or that women with complications were not adequately cared for.
79   Brown HC, Jewkes R, Levin J, Dickson-Tetteh K and Rees H. Management of incomplete abortion in South African public hospitals. BJOG 2003 April; 110(4): 371-7, p. 375.

detected earlier, making their management more successful."[80] Parkhurst and colleagues quote the 1999-2001 Enquiry into Maternal Deaths that "problems in the care of women by health care workers occurred in more than half of the maternal deaths."[81] They also note that "common problems were poor diagnosis, and poor monitoring of patients, as well as failure to follow standard protocols. [...] This suggests that the context in which staff work, the quality of human resource management, and issues around health care worker motivation are as important as whether staff are present or not."[82] In other words, the gains in maternal mortality may be attributable to better management of abortion complications, *not* necessarily to supposedly safer abortion practices produced by legalization.

Furthermore, a decreased MMR depends on a variety of interdependent factors. An analysis by Buor and colleagues in 2004 of the most important factors in reducing MMR in sub-Saharan Africa found that skilled birth attendance was at the top of the list, with female literacy, health expenditure, Gross National Product, and a high life expectancy all holding a strong, but not as conclusive a relationship with a lowered MMR.[83] Significantly, the study looks at MMR in general, not specifically its relation to abortion, and the analysis does *not* include provision of abortion as a factor. South Africa has a high skilled birth attendance rate of 86 per cent, yet has seen increases in its MMR over the past twenty years, indicating that skilled birth attendance is not enough.[84] Fawcus and colleagues also cite the development of midwifery in the home, the introduction of an ambulance service specifically for obstetric emergencies, and general improvements in the management of hypertensive disorders as contributing to the long-term decline in the MMR. They further note that developed countries have achieved declines in MMR thanks to the "ready availability of safe blood transfusions, antibiotics and oxytocics, as well as the improvement in general living standards…"[85] As for the *increase* in MMR from the late 1980s to today, they blame the HIV/AIDS epidemic, as well as "stringent financial cutbacks in health service facilities, and a continuing exodus

---

80   Mbele et al. See n. 72, p. 1198.
81   Parkhurst JO, Penn-Kekana L, Blaauw D, et al. Health systems factors influencing maternal health services: a four-country comparison. Health Policy 2005 August; 73(2): 127-38, p. 131.
82   Ibid.
83   Buor D and Bream K. An analysis of the determinants of maternal mortality in Sub-Saharan Africa. Journal of Women's Health 2004 October; 13(8): 926-38, p. 927.
84   Parkhurst et al. See n. 81.
85   Fawcus et al. See n. 74, p. 1262.

of trained midwives."[86] Thus, the evidence continues to accumulate that South Africa's troubles in maternal health have to do with problems in the health care system (not forgetting the importance of HIV/AIDS).

To their surprise, the Fawcus team also found that the Maternal Mortality Ratio attributable to abortion tumbled from thirteen per 100,000 live births in 1954-1956 to three in 1981-1983, a more than 75 per cent decline. The decrease in abortion-related deaths occurred *prior* to abortion's legalization. Their explanations for the stunning drop are not convincing— "illegally induced abortions were performed more safely in the Western Cape and also that women presented earlier with complications."[87] They furnish no evidence for either explanation, but merely present them as suggestions. Yet the fact that the decrease in abortion-related deaths occurred simultaneously with an overall improvement in the health care system suggests a linkage. An argument could perhaps be made that, if this linkage were real, abortion deaths should have risen again along with the HIV/AIDS epidemic and health cutbacks, but that they did not—thanks to abortion legalization. There are two problems with this line of reasoning. The first is that it still does not explain why, if legalization is so important in reducing maternal mortality from abortion, maternal deaths from abortion decreased so sharply for nearly three decades *prior* to its legalization? Second, the Fourth Report on Confidential Enquiries into Maternal Deaths found a *nationwide* increase in abortion deaths. If the HIV/AIDS epidemic is taken into account, there was a 44 per cent increase in deaths due to abortion in 2005-2007, from 136 to 194.[88] This is what we would expect if maternal mortality from abortion is associated not so much with "safe and legal" abortion practice, as with the strength of the general maternal health system.

RELATIONSHIP BETWEEN LEGALIZED ABORTION AND UNSAFE ABORTION

Conventional wisdom states that legalizing abortion will reduce the prevalence of illegal abortions. However, the evidence suggests that this is not always the case. Buchmann and colleagues found that deaths due to septic abortion in South Africa increased by 20.4 per cent from 1998-2001, and then decreased only slightly (2.2 per cent) in the next triennium (2002-

---

86   Ibid.
87   Ibid.
88   National Committee on Confidential Enquiries into Maternal Deaths. See n. 77.

2004).[89] No explanation is attempted for the dramatic increase after 1998, but the data still indicate that the decline in maternal deaths from abortion between 1994 and 1998 has stopped. In addition, contrary to the early findings at single hospitals, a later, much larger study found no significant decrease in the incidence of incomplete abortion.[90] What this and other research points to is what we have already noted: the continued prevalence of abortion outside accredited facilities, i.e., illegal abortions.

The fact that maternal *deaths* due to abortion *seem* to have decreased, while maternal *injuries* due to abortion have not, indicates that factors other than the legalization of abortion must be at work. If abortion has had the positive effect claimed, both mortality *and* morbidity ought to have decreased. As one group of authors comments: "In the light of this reduction in mortality, it is surprising that the incidence of incomplete abortion should be unchanged."[91] Another study notes the same discrepancy: despite the reduction in deaths from abortion, "the proportion of critically ill patients with complications due to abortion has remained constant."[92]

One reason could be that legalizing abortion appears to have generated increased demand, while large numbers of women still abort outside government facilities. As the authors of one study note, "If many of the 40,000 legal terminations each year reflected women who would have previously aborted illegally and attended hospital with an incomplete abortion, a substantial reduction in incidence of incomplete abortion would have been expected. This was not seen."[93] The 40,000 legal abortions referred to in this study likely represent close to 40,000 *additional* abortions rather than 40,000 illegal abortions moving to legal facilities. What this suggests is that the numbers of women seeking illegally-induced abortions has remained constant, despite legalization. This is what Jewkes and colleagues found, in a study that explicitly excluded complications from legally-induced abortions.[94] Similarly, another study suggests that abortion is being used for contraceptive purposes, despite its explicit prohibition in the Choice on Termination of Pregnancy Act.[95] Doctors and nurses are also involved in

---

89 Buchmann et al. See n. 68, p. 191.
90 Jewkes, Rees, Dickson, et al. 2005. See n. 72, p. 355; Mbele et al. See n. 72.
91 Jewkes, Rees, Dickson, et al. 2005. See n. 72, p. 358.
92 Mbele et al. See n. 72, p. 1197.
93 Jewkes, Rees, Dickson, et al. 2005. See n. 72, p. 358.
94 Ibid., p. 356.
95 Patel CJ and Kooverjee T. Abortion and contraception: attitudes of South African university students. Health Care for Women International 2009 June; 30(6): 550-68, p. 553.

illegal abortion activities despite legalization, some of them for profit.[96]

However, much of the research literature ignores the distinction between legal and illegal abortion. The 1994 study, which was crucial in helping to legalize abortion, specifically excluded women presenting for complications from abortion if the women said they had received a legal abortion. The 2002 Jewkes study of morbidity and the 2005 Jewkes repeat of the 1994 study also excluded women who had undergone legal abortions. In other words, all three studies were assessing the health burden of *illegal* abortions. Not one of them tells us how many women suffered complications from *legal* abortions.

One other study does, however. Analyzing the records of women presenting with complications at King Edward VIII Hospital, Moodley and Akinsootoo found that "spontaneous abortion accounted for 49.5 per cent, certainly induced abortion for 17.8 per cent, probably induced abortion 10.1 per cent, possibly induced abortion 18.3 per cent, and legally induced abortion 4.3 per cent."[97] While the authors do note a decrease in the number of women admitted for abortion complications, they do not provide a breakdown of the decrease in each of these categories. However, the numbers indicate that women do suffer complications from legal abortion, though at an apparently lower rate than from illegal abortion.

There is a puzzling silence about the complications from legal abortions in many of the studies. Jewkes and colleagues excluded from their analysis women with complications from legal abortions, meaning that the numbers presented are solely from illegally-induced or spontaneous abortions.[98] They note that 46 out of 151 women presenting to one hospital with complications from abortion had had illegal abortions.[99] No mention is made of the other 105 women—did they all have spontaneous abortions? Was it uncertain whether their abortions were legal or illegal? The authors do not say. As a result of the silence here and elsewhere, it is difficult to determine whether the abortion complications are from legal or illegal abortions. That some of them are from legal ones is clear, but how many is less certain. The *Fourth Report on Confidential Enquiries into Maternal Deaths*, for instance, simply lists deaths due to abortion; it does not distinguish between abortions that are spontaneous or induced, and if induced, between legal and illegal.

---

96   Moodley et al. See n. 55, p. 36; Jewkes, Rees, Dickson, et al. 2005. See n. 72, p. 356.
97   Moodley et al. See n. 55, p. 36.
98   Jewkes, Rees, Dickson, et al. 2005. See n. 72, p. 356.
99   Jewkes, Gumede, Westaway, et al. 2005. See n. 69, p. 1237.

To summarize, since the legalization of abortion in South Africa, complications resulting from abortions have not decreased, while maternal mortality due to abortion apparently has. Illegal abortion seems to be just as widespread as it always was, judging by the persistence of complications from illegal abortions.

THE 1994 AND 2000 STUDIES: SOME PROBLEMS

It is worth scrutinizing both the 1994 study (published in 1997) that was so influential in changing the law in South Africa, and the 2000 study (published in 2005) that sought to determine the effects of the change. The first study uncovered three deaths from induced abortion during a two-week period. The authors used this finding to estimate the number of deaths from induced abortion for the whole year at 425, and the number of complications at 12,847. Evidence from a two-week period is a very narrow base on which to calculate a yearly rate. More troubling, three deaths in two weeks, if typical, are equivalent to 78 over a year, not 425 as the authors claim.[100] Such a bloated estimate may simply reflect the authors' transparent political agenda: "the goal of safe abortions for all," and using their findings "for countering arguments about costs of legislative change."[101] Careful analysis reveals statements and conclusions that are at odds with actual findings.

However, basing itself on these highly suspect extrapolations, the 2005 study attempted to assess the impact of the new abortion law.[102] This study looked at a very short, three-week period; what is more, only illegal and spontaneous abortions were included in the survey—all legal abortions were excluded from its purview. Thus, only an incomplete picture of the effect of legislation on abortion safety can arise from this analysis.

In reality, the 2005 study found very little decrease in the number of women being admitted with complications from illegal and spontaneous abortions. Clearly then, legalizing abortion, far from eliminating illegal

---

100 To convert a two-week sample into an estimate for a full year, the figure of 3 needs to multiplied by 26, giving 78. Even taking into account the 92 per cent (p. 435) participation rate (elsewhere the authors state that data were collected from all 61 public hospitals in South Africa responsible for treating women with gynaecological problems), the estimate of 78 should only rise to 84—a far cry from the 425 claimed by the authors. Rees H, Katzenellenbogen J, Shabodien R, et al. The epidemiology of incomplete abortion in South Africa. National Incomplete Abortion Reference Group. South African Medical Journal 1997 April; 87(4): 432-7, p. 433.
101 Jewkes, Fawcus, Rees, et al. 1997. See n. 55, p. 231.
102 Jewkes, Gumede, Westaway, et al. 2005. See n. 69, p. 1236; Jewkes, Rees, Dickson, et al. 2005. See n. 72, p. 356.

abortions, has actually dramatically increased the total number of abortions. This finding belies the "expected reduction in cases of 'certainly induced' and unsafe abortions and deaths from these procedures."[103]

Regarding the claimed dramatic reduction in deaths due to abortion, this argument is based not on the 2005 study (which recorded no deaths in three weeks), but on the national inquiries into maternal deaths. As noted above, in the triennium 2005-2007, there were 45 deaths due to abortion per year, which looks like a massive reduction from the 425 estimated in the 1994 study. However, as already mentioned, the figure 425 is highly suspect, and should probably be reduced to 78. Deaths due to abortion in South Africa have actually risen recently by one-quarter, from 32 per year in the 1998 survey to 40 in 2007, even as legal abortion services have increased.[104]

In sum, then, the very data on which the argument for an improvement due to legal change is based are suspect and highly speculative. This means that the touted gains in maternal mortality due to abortion are much less than claimed; moreover, complications from abortion remain high despite greater access to legal abortion. Thus, while the Union of South Africa has been presented as a poster child for the benefits of legal abortion in Africa, the country's actual experience hardly inspires confidence that legal abortion is an unalloyed benefit for maternal health.[105]

SUMMARY: THE EXPERIENCE OF THE THIRD WORLD

Not long ago, E. Papiernik carried out a sweeping historical survey of maternal mortality in industrialized countries from 1750 to the end of the last century.[106] What he found was that a decrease in maternal mortality

---

103   Jewkes, Fawcus, Rees, et al. 1997. See n. 55, p. 234.
104   Jewkes R and Rees H. Dramatic decline in abortion mortality due to the Choice on Termination of Pregnancy Act. South African Medical Journal 2005; 93(4): p. 250; National Committee on Confidential Enquiries into Maternal Deaths. See n. 77.
105   The experience of two other African countries appears to reinforce the conclusion that legalizing abortion does little to improve maternal health. Kenya and Ethiopia are among the poorest countries in the world. Kenya continues to have a restrictive abortion law. Despite a chaotic and impoverished health system maternal mortality is reported to have declined by close to one-third between 1989 and 2003 (Central Bureau of Statistics (CBS) [Kenya], Ministry of Health [Kenya], and ORC Macro. Kenya demographic and health survey 2003, p. 237). In Ethiopia it has been difficult to discern trends in deaths from abortion, although one hospital experienced a significant *increase* in abortion fatality after abortion was legalized in 2005 (Gebrehiwot Y and Liabsuetrakul T. Trends of abortion complications in a transition of abortion law revisions in Ethiopia. Journal of Public Health 2008; 31(1): p. 81).
106   Papiernik E. The role of emergency obstetric care in preventing maternal deaths: an historical perspective on European figures since 1751. International Journal of Gynecology and Obstetrics 1995 October; 50(Supplement 2): S73-S77.

coincided with an increase in modern caesarian sections and in the percentage of women giving birth in hospitals. From this he deduced that progress in these two fronts holds out the best hope of realizing swift improvement in maternal mortality in the world's developing regions.

His argument is borne out by the analysis of this chapter. The factors that most strongly correlate with improvements in maternal mortality are provision of emergency obstetric care (such as caesarean sections), skilled attendance at birth, and the education of women. Additional factors are community outreach, and efforts to improve referral systems and transportation for emergency care.

Abortion is not a necessary component of any effort aimed at reducing maternal deaths. Chile, El Salvador, Nicaragua, and Egypt have all witnessed impressive improvements in maternal health, including health after abortion, while maintaining stringent legal restrictions on abortion. While Uganda as a whole cannot boast the same success, efforts in the Soroti district prove that such success can be within the reach of even the poorest regions. All these examples show that the main factors affecting maternal mortality can and have been addressed without legalizing abortion. Incomplete data from Kenya and Ethiopia also appear to support this conclusion.

Further, it has been seen how South Africa, hailed by many as an example of the positive effects of legalizing abortion, has not actually seen dramatic benefits from the liberalization of its abortion law. Unlike Chile, which boasts ongoing improvements in maternal health after banning abortion, South Africa has enjoyed no such gains, and even the touted reduction in maternal mortality has been much exaggerated.

The leading causes of maternal death worldwide are hemorrhage and hypertension. The interventions required to improve maternal health are known, and affordable. Proposing abortion as a solution for the developing world in its fight to reduce maternal mortality is not justified by the evidence, nor does it take into consideration the experience of those countries that have made significant gains in maternal health while declining to legalize induced abortion. Given that legalized abortion has had such an indifferent record, it would make far better sense to concentrate on those measures which have enjoyed proven success in reducing maternal mortality and improving maternal health.

EUROPEAN COMPARISONS

In Europe, there are two countries where induced abortion is not permitted: Ireland and Poland. The Polish Parliament banned abortion in 1989, shortly after the fall of communism. Since that time, maternal mortality in that country has plunged by nearly three-quarters, infant mortality is down by almost two-thirds, and the rate of premature births has dropped by well over a half.[107] Poland's maternal mortality is four to five times lower than its immediate neighbours, Hungary and Russia, both of which have very high rates of induced abortion.

Table 2.1 **Maternal Mortality per 100,000 live births in Eastern Europe**

Year	Poland	Hungary	Russian Federation
2006	3.0	8.0	23.8
2007	2.8	8.2	22.1
2008	4.6	17.2	21.0
2009	2.0	18.7	22.02
2010	Unavailable	16.0	Unavailable

Source: European Health for all Database (HFA-DB), World Health Organization, Regional Office for Europe (Copenhagen, Jan. 2011).

The reduction in premature births is significant, since premature children are prone to all sorts of medical and social afflictions. The most serious of these is a higher chance of being born with cerebral palsy than full-term babies. In the late 1980s, around a hundred children per year were dying before the age of five from cerebral palsy in Poland. By 2006, the number was down to five or ten per year—a greater than 90 per cent drop.

In the United States, by contrast, the preterm birthrate has jumped in recent years from 8.9 per cent to 12.2 per cent of all births, pointing to a corresponding increase in the incidence of cerebral palsy.[108] No Canadian

---

107　In 1989, Poland's MMR was 10.6 per 100 000 live births. By 2006, that number dropped to 2.9. Poland's infant mortality rate was 19.1 per 1000 live births, which has since dropped to 6.0 by 2006.
108　Rooney B, Calhoun BC and Roche LE. Does induced abortion account for racial disparity in preterm births, and violate the nuremberg code? Journal of American Physicians and Surgeons 2008; 13(4): 102-4, p. 102; Kochanek KD, Kirmeyer SE, Martin JA, Strobino DM and Guyer B. Annual summary of vital statistics 2009. Pediatrics 2012 January; 129(2): 338-48.

figures are available.

A woman who has one or more induced abortions significantly increases her risk of subsequently bearing a preterm baby, which in turn hugely increases the risk that that baby will be afflicted with cerebral palsy (see Chapter 15, pp. 238-9). Measures that can reduce the incidence of cerebral palsy must be welcomed on both social and financial grounds.

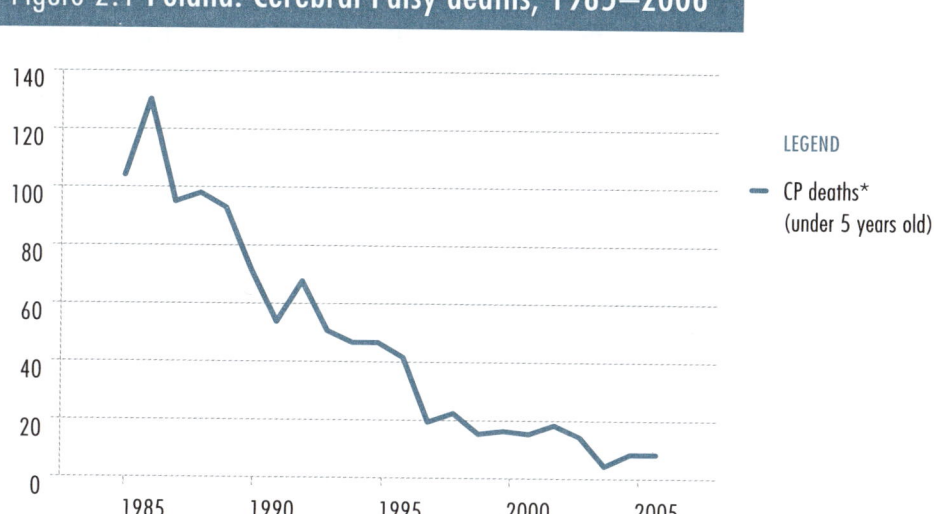

Figure 2.1 Poland: Cerebral Palsy deaths, 1985–2006

Source: Cerebral Palsy deaths in Poland, 1985-2006, Poland Central Statistical Office.

Why has Poland made such strides in cutting the incidence of cerebral palsy deaths over the past two decades? Certainly not by pumping a lot of extra money into its healthcare system. As one of the poorest countries in Europe, it lacks the resources for an extensive program to improve infant health. The only change that could have produced such dramatic improvement since 1989 is the documented decline in the abortion rate. Poland's infant mortality has also declined to the point that it is now lower than the US—six compared to seven per thousand.[109] Interestingly, Poland's immediate neighbour, Russia, which has a very high rate of abortion, also has a significantly higher rate of infant mortality, although Hungary, which also has a high abortion rate, has the same rate of infant mortality as Poland. Yet Hungary is a significantly richer country than Poland, and

---

109   UNICEF, The State of the World's Children (2009). Colorcraft of Virginia Inc., and Prographics Inc., 2010; pp. 9, 11.

might otherwise be expected to have a lower rate of infant mortality than its poorer neighbour.[110]

Table 2.2 **Infant mortality per 1000 births**

Year	Poland	USA	Russia	Hungary
1990	16	unavailable	unavailable	unavailable
2000	8	unavailable	unavailable	unavailable
2008	6	7	10	6

Sources: UNICEF, unicef.org/infobycountry/poland_statistics.html (2 March 2010); Globalis, UN Common Database/UNICEF (2002), UNICEF, The State of the World's Children (2009), Table one.

Ireland, like Poland, does not allow induced abortion.[111] But unlike Poland, it has never allowed it. Therefore it is not possible to compare Ireland's experience before and after banning abortion. It is striking, however, that Ireland continues to have among the lowest rates of maternal and infant mortality in the world, despite being far from among the richest countries in the world. Indeed, its next-door neighbour, the United Kingdom, a richer country where abortion is available upon request (except in Northern Ireland), has a significantly worse record on both counts. Maternal mortality is more than twice as high, while infant mortality is nearly 50 per cent higher than in Ireland.

Table 2.3 **Ireland and the United Kingdom: maternal mortality per 100,000 live births; infant mortality per 1000 live births**

	Year	Maternal Mortality	Infant Mortality
Ireland	2009	4.0	3.2
United Kingdom	2009	9.4	4.7

Source: European Health for all Database (HFA-DB), World Health Organization, Regional Office for Europe (Copenhagen, Jan. 2011).

---

110   National Center for Health Statistics. *Health, United States, 2007.* Hyattsville, MD: Chartbook on Trends in the Health of Americans, 2007; p. 172.
111   At the time of writing the Irish parliament was considering a limited legalization of abortion.

Conclusion

Wherever we look—Latin America, Africa, Europe—we find next-to-no evidence to support the proposition that legalizing abortion leads to improved maternal and infant health. On the contrary, we find that those countries who do not permit abortion, or who have banned it in the past two decades, have a consistently better record in caring for mothers and newborns. This puzzling finding is contrary to what people have been led to expect. How are we to explain it? Perhaps countries that do not permit abortion devote greater effort to protecting and improving the health of their mothers and infants. This is clearly evident in Chile, Poland and Ireland, and it may be true of other countries as well, such as El Salvador, Nicaragua, Egypt and Uganda. What is beyond dispute is that countries that have made strides in improving the education of women, in emergency obstetric care (such as caesarean sections), in skilled attendance at birth, as well as community outreach, improved referral systems and transportation for emergency care—most notably Chile, Uganda and Egypt—have been rewarded with greatly improved maternal and infant health. Can it be an accident that these are also countries where abortion is not permitted?

Chapter 3

So many missing girls: Abortion and sex selection

KEY POINTS

- In the past 20 to 30 years it has become known that the practice of sex-selective abortion is widespread in many countries, resulting in skewed sex ratios at birth.

- Overwhelmingly, the practice of sex-selective abortion reflects the preference for male children over female children in the countries where it is practised.

- Sex-selective abortion may be as much a consequence of western pressure for population control as it is a reflection of traditional religious or cultural prejudice against females.

- Sex-selective abortion is the ironic, unforeseen consequence of the triumph of "a woman's right to choose", since it has led to the intentional death of millions of female unborn children.

- Strong ethical objections have been advanced against the practice of sex-selective abortion.

- The social and cultural consequences of sex-selective abortion are also a source of great concern.

- At least one country (South Korea) has succeeded in reversing the practice of sex- selective abortion.

> "I had two daughters and I was desperate for a boy. So when I got pregnant I had an ultrasound and it was another girl. I knew my husband would not accept another girl, so I had an abortion. There was no choice."[1]

INTRODUCTION

According to J.M. Milliez, "sex selection of the future offspring is usually regarded as acceptable when medically indicated, in order to avoid the transmission of severe sex-linked genetic diseases."[2] Yet it has been noted that the practice of aborting after prenatal diagnosis for genetic anomalies paved the way for aborting for non-medical reasons. People often scoff at the 'slippery slope' argument, but it is undeniable that "sex-selective abortion has been made possible by prenatal diagnosis."[3] As Wachbroit and Wasserman warned in the 1990s, the "real threat" of prenatal diagnosis "comes from the identification of an increasing number of genetic markers associated with conditions that are not life-threatening, but impairing or socially undesirable, such as hyperactivity, homosexuality, and obesity. The availability of prenatal tests for these conditions threatens to make pregnancy ever more tentative and to stigmatize further those with the conditions tested for."[4] What has been the impact of sex-selective abortion on women and on the world?

STATISTICS

At the beginning of the 1990s, Nobel Laureate Amartya Sen made an astonishing pronouncement: over 100 million girls were missing in Asia and North Africa.[5] As early as the mid-eighties, researchers had begun to

---

1   Zhou C, Wang XL, Zhou XD, and Hesketh T. Son preference and sex-selective abortion in China: informing policy options. International Journal of Public Health 2012; 57(3): 459-65.
2   Milliez JM. Sex selection for non-medical purposes. Reproductive BioMedicine Online 2007; 14(Supplement 1): pp. 114-17, p. 114.
3   Dahl E. Procreative liberty: the case for preconception sex selection. Reproductive BioMedicine Online 2003; 7(4): p. 380.
4   Wachbroit R and Wasserman D. Patient autonomy and value-neutrality in nondirective genetic counselling. Stanford Law & Policy Review 1995; 6(2): 103-11.
5   Sen A. More than 100 million women are missing. New York Review of Books, December 20, 1990. http://www.nybooks.com/articles/archives/1990/dec/20/more-than-100-million-women-are-missing/.

realize that such gender imbalance was due in large part to "gendercide" via sex-selective abortion, the systematic killing of females before birth.

The normal sex ratio at birth (SRB)—the number of male births for every 100 female births—ranges from 103 to 107, i.e. 105 plus or minus two. It is now common knowledge that, with spiraling SRBs that have peaked as high as 160 and 200 in some regions,[6] over 160 million girls have gone missing worldwide. The explanation for this phenomenon is straightforward: with the technological advancements of ultrasound and amniocentesis came the possibility of aborting the unborn according to their sex. As UNICEF explains, "Where there is a clear economic or cultural preference for sons, the misuse of these techniques can facilitate female foeticide."[7]

In many Asian countries, the sex ratio at birth (SRB) increases with each subsequent birth, meaning that sex-selective abortion becomes increasingly likely with each additional pregnancy, especially if the first child is female. For example, in China, "the SRB across the country for first-order births is 108, for second-order births it is 143 and for the (albeit rare) third-order births it is 157."[8] A large study in India showed that "for second births with one preceding girl the SRB is 132, and for third births with two previous girls it is 139, whereas sex ratios are normal where the previous child was a boy."[9]

SEX-SELECTIVE ABORTION IN CHINA

The preference for sons in China stems from its traditional "lineage-based kinship systems, which effectively ensure that only boys can continue the household and lineage and care for their parents in their old age."[10] The cultural preference for sons is evident in such Chinese sayings as "eighteen

---

6   Das Gupta M, Chung W and Shuzhuo L. Evidence for an incipient decline in numbers of missing girls in China and India. Population and Development Review; 35(2): p. 412.
7   UNICEF. State of the world's children 2007: women and children: the double dividend of gender equality. New York: UNICEF House, 2006. Online edition: http://www.unicef.org/sowc07/report/report.php.
8   Hesketh T, Li L and Zhu WX. The consequences of son preference and sex-selective abortion in China and other Asian countries. CMAJ 2011; 183(12): p. 1375.
9   Ibid., p. 1374.
10   World Bank. Promoting gender equality and women's empowerment. *Global monitoring report: confronting the challenges of gender equality and fragile states.* Washington, DC: The World Bank, 2007: 105-38, p. 124. http://siteresources.worldbank.org/INTGLOMONREP2007/Resources/3413191-1179404785559/Chp3-GMR07_webPDF-corrected-may-14-2007-6.pdf.

goddesses are less valuable than even a single hunchbacked boy" and "raising a girl is like watering the field of the neighbour."[11]

According to China's 2010 census, the country's sex-ratio at birth (SRB) was 118, soaring as high as 135 in some rural areas.[12] To understand the effect of such distorted sex ratios, consider the fact that in 2005, "males under the age of twenty exceeded females by more than 32 million in China, and more than 1.1 million excess births of boys occurred."[13] A prominent Chinese demographer has described the severely distorted sex ratio as "the crime of the twentieth century against the twenty-first."[14]

Researchers confirm that "it is sex-selective abortion, rather than female infanticide or under-reporting, that is actually behind the rise in China's SRB."[15] The Chinese cultural preference for male children combined with China's attempt at population control, commonly known as the one-child policy, has led to the distorted SRB.[16] Most Chinese couples desire a son, and if only one pregnancy is allowed to be carried to term, many will use sex-determining technology to abort female fetuses and ensure that they get their son.

Even the increasing number of Chinese couples who qualify to have two children, partly in an attempt to correct the skewed sex ratio at birth, often feel that they must terminate additional pregnancies. Female deaths will inevitably result from this infringement on human freedom. Moreover, the "variant of the one child policy, which allows a second child if the first is a girl, leads to the highest sex ratios."[17] In other words, following the pattern of SRB increase after each subsequent birth, a Chinese couple is more likely to abort a female fetus if they already have a daughter than if they have no child.

---

11   Milliez. See n. 2, p. 115.
12   Zhou, Wang, Zhou and Hesketh. See n. 1.
13   Zhu WX, Li L and Hesketh T. China's excess males, sex selective abortion, and one child policy: analysis of data from 2005 national intercensus survey. BMJ 2009 April; 338(b1211): p. 1.
14   Quoted in Nie JB. Limits of state intervention in sex-selective abortion: the case of China. Culture, Health & Sexuality 2010; 12(2): p. 207.
15   Li S. Imbalanced sex ratio at birth and comprehensive intervention in China. *Hyderabad, India: 4th Asia Pacific conference on reproductive and sexual health rights*, October 29-31, 2007: p. 5. http://www.unfpa.org/gender/docs/studies/china.pdf.
16   Ebenstein A and Leung S. Son preference and access to social insurance: evidence from China's rural pension program. Population and Development Review 2010; 36(1): p. 53.
17   Zhu, Li and Hesketh. See n. 13.

SEX-SELECTIVE ABORTION IN INDIA

Indian culture has also demonstrated a preference for sons that has led to an increase of selected female abortions. India is a patriarchal society in which sons work to provide income and care for elderly parents, and preserve the family name. In Hindu belief it is sons who must light their parents' funeral pyres to ensure their spiritual salvation.[18] In addition, "The prospect of a heavy financial expenditure on the marriage of daughters [via dowry payments] is a key factor driving people to resort to sex-selective abortion in India… In fact, private clinics openly advertise their sex selection services as inducing couples to 'spend now' (on procuring the services) to 'save later' on hefty marriage and dowry expenditure in case a girl is born."[19]

Interestingly, "… selective abortion of girls is more common in educated or richer households, presumably because they can afford ultrasound and abortion services more readily than uneducated or poorer households."[20] Furthermore, although "it has long been argued that improvement in literacy rates and socio-economic development amongst women could change the adverse sex ratio for the better…it has been observed that educated mothers in Punjab are more prone to discriminate against their daughters than the uneducated ones."[21] Since "gender bias exists regardless of religion, caste and socio-economic class,"[22] curbing unbalanced sex ratios at birth may require a ban on sex-selective abortion rather than a fruitless attempt to educate the bias out of the culture.

The 2011 Indian census revealed about 7.1 million fewer girls than boys aged six or under, "a notable increase in the gap of 6.0 million fewer girls recorded in the 2001 census and the gap of 4.2 million fewer girls recorded in the 1991 census."[23] Even with infant mortality rates taken into account, the numbers are indicative of a decided increase in sex-selective

---

18   Garg S and Nath A. Female feticide in India: issues and concerns. Journal of Postgraduate Medicine 2008; 54(4): p. 277.
19   Unnithan-Kumar M. Female selective abortion—beyond 'culture': family making and gender inequality in a globalising India. Culture, Health & Sexuality 2010; 12(2): p. 157.
20   Jha P et al. Trends in selective abortions of girls in India: analysis of nationally representative birth histories from 1990 to 2005 and census data from 1991 to 2011. The Lancet 2011; 377(9781): p. 1926.
21   Garg and Nath. See n. 18.
22   Sahni M et al. Missing girls in India: infanticide, feticide and made-to-order pregnancies? Insights from hospital-based sex-ratio-at-birth over the last century. PLoS ONE 2008; 3(5): p. 3.
23   Ibid.

abortion. Although "some [Indian] states are now showing a trend towards improvement," overall, the sex ratios have been steadily worsening.[24]

SEX-SELECTIVE ABORTION IN OTHER ASIAN COUNTRIES

Researchers are beginning to detect sex-selective abortion in Vietnam: "Although in 2000, the ratio was about 106 male births per 100 female births, it increased to 112 in 2008."[25]

In Nepal, "the sex ratio at last birth…for women who claim to have completed their families or to have been sterilized is estimated at 146, suggesting that stopping behaviour among these women is driven by son preference."[26] The United Nations Population Fund (UNFPA) places the "harmful practice" of prenatal sex selection in Nepal under the heading of "gender-based violence."[27]

So far only South Korea has been able to rebalance its once skewed sex ratios: "The country had a rapid rise in sex ratio at birth, up to 116 [in the early 1990s], but managed to engineer a rapid decline over a period of about 20 years through a raft of policy reforms: government investment in social security, reinforcement of health and social insurance systems, [and] measures to benefit families having girls."[28] In addition, the status of women improved through education and employment, and laws against sex-selective abortion were strongly enforced.[29]

SEX-SELECTIVE ABORTION IN THE WEST

It is mostly because of immigration from Asia that we find sex-selective abortion being practiced in the West. In the United States, the President's Council on Bioethics has acknowledged that sex selection via sonography

---

24   Ibid. See n. 22, p. 341.
25   Chatterjee P. Sex ratio imbalance worsens in Vietnam. The Lancet 2009; 373(9699): p. 1410.
26   Leone T, Matthews Z and Zuanna GD. Impact and determinants of sex preference in Nepal. IFPP 2003; 29(2): p. 69.
27   United Nations Population Fund (UNFPA). *Delivering on the promise of equality: UNFPA's strategic framework on gender mainstreaming and women's empowerment 2008-2011.* New York, NY: UNFPA, 2008. http://nepal.unfpa.org/pdf/UNFPA%20Gender%20Strategy.pdf.
28   Chatterjee. See n. 25.
29   Frejka T, Jones GW and Sardon JP. East asian childbearing patterns and policy developments. Population and Development Review 2010; 36(3): p. 602.

and abortion is on the rise there.[30] While most Americans prefer gender balance[31]—i.e. at least one male and one female child—a small 2011 study of Indian immigrants to the US found strong son preference and heavy resort to sex-selective abortion.[32]

Because it lacks any restrictions on induced abortion, Canada has been described as "a haven for parents who would terminate female fetuses in favour of having sons, despite overwhelming censure of the practice."[33] Statistics from communities with a large Asian immigrant population in Quebec, Ontario and British Columbia all show skewed sex ratios at birth.[34] The son preference characteristic of various Asian countries has migrated to the West, resulting in sex-selective abortion of females in countries that pride themselves on gender equality.

Apart from Asian biases, sex-selective abortions are sometimes obtained in the West for gender-specific genetic anomalies or medical issues. However, even in non-immigrant populations in North America, Europe and Australia there has been detected a preference for a "balanced" family, meaning at least one son and not too many daughters.[35]

The practice of sex-selective abortion is often blamed on the sexism of the country or region where it is found to exist. However, Mara Hvistendahl argues that rather than Asian prejudices making their way to the West to cause sex-selective abortion here, it is Western prejudices—particularly the adamant call for population control to reduce poverty—which first led to

---

30   George SM. Millions of missing girls: from fetal sexing to high technology sex selection in India. Prenatal Diagnosis 2006; 26(7): p. 608.
31   Dahl. See n. 3, p. 382.
32   Puri S, Adams V, Ivey S and Nachtigall RD. "There is such a thing as too many daughters, but not too many sons": A qualitative study of son preference and fetal sex selection among Indian immigrants in the United States. Social Science & Medicine 2011; 72(7): p. 1175.
33   Vogel L. Sex selection migrates to Canada. CMAJ 2012; 184(3): e163.
34   Auger N, Daniel M and Moore S. Sex ratio patterns according to Asian ethnicity in Québec, 1981-2004. European Journal of Epidemiology 2009: 24(1): pp. 17-24; Mrozec A. Canada's lost daughters. Western Standard 2006 June: 33-9; Thiele AT and Leier B. Towards an ethical policy for the prevention of fetal sex selection in Canada. JOGC 2010; 32(1): 54-7.
35   Dahl E, Beutel M, Brosig B, et al. Social sex selection and the balance of the sexes: empirical evidence from Germany, the UK, and the US. Journal of Assisted Reproduction and Genetics 2006; 23(7-8): 311-18; Kippen R, Evans A and Gray E. Parental preference for sons and daughters in a Western industrial setting: evidence and implications. Journal of Biosocial Science 2007; 39(4): 583-97.

sex-selective abortion in the East. She notes that it is not merely in places with "backward traditions" that one finds distorted sex ratios at birth today, but in countries with economies advanced enough to afford the technology that enables sex-selective abortion.[36] In a nutshell, "western governments actively promoted abortion and sex selection in the developing world, encouraging the liberalization of abortion laws and subsidizing sales of ultrasounds as a form of population control."[37] Perhaps it is less the preference for one sex over another than the desire for population control that needs to be addressed as the root of imbalanced sex ratios.

THE ETHICS OF SEX-SELECTION

Sexism and Women's Rights[38]

Most people who hear about the deliberate abortion of a female will label the act inherently sexist and immoral: "a human rights issue, a tangible manifestation of the ideological discrimination of a male-biased society towards girls and women [reflecting] how customary practices of female neglect are being replaced by the fact of not allowing female children to be born in the first place."[39] However, ethicists who think abortion is a woman's right argue that the practice of sex-selective abortion is the result of pre-existing sexism, not a *cause* of women's oppression; hence, banning fetal sex determination and abortion will not eliminate the oppression of women and will serve only to harm their absolute right to procreative choice. Yet they face a dilemma: "the right to procreative liberty philosophically supports gender discrimination."[40] In the minds of those who support sex-selective abortion, free choice is the good that trumps all else. Some ethicists go so far as to argue that sex-selective abortion must be allowed in order to ensure personal fulfillment via family balancing for the satisfaction of the parents and the mutual understanding of the children.[41]

---

36   Hvistendahl M. *Unnatural selection: choosing boys over girls, and the consequences of a world full of men.* (New York: Public Affairs, 2011), p. 5.
37   Pilkington E. See Section I Abstract: The Big Picture, n.1.
38   For more information, see articles such as: Suter SM. Sex selection, nondirectiveness, and equality. University of Chicago Law School Roundtable 1996; 3(2): 473-89; Steinbock B. Sex selection: not obviously wrong. Hastings Center Report 2002; 31(1): 23-28; Dahl. See n. 3, 380-4.
39   Unnithan-Kumar. See n. 19, p. 154.
40   Milliez. See n. 2, p. 115.
41   Pennings G. Ethics of sex selection for family balancing. Human Reproduction 1996; 11(11): 2339—45.

In contrast, the International Federation of Gynecology and Obstetrics' ethical guidelines on sex selection for non-medical purposes state that "while procreative liberty warrants protection, *this is limited when its exercise results in sex discrimination*, and that the individual right to procreative liberty needs to be balanced by the communal need to protect the dignity and equality of women and children"[42] Ethicists who oppose sex-selection, therefore, consider the practice to be inherently sexist, and acknowledge the existence of goods greater than women's right to procreative freedom.

Even if free choice is assumed to be the highest good, it has been observed that women undergoing sex-selective abortions are not always truly autonomous. Researchers at the University of California write that "technological advances can actually decrease the scope of women's reproductive choice" so they feel increased "pressure and even obligation to use it."[43] They found that US Indian immigrants often felt coerced into sex selection.[44] China's enforced family planning policy is even more at odds with procreative liberty, and is one of the main causes of that country's increasingly skewed sex ratio.

Some ethicists have argued that intentionally aborting females is actually doing a favour for women. This is a common argument in India: "Is it not better to kill a female before she takes any form than give birth to a girl and either kill her soon after or subject her to life-long torture, misery and harassment at the hands of the husband, in-laws and society at large?"[45] Similarly, some ethicists have suggested that having fewer women will increase their value and diminish sexism. On the contrary, as we will see, a shortage of women has actually led to their greater objectification and abuse.

The Consequences of Sex-Selective Abortion

The social effects of sex-selection abortion are still unfolding. Since "the large cohorts of surplus young men have only now started to reach reproductive age...the consequences of this male surplus in

---

42   FIGO. Resolution on 'sex-selection for non-medical purposes'. London: March, 2005. http://www.figo.org/projects/sex_selection. Emphasis Added.
43   Puri S et al. See n. 32.
44   Ibid., pp. 1169-1176.
45   Kusum K. Sex selection. In *Ethical aspects of human reproduction*. Claude Sureau & Francoise Shenfield, eds. Paris: John Libbey Eurotext, 1995: p. 304.

the reproductive age group are still largely speculative."[46] However, certain outcomes have already become apparent. For example, there is a "marriage squeeze" in populations with distorted sex ratios: many males of marriageable age are unable to find a wife because of the shortage of women. Hence, in Asia, "girls are now abducted for criminal traffics and sold for marriage in remote rural regions."[47] One researcher reports in detail:

> From Taiwan and Korea, where we had sex selection early and men now can't find wives, bachelors go on marriage tours to Vietnam. They pay $10,000 and that covers the flight to Ho Chi Minh City and room and board. Once they arrive they go to a hotel and the women are basically village women who are sold by their parents and they're lined up for the men to pick from…As for forced marriages, there are stories of women being forced to marry multiple brothers, of girls being bought very young and families who raise them until they're old enough to marry their sons.[48]

A sex imbalance at reproductive age may also lead to "enforced celibacy, polyandry, homosexuality, prostitution, rape and other sexual crimes,"[49] as well as an "increase in sexually transmitted diseases and gender-based violence [and] decreasing female participation and political weight."[50] Some researchers have argued that "an imbalanced sex ratio perpetuates gender discrimination against women [and] contributes to poor health in women."[51]

The obvious demographic consequence will be a decline in fertility: "Even if all women continue to have the same number of births as previously, the reduction in the number and share of females in the total population

---

46   Hesketh, Lu and Xing. See n. 8.
47   Milliez. See n. 2, p. 115.
48   Hvistendahl M, interview by Brian Bethune. The women shortage: how sex selection of babies has led to a huge surplus of men and why that's bad for all of us. *Maclean's*. June 2011. http://www2.macleans.ca/2011/06/14/how-sex-selection-of-babies-has-led-to-a-huge-surplus-of-men-and-why-that%E2%80%99s-bad-for-all-of-us/.
49   Dahl. See n. 3, p. 380.
50   Adhikari N, Ghimire A and Ansari I. Sex preference in urban Nepal. Journal of the Institute of Medicine (Online). 2008 August; 30(2): 1-22.
51   Lamichhane P, Harken T, Puri M, et al. Sex-selective abortion in Nepal: a qualitative study of health workers' perspectives. Women's Health Issues 2011; 21(Supplement 3): p. S37.

will lead to a reduction in total births [and] smaller future cohorts will lead to a rapid slowdown in...population growth."[52] It is also predicted that distorted sex ratios "will ultimately present a threat to long-term stability and the sustainable development" of a society.[53]

Societies in the past have occasionally experienced the consequences of distorted sex ratios. Examples include the 1800's American Wild West, 1930's Shanghai, and Australia in the eighteenth and early nineteenth centuries. Based on their experiences, it is not implausible to predict that a large deficit of women leads to increased violence and crime. In fact, the Chinese government "has openly expressed concerns about the consequences of large numbers of excess men for societal stability and security."[54]

The consequences of distorted sex ratios on men, besides obliging them to go to extremes to find a wife, often include social isolation, resort to commercial sex, and an increased chance of acquiring a sexually-transmitted disease.[55] Beyond that, a recent Chinese study found that a "very high local sex ratio was the strongest independent determinant of depression in men."[56]

Other Methods of Sex Selection

Technology is developing to the point that abortion need not be relied upon for sex selection. Sperm can be sorted so as virtually to guarantee the conception of the desired sex. Although post-abortive damage to women is not a factor in these circumstances, underlying ethical questions remain.

Conclusion

The well-known distorted sex ratios in China, India and other countries point to the widespread practice of sex-selective abortion of females. The loss of over 160 million girls is not only a direct, sexist attack on the female half of the human race, but has left the remaining women more vulnerable as men begin to confront the marriage squeeze.

---

52   Attané I. The demographic impact of a female deficit in China, 2000-2050. Population and Development Review 2006; 32(4): pp. 755-6.
53   Li. See n. 15, p. 1.
54   Zhu, Li and Hesketh. See n. 13, p. 6.
55   Merli MG and Hertog S. Masculine sex ratios, population age structure and the potential spread of HIV in China. Demographic Research 2010; 22(3): p. 64.
56   Zhou XD, Li L, Yan Z and Hesketh T. High sex ratio as a correlate of depression in Chinese men. Journal of Affective Disorders January 2013; 144(1/2): p. 79.

There is also evidence that sex-selective abortion is being practised in countries that previously preferred gender balance. Even if there were no negative demographic consequences, would it still be inherently wrong to abort on the basis of sex? If procreative autonomy is the highest good, then sex-selective abortion is justified and beyond reproach. But if the right of females to be born and the wellbeing of society are higher goods, then sex-selective abortion cannot be justified. Until we agree on which of these two fundamentally opposed positions is right, adequately addressing the problem of skewed sex ratios will be a long time coming. Although abortion rights advocates insist that raising the status of women will eradicate sexism and eliminate the destruction of females in the womb, there is ample counter-evidence that even women with higher education or income do *not* refrain from selectively aborting their female children.

Another consideration is that since sex cannot be detected early in pregnancy, sex-selective abortion is almost always late-term abortion. Of course, for those who uphold abortion as an absolute right, age of gestation is irrelevant. But most people regard abortions at later gestation as morally objectionable. They are also much more dangerous for the women undergoing them.

Sex-selective abortion presents a dilemma for everyone. Do we countenance the continuing, intentional destruction of millions of unborn females in the name of a woman's right to choose? Or should we support the limiting of abortion, as South Korea has done, in order to protect the lives of females in the womb? Which is the bigger affront to women? The answer to that question holds ideologies and lives in the balance.

Chapter 4

Has abortion reduced the crime rate?

KEY POINTS

- Two American economists have argued that the complete legalization of abortion in the US between 1967 and 1973 resulted in a significant drop in the crime rate from the 1990s onward.

- This argument has been challenged by other economists who observe that the drop in the crime rate can also be linked to the decline of the crack-cocaine epidemic during the same period.

- Other researchers have also noted that the great increase in the number of abortions has resulted in a significant increase in single motherhood. The children of single-parent families are more likely to end up with a criminal record than the children of two-parent families.

- Other researchers have pointed out that in the UK, since abortion was legalized, crime rates have risen rather than declining.

Introduction

In 2001, economists John Donohue and Steven Levitt published an article linking the decrease in crime in the United States since the early 1990s to the legalization of abortion in 1973.[1] This article unleashed a storm of controversy. It was criticized by those who oppose abortion because of the implication that "abortion could be construed as a crime-fighting tool,"[2] and by social justice advocates, on the grounds that the evidence targeted black and poor women. Levitt later published his claims before a much broader audience in a chapter of his best-selling book *Freakonomics*. This chapter offers a critique of Donohue and Levitt's argument in light of subsequent research.

Donohue and Levitt's Hypothesis

The two authors point to the sharp decline in crime rates during the 1990s. Although they acknowledge that several factors may have contributed to this decline, they hypothesize that a significant, if not the most important factor, was the legalization of abortion. "Legalized abortion," they submit, "may account for as much as one-half of the overall crime reduction" witnessed in the 1990s.[3]

Abortion, they argue, lowers crime for two principal reasons: First, it reduces the overall number of births for each cohort born after the legalization of abortion.[4] Simply put, if there are fewer people in a given age group, there will be fewer criminals. Secondly, abortion reduces the number of people born in groups that would be considered high risk for developing criminal behaviour.[5] High-risk groups can be defined using factors such as the age of the mother, marital status, education level, and poverty. The authors further hypothesize that abortions are more likely to be obtained by women who do not want the child and would, if the child were born, not give it the proper care needed for healthy development.[6]

---

1   Donohue III JJ and Levitt SD. The impact of legalized abortion on crime. Quarterly Journal of Economics 2001; 116(2): 379-420.
2   Dubner SJ. The probability that a real-estate agent is cheating you (and other riddles of modern life): inside the curious mind of the heralded young economist Steven Levitt. *New York Times Magazine*. August 3, 2003. In: *Freakonomics: a rogue economist explores the hidden side of everything*. New York: William Morrow; 2006: p. 200.
3   Donohue and Levitt. See n. 1, p. 414.
4   Ibid., p. 381.
5   Ibid., p. 381.
6   Ibid., p. 381.

Summarizing these arguments in *Freakonomics*, Levitt and Dubner write that, "legalized abortion led to less unwantedness; unwantedness leads to high crime; legalized abortion, therefore, led to less crime."[7]

The first body of evidence that demonstrates why abortion has contributed to lower crime rates, according to Donohue and Levitt, is that the time during which the United States saw a decrease in crime coincides precisely with the time when those conceived during or just after the 1973 legalization of abortion would have been reaching their "peak ages for violent crime" — "roughly 18-24."[8] Legalized abortion eliminated many of the would-be criminals who would have begun to surface during the early 1990s, they argue; hence, the dramatic decrease in crime during the early 1990s and in subsequent years. Since there were "fewer young males in their highest-crime years," there was a decrease in crimes being committed.[9] In short, there was a decrease in crime during the 1990s because there were fewer criminals to commit crimes, thanks to legalized abortion.

The authors further contend that in states where more abortions were performed, there was a significant decrease in crime fifteen to seventeen years later, precisely when those would-be criminals would have been reaching their peak crime years. They show that crime rates fell in the five states (New York, Washington, Alaska, Hawaii and California) that legalized abortion before the 1973 Supreme Court *Roe v. Wade* decision, and before crime rates fell in the rest of the country. This, they argue, demonstrates that abortion and crime are strongly linked.[10]

Finally, Donohue and Levitt argue that the constant decrease in crime that occurred between 1991 and 1999 is a result of the smaller cohort size of high-risk groups. As they explain: "The continual decrease in crime between 1991 and 1999 is also consistent with the hypothesized effects of abortion. With each passing year, the fraction of the criminal population that was born post-legalization increases."[11] From this, they predict that we have not yet witnessed the full impact abortion will have on reducing crime.[12]

---

7   Levitt SD and Dubner SJ. *Freakonomics: a rogue economist explores the hidden side of everything*. New York: William Morrow; 2006: p. 127.
8   Donohue and Levitt. See n. 1, p. 382.
9   Ibid., p. 381.
10   Ibid., p. 384.
11   Ibid., p. 394.
12   Ibid., p. 415.

COUNTER ARGUMENTS AND EVIDENCE:

Responding to Donohue and Levitt's initial paper, economists Christopher Foote and Christopher Goetz noted a number of errors in their calculations and overall findings.[13] Taking these mistakes into account and recalculating the abortion-crime link, Foote and Goetz found that there was "no compelling evidence that abortion has a selection effect on crime."[14]

Responding to this criticism of their work, Donohue and Levitt admit they made mistakes, but that after factoring in "better data" than they "initially had available and a more thoughtfully constructed abortion proxy," the results "are in many cases stronger" than those initially reported, "even after the issues raised by Foote and Goetz are addressed."[15]

Crack Epidemic

Another economist, Ted Joyce, dismissed the abortion-crime link because Donohue and Levitt failed to take adequate account of the fact that the period they used for their calculations was also the period that witnessed the rise and decline of the crack-cocaine epidemic that swept across the United States from the mid- to late-1980s, after which it began to fall. This epidemic was linked in the view of many observers to the spread of guns and the unprecedented increase in youth violence.[16] Joyce argues that a lower crime rate is likely not so much a result of the legalization of abortion, as it is of the decline of the crack-cocaine epidemic.

Aggregate Crime Rates

John Lott and John Whitley also accuse Levitt and Donohue of erroneous calculations, this time on account of their use of aggregate crime statistics, rather than data that separate the criminals into age categories. They argue that this is essential because the crux of Levitt and Donohue's argument rests on proving that crime rates fell within the age groups that would have been affected by the legalization of abortion. Lott and Whitley use the *Supplemental Homicide Reports* rather than the *Uniform Crime Reports*, used

---

13   Foote CL and Goetz CF. The impact of legalized abortion on crime: comment. Quarterly Journal of Economics 2008; 123(1): p. 421.
14   Ibid., p. 422.
15   Donohue and Levitt. See n. 1, pp. 428-39.
16   Joyce T. Did legalized abortion lower crime? Journal of Human Resources 2004; 39(1): 1-28, pp. 2-4.

by Levitt and Donohue, because "they allow us to much more accurately disaggregate the number of murders committed by each age for each state."[17] Hence, they are able "to move beyond these aggregate crime and abortion numbers and directly link the age of the murderer with the year in which the crime occurs."[18]

By using the *Supplemental Homicide Reports* from the Centers for Disease Control (CDC), Lott and Whitley come up with a startling finding. Rather than a decrease in murders starting with the youngest age category—those who would be the ones affected by the legalization of abortion—there is a larger decrease in murder amongst the oldest age group. This demonstrates that, rather than crime decreasing among cohorts born after the legalization of abortion, *it has actually been increasing in this age category*.[19]

According to Lott and Whitley, far from reducing crime and victimization costs as Donohue and Levitt have claimed, total annual "victimization costs" rose by at least $3.2 billion as a result of abortion.[20] Why should this be so? They attribute it in part to the increase in births outside of marriage: "With about 1.6 million abortions taking place a year from around 1980 on that implies about 9600 more out-of-wedlock births annually. The linear estimates for abortion implied that legalization resulted in around 700 more murders annually in 1998, about four per cent of a year's worth of out-of-wedlock births."[21]

Abortion, Fertility, and "Unwanted" Children

As we have seen, part of Donohue and Levitt's hypothesis is that abortion lowers crime because it reduces the number of children born into high-risk categories who, they conjecture, are more likely to become criminals later in their lives. For this hypothesis to be correct, however, two assumptions made by Donohue and Levitt need to be explored: First, have there actually been fewer unwanted children born since the legalization of abortion? Second, is it really true that children born in high-risk categories are more likely to engage in criminal behavior later in life?

In *Freakonomics*, Dubner and Levitt note that since the legalization of

---

17   Lott JR and Whitley J. Abortion and crime: unwanted children and out-of-wedlock births. Economic Inquiry 2007; 45(2): p. 308.
18   Ibid., p. 313.
19   Ibid., pp. 308-10.
20   Ibid., pp. 322-3.
21   Ibid., p. 323.

abortion, conceptions in the United States "rose by nearly 30 percent" while "births actually *fell* by six per cent."[22] One explanation for this increase in conceptions and abortions, according to Ramesh Ponnuru, is that an "effect of legalized abortion was to increase the rate of careless conceptions. Its availability made it easier for people to have casual sex and to dispense with contraceptives."[23] Or, as Dubner and Levitt suggest, the numbers indicate "that many women were using abortion as a method of birth control."[24] In short, while the birth rate fell, there were also more conceptions as a result of legalized abortion. As Joyce puts it, "Some pregnancies that were aborted in the mid-to-late 1970s may not have been conceived had abortion remained illegal."[25] Commenting on this phenomenon, Ponnuru states, "it stands to reason that some of those extra conceptions made it through to birth. Some kids, paradoxically, would not have been born if not for legal abortions."[26] Regarding the number of children born outside of marriage, Lott and Whitley report that between "the 1960s through to the late 1980s . . . there has been a tremendous increase in the rate of out-of-wedlock births. On average between 1965 and 1969, only 4.8 per cent of whites were born out of wedlock, rising to 16.1 per cent twenty years later (1985-1989). For blacks, the numbers rose from 34.9 per cent to 61.8 per cent."[27] These figures indicate that the assumption made by Donohue and Levitt that legalized abortion reduced the number of unwanted children requires further research and evidence, as it is equally reasonable to assume that legalized abortion increased the number of children being born into undesirable circumstances, since without legalized abortion they might never have been conceived in the first place.

One persuasive explanation as to why legalized abortion may have led to an increase in conceptions and unwanted child births is put forward by George Akerlof, Janet Yellen, and Michael Katz. They argue that the legalization of abortion reduced a woman's ability to withhold premarital sexual favours from men. Women who are willing to obtain an abortion are more likely to engage in premarital sexual activity without a promise of marriage should pregnancy occur. However, other women who are unwilling to obtain an abortion face competition from women who are

---

22 Levitt and Dubner. See n. 7, p. 127.
23 Ponnuru R. *The party of death: the democrats, the media, the courts, and the disregard for humanlLife*. Washington, DC: Regnery Publishing, Inc.; 2006, p. 69.
24 Levitt and Dubner. See n. 7, p. 127.
25 Joyce. See n. 16, p. 6.
26 Ponnuru. See n. 23, p. 209.
27 Lott and Whitley. See n. 17, p. 305.

willing to do so, as men "'seek satisfaction elsewhere'."[28]

In summary, legalized abortion led to an increase in premarital sex, which in turn led to an increase in the number of conceptions (and abortions), which presumably led to children being born who would never have been conceived if not for legalized abortion. Donohue and Levitt's assumption, therefore, that legalized abortion has lowered the number of unwanted children is highly dubious. Further doubt is cast on their theory by the evidence that, since abortion was legalized, more children are being raised by single parents. This is a high-risk category that Donohue and Levitt identify as contributing to unwantedness and subsequent criminal behaviour. Statistics show that as abortion numbers have increased, so too have births outside of marriage. As Ponnuru comments, "abortion and illegitimacy rates rose in tandem during the 1970s and have fallen in tandem since the 1990s."[29] In part, this is due to the increase in premarital sexual activity since the legalization of abortion, as work by Akerlof and colleagues explains.[30] Those women who are unwilling to obtain an abortion are left as single mothers. Commenting on why there has been such an increase in the number of single mothers, Akerlof and colleagues raise the point that abortion made "shotgun" weddings unnecessary. Prior to the legalization of abortion, if a young woman was found to be pregnant there was far more pressure on the father to marry her and take responsibility for the child. With abortion easily obtainable, fathers of children were less likely to feel pressured into marrying the mother because if she was unwilling to have an abortion, there was less social expectation of him to make the sacrifice of marrying her and caring for the child. Akerlof and colleagues reflect that the "fact that the birth of the baby is now a *choice* of the mother has implications for the decisions of the father. The sexual revolution, by making the birth of the child the *physical* choice of the mother, makes marriage and child support a *social* choice of the father."[31]

As we have seen, Donohue and Levitt assume that there are fewer children born into high-risk categories as a result of legalized abortion. However, this assumption is undermined by statistics showing a drastic increase in the number of children raised by a single mother since the legalization of abortion. This is in part due to the fact that fewer fathers

---

28 Akerlof GA, Yellen JL and Katz ML. An analysis of out-of-wedlock childbearing in the United States. Quarterly Journal of Economics 1996; 111(2): 277-317, pp. 296-7.
29 Ponnuru. See n. 23, p. 71.
30 Akerlof, Yellen and Katz. See n. 28.
31 Ibid., p. 281.

are willing to marry the woman carrying their unborn child. It is also in part due to the decrease in children placed for adoption. Prior to the legalization of abortion, "unmarried women used to be much more likely to put up their children for adoption. In 1969 only about 28 per cent of children born out of wedlock were being raised by mothers who were still unmarried within three years. By 1984, that same fraction doubled to 56 per cent. Hence, before legalized abortion most of the children born out of wedlock ended up in families with a father."[32] These numbers would suggest, therefore, that prior to abortion's legalization there were fewer children growing up in the high-risk category of being raised by a single mother. Since the legalization of abortion then, more and more children are growing up in a home without a father.

Another of Donohue and Levitt's questionable assumptions is that those who are in what they identify as high-risk categories (poor, uneducated, single, teenage) are more likely to resort to legalized abortion than their low-risk counterparts. Joyce notes that in reality "pregnant teens with better grades, more completed schooling, and not on public assistance were much more likely to abort than their poorer, less academically oriented counterparts."[33] The same holds true not only for teens but also for unmarried women. Those with more education and better financial situations are *more* likely to abort than those who are on social assistance and have lower education levels.

If abortion had reduced the number of children born in high-risk categories, then there should have been a clear decline in the number of births for women in those categories. Examining data from the National Center for Health Statistics from 1997 to 2003, Chamlin and colleagues found that in both of these categories there has been no clear evidence to support Donohue and Levitt's theory. For teenage mothers, there was a decline in the number of births, but the decline began about fifteen years *before* abortion was legalized.[34] In the case of unmarried women, both "the unmarried women birthrate and the percentage of all births to unmarried women time series maintain their patterns of increase after 1973—patterns that began long before the *Roe* decision."[35]

---

32   Lott and Whitley. See n. 17, p. 305.
33   Joyce. See n. 16, p. 26.
34   Chamlin MB, Myer AJ, Sanders BA, and Cochran JK. Abortion as crime control: a cautionary tale. Criminal Justice Policy Review 2008: 19(2): p. 142.
35   Ibid.

The Risk of Unwanted Children Becoming Criminals Questionable

Another questionable assumption made by Donohue and Levitt in their abortion-crime link theory is that unwanted children are more at risk of becoming engaged in criminal activity later in life. In their article, "Has Roe v. Wade Reduced US Crime Rates?" Carter Hay and Michelle Evans stress how important the accuracy of the assumption is to Donohue and Levitt's conclusions. They explain that "their interpretations of state and national trends in crime generally cannot be correct if children from unwanted pregnancies are not found to be more involved in crime."[36] Careful and thorough research needs to be done to demonstrate whether or not unwanted children are more likely to develop into criminals before Donohue and Levitt's theory can be accepted. Through their own research, Hay and Evans question whether such a link between unwantedness and crime can ever be validated.

One of Hay and Evans' points is that it is impossible to determine whether or not children who are unwanted at conception will remain so. Parents' attitudes towards their children can change: "An unwanted pregnancy may sometimes give rise to a birth that is wanted—some parents may have a change of heart as the birth nears. In other instances, parents' regrets about becoming pregnant may be countered by feelings of responsibility; thus, the unwanted pregnancy may not give rise to neglectful parenting."[37]

Nor has it been shown that bearing an unwanted child leads to neglectful parenting or bad outcomes for the child. A Czech study reported that compared to the controls, "the care of these unwanted children, as far as feeding, general health and actual state of health [was] very good; they practically did not differ from their siblings and other average children."[38] Summing up the results from five other studies, Del Campo reported that the great majority of women who were denied an abortion completed their pregnancy and experienced no greater incidence of complications than their paired controls. There was "good acceptance of the infant by the mother...and minimal to moderate psychosocial disadvantages for the child." There was no statistically significant difference in the rates of drunken misconduct, crime or "educational mental subnormality" between

---

36   Hay C and Evans MM. Has Roe v. Wade reduced US crime rates? Examining the link between mothers' pregnancy intentions and children's later involvement in law-violating behaviour. Journal of Research in Crime and Delinquency 2006; 43(1): p. 38.
37   Ibid., pp. 41-2.
38   Schüller V and Stupkova E. The unwanted child in the family. International Mental Health Research Newsletter Fall 1972; 14(3): p. 8.

the two groups.[39] Most authoritative is the Swedish study, which tracked from birth to age 35 a group of children born to women denied abortion. Measured against four major criteria, the "unwanted" children were found to be only slightly worse off than the control children, whose mothers had not sought abortion. The differences were not statistically significant. The criteria were: psychiatric consultation and hospitalization, criminal record, drunken misconduct, and dependence on public assistance. The authors concluded that whatever social-psychiatric difficulties the "unwanted" children did experience were manifested for the most part early in life and became progressively smaller later on.[40]

Hay and Evans state that the link between unwantedness and later criminal activity is small, and is confined to ages eleven to seventeen. Unwantedness had no effect at all on crime reported six years later when respondents were ages seventeen to 23. This was the case for both serious and general crime."[41] They conclude that "the modest effects... observed generally run counter to the claim that legalized abortion has had dramatic effects on the crime rate."[42] This is clearly contrary to Donohue and Levitt's pronouncement that "...abortion was one of the greatest crime-lowering factors in American history..."[43]

Legal and Illegal Abortions

Economist Ted Joyce also calls into question Donohue and Levitt's conclusions because they do not take into account the number of illegal abortions that were occurring prior to legalization: "Demographers estimate that approximately two-thirds of all legal abortions replaced illegal ones in the first year after legalization."[44] Too much should not be made of this argument, since the number of legal abortions later rose much higher than those recorded in 1973-4. That is why it is misleading to assert that two-thirds of all legal abortions replaced illegal ones. Around the time of legalization there were many exaggerated claims as to the number of abortions that were occurring illegally. The figures cited were

---

39 Del Campo C. Abortion denied: outcome of mothers and babies. CMAJ 15 February 1984; 130: pp. 361-2.
40 Forssman H and Thuwe I. Continued follow-up study of 120 persons born after refusal of application for therapeutic abortion. Acta Psychiatrica Scandinavica 1981; 64(2): pp. 147-8.
41 Hay and Evans. See n. 36, p. 59.
42 Ibid.
43 Levitt and Dubner. See n. 7, p. 129.
44 Joyce. See n. 16, p. 5.

for the most part fabrications for the purpose of advancing the campaign for legalization. It has been determined that in the USA, Canada and the UK, the number of illegal abortions was far lower than initially reported. For instance, in Canada in 1976 the number of illegal abortions was likely to have been no more than 10,000 per year in the time leading up to legalization—a far cry from the widely reported estimates of 100,000. The same is true for the United States. The most commonly quoted number of illegal abortions before 1973 was one million per year. However, these statistics were derived from highly unreliable publications, and the actual number, though impossible to determine accurately, was probably closer to 200,000. In any case, the number of abortions after 1973 could not simply have replaced the number of those occurring before legalization since their numbers rose much higher than even the highest figure quoted before legalization.[45]

The recognition that the number of abortions rose dramatically after legalization does not, however, validate the argument for a connection between the rise of abortion and the lowering of crime. As we have seen, Donohue and Levitt's theory is flawed in a number of important ways. But this is not the end of the story.

Defining "Peak Crime" Years

The way in which Donohue and Levitt choose to identify the age at which people typically enter their peak crime years—eighteen to 24[46]—is also problematic. Chamlin and colleagues point out that the "difficulties associated with identifying the age at which individuals begin to engage in serious criminality are well established in the criminological literature."[47] Since there is little agreement on when individuals reach their peak crime years, "there is little agreement among researchers with respect to selecting a point in time at which the legalization of abortion should begin to influence rates of crime."[48] Chamlin and colleagues go on to state that, "Although one can readily specify the year (1973) in which the vast majority of states had their antiabortion laws nullified . . . the point in time at which this event should have begun to affect the crime rate is less clear."[49] Donohue and

---

45   Gentles I. Good news for the fetus: two fallacies in the abortion debate. Policy Review Spring 1987; 40: 50-4.
46   Donohue and Levitt. See n. 1, p. 382.
47   Chamlin, Myer, Sanders and Cochran. See n. 34, p. 137.
48   Ibid.
49   Ibid.

Levitt, therefore, fail to consider the differing evidence on what should be accepted as peak crime years. In not taking these variations into account, it seems they have selected the findings that fit their theory. As Chamlin and colleagues explain, "Such an approach invariably capitalizes on chance variation and, thereby, has low statistical power."[50]

ABORTION AND INFANTICIDE RATES

In an article on the homicide of young children, Sorenson and colleagues conclude that the "US Supreme Court decision in *Roe v. Wade* is associated with a gradual reduction in the number of homicides of children who are one to four years old."[51] They offer three explanations for this association. "First, with fewer unwanted children, there are fewer stresses on parents who might be inclined to take out their frustrations and hostilities on their children... [Second,] familial resources... would be divided among fewer children rather than stretched to accommodate a newborn. Third, abortion reduces, theoretically, at least, unwanted children who themselves might have become targets, if not immediately then over time."[52]

Although it may be the case, as Sorenson and colleagues claim, that legalized abortion coincides with the lowering of infanticide rates, there would need to be concrete evidence that proves there are fewer children born into families with financial difficulties or fewer children within each family. If the reverse were shown, namely that legalized abortion has not coincided with a lowering of the number of children born into poverty or a reduction in the number of children in a financially volatile family, then the relationship between the lowering of infanticide rates and the legalization of abortion would not be causal but merely coincidental.

THE EXPERIENCE OF OTHER COUNTRIES

United Kingdom

Another way in which Donohue and Levitt's hypothesis and conclusions can be tested is by investigating whether other countries that have legalized abortion have also seen a decline in crime. The United Kingdom, for

---

50   Ibid.
51   Sørenson SB, Wiebe DJ and Berk RA. Legalized abortion and the homicide of young children: an empirical investigation. Analyses of Social Issues and Public Policy 2002; 2(1): p. 239.
52   Ibid., pp. 250-1.

example, has experienced no such decline.

> ... the United Kingdom legalized abortion in 1968, some years before most other Western countries; as a result, we have a longer time period over which to examine any possible impacts on crime. More importantly, a particular feature of the UK legislation is that there is a statutory requirement for every abortion to be reported. A consequence of this is that abortion data are of very high quality. In contrast, the analyses of abortion and crime in the United States have had to rely on survey data that are incomplete and, in some cases, of questionable quality. In addition to the abortion data in the UK being complete, much more detail is available than from most other countries. Abortion data are available broken down by age of mother, marital status and whether or not the mother had to travel outside her area of residence to obtain the abortion.[53]

The authors of the UK study go on to point out that

> ... the 1967 Abortion Act did not apply in Northern Ireland. Similarly, no comparable legislation was passed in the Republic of Ireland ... If legislation of abortion reduces crime, we might expect that crime in England/Wales and in Scotland decreases relative to the other two areas from the mid-1980s onwards. In fact, if anything the graph suggests a relative increase in crime, at least at the start of the period, in the areas affected by abortion legalization.[54]

The finding that crime did not decrease in the areas that legalized abortion, but in fact increased, further undermines the Donohue and Levitt theory.

In their conclusions, Kanane and colleagues remark, "... we are unable to say that abortion legalization in the United Kingdom significantly reduced crime in England and Wales some twenty years thereafter. We come to this

---

53 Kahane LH, Paton D and Simmons R. The abortion-crime link: evidence from England and Wales. Economica February 2008; 75(297): p. 2.
54 Ibid., p. 8.

conclusion by first noting... that total recorded crime in the United Kingdom began to decrease at about the same time as in the United States, despite the fact that abortion legalization occurred here about five years earlier. Thus, we have a discrepancy in the timing of the potential effect of abortion on crime between the United States and the United Kingdom." Equally, crime in England and Wales did not decrease relative to Northern Ireland and the Republic of Ireland, where abortion remained illegal throughout the period in question. In sum, "...our results are mixed and indicate either no relation between abortion and subsequent crime, or a positive one in cases where London is excluded from the analysis—these latter results being opposite to those results found in Donohue and Levitt."[55]

Australia

In Australia, Leigh and Wolfers also discovered a causal link between abortion and lower crime rates. Their study, however, focused exclusively on homicide data, rather than the three crime categories used by Donohue and Levitt. Like the US, Australia saw a steady decrease in crime beginning in 1988 and continuing throughout the 1990s.[56] This coincides, according to Leigh and Wolfers, with the legalization of abortion in Australia, as "for over two-thirds of the Australian population, the change occurred in the late-1960s or early-1970s—or about twenty years before the drop in crime rates."[57] In addition to the timing of the drop in crime, Leigh and Wolfers find some evidence that suggests that the states in Australia that legalized abortion before other areas did witness an earlier drop in crime rates. However, as with Donohue and Levitt, they fail to distinguish among various age groups, lumping them all together, when they ought to have focused on the seventeen- to 24-year olds, whose crime rate may legitimately be said to have had something to do with the earlier legalization of abortion. Moreover, while some areas indicate a causal link between abortion and lower crime, Leigh and Wolfers also note that "the evidence for other regions does not support this proposition," and that, "at best, we can say that this part of the theory holds for the states where most Australians live."[58]

Although Leigh and Wolfers find a positive link between legalized

---

55 Ibid., p. 17.
56 Leigh A and Wolfers J. Abortion and crime. Australian Quarterly August—September 2000; 72(4): p. 29.
57 Ibid.
58 Ibid., p. 30.

abortion and lower crime in the two tests above—in the time of the lowering of crime and the instances where crime rates dropped earlier in the states that legalized earlier—in two other tests that are part of Donohue and Levitt's theory they are unable to find any evidence supporting the link. Without the data and evidence to support a positive link between abortion and crime in these two crucial areas, it is impossible to draw any conclusions. To say that the Australian experience demonstrates a causal link between legalized abortion and the lowering of crime and proves Levitt and Donohue's theory correct ignores the inconclusive evidence in other important areas. Before Australia can be used either to support or oppose the abortion-crime link, more thorough and complete research needs to be conducted.

Canada

Although the Australian experience provides a weak validation of the link between legalized abortion and lower crime, Anindya Sen's application of the theory to Canada seems strongly to support Donohue and Levitt. Canada provides a good test for the theory, argues Sen, because "unlike the US, the incidence of the crack-cocaine and gun 'epidemics' were much more limited in Canada, thus minimizing the possibility of confounded empirical estimates of the impact of abortion on crime."[59]

Sen focused his research on teenage abortion rates.[60] He explains:

> Specifically, while general fertility rates are insignificantly correlated with crime, corresponding estimates of teen fertility are positive and statistically significant, substantiating empirical estimates of the impacts of abortion on crime. These estimates suggest that abortion legalization ultimately results in a drop in crime through a corresponding decrease in teenage or unwanted childbearing (selection effects) rather than lower cohort size. Further, these results are important as they are slightly more refined than strategies adapted by other studies.[61]

---

59   Sen A. Does increased abortion lead to lower crime? Evaluating the relationship between crime, abortion, and fertility. The B.E. Journal of Economic Analysis and Policy September 2007; 7(1): p. 3.
60   Ibid., p. 4.
61   Ibid., p. 4.

Sen finds that there is a "statistically significant and negative association between violent crime" and teenage abortions. "The drop in these abortion rates, account for nearly a quarter of the decline in violent crime during the nineteen-nineties," a result that parallels evidence offered by Donohue and Levitt. Further, the corresponding decline in teenage fertility was responsible for more than half the decline in violent crime over the specific time period.[62]

Romania

Christian Pop-Eleches tries to understand the relationship between abortion and lower crime rates by looking at the effects of a policy directly opposite to that which was introduced in the US. He examines what happens when a country that had one of the most liberal abortion policies in the world suddenly adopts the most severe limitations on abortion. When Romania's abortion law was completely reversed in 1966 to outlaw almost all abortions, there was an immediate, if short-lived increase in the country's birth rate. According to Pop-Eleches, "the total fertility rate increased from 1.9 to 3.7 children per woman between 1966 and 1967."[63] Given the drastic increase in births in Romania as a result of the banning of abortion, Pop-Eleches tries to examine the effects in terms of socioeconomic outcomes for the children born during this period. He finds that "children born in 1967 just after abortion became illegal display *significantly better* educational and labor market achievements than children born just prior to the change."[64] This finding would seem to discredit the abortion-crime theory, yet Pop-Eleches overturns his own finding by explaining that a number of educated, wealthy women were now giving birth. This is important, he says, because "urban, educated women were more likely to have abortions prior to the policy change, so a higher proportion of children were born into urban, educated households after abortions became illegal."[65] By this reasoning Pop-Eleches is able to arrive at the opposite conclusion, namely that "children born after the abortion ban had *worse* schooling and labor market outcomes".[66] Here we have another remarkable example of a researcher drawing a conclusion that completely contradicts his findings.

---

62   Ibid., pp. 24-5.
63   Pop-Eleches C. The impact of an abortion ban on socioeconomic outcomes of children: evidence from Romania. Journal of Political Economy August 2006; 114(4): p. 745.
64   Ibid.
65   Ibid.
66   Ibid.

CONCLUSION

Because Donohue and Levitt's theory has far-reaching social, political and moral implications, it cries out for rigorous scrutiny. Our analysis demonstrates that, although the abortion-crime theory has gained widespread attention, there are compelling reasons for regarding it with skepticism. It fails to acknowledge other reasons why crime may have declined in the US in the 1990s. It fails to recognize that by contributing to the rise of single motherhood, abortion may have resulted in worse parenting for a growing percentage of children. Its assumption that if children are unwanted they are more likely to fall into crime is not supported by research findings from Europe. The United Kingdom, which legalized abortion five years before the US, has experienced no significant drop in the crime rate. On the contrary, in Northern Ireland, where abortion remains illegal, the crime rate is significantly lower than in the rest of the UK. In sum, much of the research done in the past decade casts doubt on whether Donohue and Levitt's supposed link between abortion and falling crime rates exists at all.

Chapter 5

Informed consent: A woman's right

KEY POINTS

- It is a longstanding legal principle that patients may not be subjected to medical procedures without their consent.

- The principle of 'informed consent', meaning that the patient has the right to be told of the risks involved in a given medical procedure, has emerged over the past several decades.

- It is still difficult to prosecute a physician for failing to obtain a patient's informed consent to a medical procedure, abortion in particular.

- Several jurisdictions in the US have introduced 'Right-to-Know' laws that make physicians legally liable for failing to inform their abortion patients about the risks involved in induced abortion, and the alternatives to it.

- In the past few years, several abortion providers have been successfully sued for their failure to inform patients of the risks of abortion, in particular the increased risk of breast cancer.

INTRODUCTION

The phrase "informed consent" was originally coined in a law case in the United States in 1957.[1] It represented a new set of obligations on physicians above and beyond the requirement to obtain mere consent that existed before that time. Rather than just gaining the acquiescence of the patient to perform a procedure, the physician now has what is called an "affirmative duty of disclosure".[2] In other words, unless the right to be informed is specifically waived or is impossible to fulfill, the physician is obliged to provide patients with information on the risks of the proposed procedure before undertaking it.

Though affirmative disclosure is now an ethical and legal obligation throughout most of the Western world, its application to abortion cases has been controversial. As we shall see in later chapters, both the number and the scope of risks are in dispute. However, even the risks that are known and accepted are not always disclosed. Part of the reason for this is that informed consent codes are difficult to enforce with respect to abortion. We shall now discuss the reasons for these difficulties, and examine some of the laws that American states have enacted in order to resolve them.

ETHICAL CODES

Code Texts

Both the American and Canadian Medical Associations require their members to provide patients with information concerning risks and alternatives before asking them to consent to a medical procedure. The AMA states:

> The patient's right of self-decision can be effectively exercised only if the patient possesses enough information to enable an informed choice. The patient should make his or her own determination about treatment. The physician's obligation is to present the medical facts accurately to the patient or to the individual responsible for the patient's care and to make recommendations for management in accordance with good medical practice.

---

1   Salgo v Leland Stanford Jr. University Board of Trustees: Ruth R. Faden and Tom L. Beauchamp. *A history and theory of informed consent.* Oxford: Oxford University Press, 1986, p. 125.
2   Berg JW, Appelbaum PS, Lidz CW and Parker LS. *Informed consent: legal theory and clinical practice.* Oxford: Oxford University Press, 2001: pp. 43-4.

The physician has an ethical obligation to help the patient make choices from among the therapeutic alternatives consistent with good medical practice. Informed consent is a basic policy in both ethics and law that physicians must honor, unless the patient is unconscious or otherwise incapable of consenting and harm from failure to treat is imminent. In special circumstances, it may be appropriate to postpone disclosure of information (see Opinion E-8.122, "Withholding Information from Patients").

Physicians should sensitively and respectfully disclose all relevant medical information to patients. The quantity and specificity of this information should be tailored to meet the preferences and needs of individual patients. Physicians need not communicate all information at one time, but should assess the amount of information that patients are capable of receiving at a given time and present the remainder when appropriate (I, II, V, VIII)[3].

The CMA includes the following principles in its Code of Ethics:

21. Provide your patients with the information they need to make informed decisions about their medical care, and answer their questions to the best of your ability.

22. Make every reasonable effort to communicate with your patients in such a way that information exchanged is understood.

23. Recommend only those diagnostic and therapeutic services that you consider to be beneficial to your patient or to others. If a service is recommended for the benefit of others, as for example in matters of public health, inform your patient of this fact and proceed only with explicit informed consent or where required by law.

24. Respect the right of a competent patient to accept or reject any medical care recommended.[4]

---

3   American Medical Association (AMA), Council on Ethical and Judicial Affairs. *Code of medical ethics: current opinions with annotations*. Chicago: AMA Press, 2007: Opinion 8.08.
4   Canadian Medical Association (CMA). CMA code of ethics (update 2004): p. 2. http://policybase.cma.ca/PolicyPDF/PD04-06.pdf.

Both codes are largely consistent with the legal obligations for informed consent that have arisen in common law. In fact, both ethical codes go beyond the common law in these important respects:

- The American code includes the requirement that physicians make recommendations in accordance with good medical practice. Informed consent law says nothing of recommendations, only of risks and alternatives.

- The Canadian code requires that patients be made aware of who the intended beneficiary is of a medical treatment, if the beneficiary is not the patient him- or herself.

- Both require not only disclosure, but also that the disclosure be *understood* by the patients. By contrast, the common law focuses almost entirely on what was actually disclosed and not the understanding of those who heard the disclosure. This is likely because such understanding, or lack of it, would be difficult to demonstrate in a courtroom.

Disciplinary Actions

Disciplinary actions within the medical profession are handled within state and provincial, not national, professional associations. Hence, the rules governing disciplinary actions for discipline for violation of ethical codes varies from state to state and province to province. Despite these variations, some observations can be made:

- Definitions of professional misconduct are generally very narrow. In order to be disciplined, a physician must engage in actual professional misconduct, not merely fail to live up to one of the expectations of the code.
- Failure to disclose rarely provides grounds for a finding of professional misconduct. For instance, in the Province of Ontario the only violation of the Code of the College of Physicians and Surgeons regarding consent that will give rise to a finding of professional misconduct is, "performing a professional service for which consent is required by law without consent".[5]

---

[5] The College of Physicians and Surgeons of Ontario (CPSO). CPSO policy statement: consent to medical treatment. Policy #4-05. 2006: p. 8. Note that this part of the policy statement is a restatement of the Health Care Consent Act, 1996; Ontario Regulation 853/93, as amended (made under the Medicine Act, 1991).

Failure to inform a patient appropriately of risks does not constitute professional misconduct. Rather, the code envisions cases where patients are treated without any consent. Physicians are obliged to disclose risks and alternatives to patients according to ethical codes that are more demanding than the common law. However, the professional disciplinary codes do not provide patients with redress for a physician's failure to disclose. While it is true that a physician who fails to inform a potential abortion patient of the risks is acting unethically, there is usually no redress within the profession's disciplinary code.

THE LEGAL FRAMEWORK

Elements of Informed Consent Cases

In virtually all cases, failures to obtain informed consent are handled under tort (or civil) law, rather than criminal law. The obligation in tort law to obtain consent and disclose risks and alternatives developed under two separate torts, *battery* and *negligence*:

Battery

Until the mid-twentieth century, law suits concerning lack of consent were largely resolved under the tort of battery.[6] According to the tort of battery, a person has a right to *bodily integrity*, that is, the right not to be touched without his or her consent. Physicians who failed to inform their patients sufficiently concerning a medical treatment were thought to vitiate the consent of the patient, thereby invalidating the consent and making any physical contact a battery. Battery is an *intentional tort*, which is not covered by most physicians' malpractice insurance.[7]

However, almost no North American jurisdiction treats failure to obtain *informed* consent under the tort of battery. Like the professional misconduct mentioned above, the tort of battery normally applies when physicians fail to get their patients' consent for a procedure *at all*, rather than when they simply fail affirmatively to disclose information.[8] In order

---

[6] American Medical Association (AMA). Patient physician relationship topics: informed consent. AMA. 2011. http://www.ama-assn.org/ama/pub/physician-resources/legal-topics/patient-physician-relationship-topics/informed-consent.page.
[7] Ibid.
[8] Note that this assumes that consent can be obtained at all. In the case of an emergency where consent cannot be gained, physicians do not need to attain the explicit consent of their patients.

to sue under the tort of battery, a patient needs to show that the physician either failed to obtain consent before performing a procedure, or obtained it by misrepresentation or fraud.

Negligence

In the mid-twentieth century, the primary tort under which physicians were obliged to inform patients increasingly became the tort of negligence rather than battery. From the mid-1970s in the US, only Pennsylvania has continued to use the tort of battery in cases of failure to disclose.[9] In 1980 in Reibl v Hughes, Canada's Supreme Court also moved towards including informed consent under the tort of negligence rather than battery.[10] Under the tort of negligence, a physician can be sued for not providing due care to patients.

The requirements of the tort of negligence make it more difficult to sue a physician for failure to inform. To sue successfully for negligence on account of failure to disclose, a patient must demonstrate five elements of the negligence:[11]

1. *Duty*: The patient must show that the physician actually had the duty to inform the patient.
2. *Breach of Duty*: The patient must show that the physician breached the standard of care in not disclosing information.
3. *Decision-Causation*: The patient must show that, had the relevant risks been disclosed, a different decision would have been made by either:
    a. The patient him/herself (a subjective standard)
    b. A reasonable patient (an objective standard)
4. *Injury*: The patient suffered a physical injury as a result.
5. *Injury-Causation*: The patient must show that the risk of which he or she was not informed actually came to fruition or that an undisclosed alternative would have prevented an injury

All five elements of negligence must be shown before a physician can be sued for failure to inform a patient.

---

9 Because of this difference, informed consent applies only to surgery in Pennsylvania, not to medication or any other treatment that does not involve touching. See Morgan v. MacPhail, 550 Pa. 202, 704 A.2d 617 (1997).
10 Reibl v. Hughes, [1980] 2 S.C.R. 880.
11 Faden and Beauchamp: See n.1, p. 29.

Note that failure to inform a patient of a risk or possible alternative does not constitute an injury in itself. While patients have successfully sued for pain, and suffering-related worry brought on by risks of which they should have been informed, no one outside of Pennsylvania has successfully sued for the dignitary damages involved in not being informed *per se* in over 30 years.

Duty and Breach of Duty

The first two elements of a successful law suit in a case of informed consent are duty and breach of duty. The duty at issue in informed consent concerns the risks and alternatives a physician is obliged to disclose to a given patient. Regarding abortion, the risks at issue may include some of those discussed in this book. Although the Salgo case that coined the term "informed consent" originally called for "full disclosure", this ultimately became impractical. Instead, three different types of standards for disclosure have been developed:

Professional Practice: Under the professional practice standard, the physician is expected to provide the risks and alternatives that a typical physician usually discloses in such a situation. This was the first standard to be applied, and is still used in about half of the US states.[12] In the case of abortion, professional practice standards have been especially problematic in ensuring that physicians inform women of the risks of abortion. Since under this standard physicians are only obliged to disclose what physicians normally disclose, there is no way to improve the disclosure habits of physicians as a whole. Furthermore, in states with a professional practice standard, patients pursuing a law suit must find a physician who will serve as an expert witness, something that can be quite difficult.

Reasonable Person: Under the "reasonable person" standard, the physician is expected to disclose the risks and alternative that a hypothetical "reasonable person" would wish to know. The "reasonable person" is a legal construct who represents the interests of an average person. This standard is used in Canada and about half of the US states.[13]

The problems with professional practice standards led to the transition to the "reasonable person" standard. Note, however, that this standard is not a subjective one. In other words, it does not ask the question, whether *this* patient would want to know such a risk, but whether an *average* patient

---

12 Berg, Appelbaum, Lidz and Parker. See n. 2, pp. 46-7.
13 Ibid., pp. 48-51.

would want to know such a risk. In cases of abortion, differences in values tend to cause the "reasonable person" construct to break down. Thus a woman may find herself in a situation where she might have wanted to know a risk about which the average person was judged not to care about knowing, and so lose her case.

Statutory Standards: In several US states, including prominently Texas and Florida, the state government has intervened to state exactly which risks must be disclosed in the case of certain medical treatments. In those states, the statutorily disclosed risks trump the professional practice and "reasonable person" standards for the procedures covered under the statutes. When a course of treatment is not covered by statute, cases will instead be handled by professional practice or "reasonable person" standards, depending on the jurisdiction.

Right-to-Know Laws: "Right-to-Know" laws have been introduced in a number of US states over the last few decades. These laws often focus on abortion, but many are folded into general statutory standards of disclosure. They create a number of different legal requirements:

- Some laws make provisions about the manner in which the information must be delivered, such as by face-to-face conversation. They may also require that a form be signed indicating that the information has been conveyed.
- Some laws require that specific literature be distributed to women seeking an abortion.
- Some laws require that information about alternatives to abortion also be discussed.
- Some laws require that an ultrasound of the fetus be taken and shown to the mother.

In all cases, Right-to-Know laws establish that failure to follow their guidelines provides a *prima facie* case that the duty to inform has been breached. In addition, many Right-to-Know laws add enforcement mechanisms above and beyond that of suing the physician:

- In some jurisdictions, (such as Ohio), failure to follow a Right-to-Know law can result in the physician's license being revoked.[14]
- In some jurisdictions, failure to follow a Right-to-Know law may

---

14   Ohio Revised Code. Title [47] XLVII Occupations—professions. Chapter 4731: Physicians; Physicians; Limited practitioners.

result in fines. For example, in Oklahoma, for a third-time offence, the fine is $100,000.[15]
- In some jurisdictions (such as Indiana)[16], failure to follow the law may be a misdemeanor; in others a criminal offence (as in South Carolina).[17]
- In some jurisdictions (such as Tennessee)[18], physicians may be imprisoned for failure to follow the law. No jurisdiction, however, imposes a mandatory minimum term of imprisonment for a first offence.

Right-to-Know laws, therefore, seek to circumvent some of the difficulties with "professional and reasonable person" standards by setting strict guidelines for abortion. In addition, many include stronger enforcement mechanisms than those provided by the right to sue.

Decision-Causation

Decision-causation may also be difficult to show in an informed consent case. Decision-causation means that, had a given risk been disclosed, the patient would not have undergone the procedure. Notice what this implies. A patient cannot simply sue for not having been informed. If a patient was not informed, but the information that she lacked would not have changed her mind about the procedure, then she will lose her case. Decision-causation can be difficult to establish, especially given people's capacity for distorted hindsight. Moreover, there are two different standards in place:[19]

- *The Objective Standard*: Under an objective standard, the question is whether a reasonable person would have undergone the procedure had she known the risks. The problem with this standard for abortion (or for almost any common medical procedure) is that, since average informed people do undergo abortions while aware of the risk, decision-causation is difficult to establish.
- *The Subjective Standard*: Under a subjective standard, the question is whether this patient would have changed her mind had she known

---

15 Oklahoma Statutes §63-1-738.3b.E.
16 Indiana General Assembly. Chapter 2: requirements for performance of abortion; criminal penalties. Indiana Code. Title 16. Article 34. http://www.in.gov/legislative/ic/code/title16/ar34/.
17 South Carolina Code of Laws. Section 44-41-10.
18 Tennessee Code. 39-15-202.
19 Berg, Appelbaum, Lidz and Parker. See n. 2, pp. 138-40.

the risks. In some ways this is easier to establish than the objective standard, but it can also be difficult to demonstrate one's mental state adequately to a jury.

Injury and Injury-Causation

In addition to demonstrating that the physician had an obligation to disclose the risk and that this or an average patient would have acted otherwise, the plaintiff must also show that injury was actually caused by the procedure. This is called "injury-causation". Even if the gravest and most common risks are not disclosed, unless the failure to disclose causes actual physical or emotional harm, she cannot sue.

One serious difficulty with showing injury-causation is that risk alone is not recoverable; the patient must establish actual harm. Injury-causation must be established by the preponderance of evidence; that is, it must be likely that the injury was caused by the procedure. To take an example from this book let us assume that all parties are agreed that risk of bearing a premature child is increased by a minimum of 25 to 27 per cent for women who have had abortions.[20] A woman had an abortion and was not informed of this risk (duty and breach of duty). She would have chosen otherwise had she known (decision-causation). Even if she subsequently bears a premature child, she still cannot demonstrate injury-causation. Because her abortion increased her risk of a subsequent premature birth by less than 50 per cent, there is a *greater* than 50 per cent chance that her premature birth would have occurred even if she had not had the abortion. Since the threshold for preponderance of evidence is 50 per cent, injury causation cannot be established.

For injuries where injury-causation is obvious, such as a perforated uterus, this fourth element of a law suit may be easy to establish. However, for any risks that are simply increases in risk below a preponderance of evidence, injury-causation may prove impossible to establish, even if those increases are widely known and uncontroversial.

FURTHER CHALLENGES IN CONSENT LAW

Finding Those Willing to Sue

As with any other case of negligence, there is no official body whose role it

---

20   See Chapter 15, p. 236.

is to enforce informed consent. In order for such cases to be brought to trial, individuals must be willing to sue. This means that without women both willing and informed enough to bring lawsuits against their physicians, there is no enforcement mechanism for informed consent.

Here are several reasons why few women are willing to bring lawsuits against physicians for damages related to informed consent in abortion:

- Feelings of guilt surrounding the abortion.
- Feelings of embarrassment arising from being injured during an elective procedure (similar problems arise, for example, in elective plastic surgery).
- Lack of knowledge on the part of most patients as to their legal rights to informed consent and the means of redress.
- The enormous cost of a lawsuit, together with the risk that it will fail.

For these reasons physicians have little incentive to inform their patients of the risks of induced abortion. Lawsuits on the basis of failure to disclose the risks surrounding abortion are rare in both the US and Canada.

Psychological Harm

Much of the evidence concerning the health risks of abortion concerns psychological health and the large increase of diagnosable psychological conditions after an abortion, especially depression. Nonetheless, the courts have routinely ruled that, without physical injury, failure to inform of possible psychological harm is not sufficient ground for a lawsuit. The most important case in this respect is *Humes v Clinton* (1990). The Kansas Supreme Court ruled that unless there was physical injury, a plaintiff has not met the injury criterion for a successful informed-consent suit.[21] As a result, even if there were no controversy about the possibility of psychological harm resulting from abortion, failure to inform about the possibility of psychological harm would be unlikely to provide sufficient grounds for a successful suit.

Duress

The legal definition of duress varies. Adults are assumed to be competent to make rational decisions unless it can be demonstrated otherwise. As a

---

21 Humes v Clinton. 792 P.2d 1032 (Kan. 1990).

result, informed consent laws cannot do much to ensure that women are not pressured into having an abortion. Care providers, family and fathers of the fetus may exert tremendous pressure upon a woman to have an abortion, but unless she is under *duress*, she will have no legal recourse. A woman is under *duress* only if she is subject to a threat that is itself illegal or which would cause her to break a binding contract.[22] In Canada, however, duress is defined more narrowly, as a threat of immediate physical harm.

Medical risks do not constitute duress. For example, if a woman's life is endangered by a pregnancy, that is not duress. Nor are threats to cut off financial support from an adult child or to terminate a relationship. The threat of being fired for refusal to have an abortion can constitute duress, but only in the US, not in Canada. A physician not directly complicit in such a case would not be liable. Redress for losing one's job for being pregnant is best achieved under employment discrimination law.

Informed consent law, then, cannot in its present form serve to ensure that women are not pressured into abortion, even by their physician. The standard of competence is much lower than that of a philosophical standard of autonomous decision.

In Canada in 2010 a private member's bill (Bill C-510) was introduced into the House of Commons. It would have amended the Criminal Code to prohibit coercing a woman into an abortion by physical or financial threats, illegal acts, or through "argumentative and rancorous badgering or importunity". Designed to circumvent the weakness of informed consent law to deal with cases of duress, it defined the following as coercive activity:

> (a) committing, attempting to commit, or threatening to commit physical harm to the female person, the child or another person;
>
> (b) committing, attempting to commit or threatening to commit any act prohibited by any provincial or federal law;
>
> (c) denying or removing, or making a threat to deny or remove, financial support or housing from a person who is financially dependent on the person engaging in the conduct; and
>
> (d) attempting to compel by pressure or intimidation including

---

22 "Duress." *Black's law dictionary*. Eds. Bryan A. Garner and Henry Campbell Black. 9th Edition. Saint Paul: West Group, 2009.

argumentative and rancorous badgering or importunity.

However, it would *not* have included speech protected under the Canadian Charter of Rights and Freedoms.[23] In the end, like most private members' bills, C-510 was defeated on second reading (15 December 2010), and failed to become law.

CONCLUSION

Both the law and professional codes require that physicians reveal risks and alternatives to women considering having an abortion. This is a positive duty of disclosure, something that physicians are required to do, regardless of whether they are asked. When physicians fail to disclose those risks, they violate their professional and legal obligations. Until recently, these obligations have been difficult to enforce in cases of abortion. In this century, however, some successful legal steps have been taken, in the form of various "Right-to-Know" laws in several American states. These laws are beginning to create difficulties for abortion providers such as Planned Parenthood. In Kansas, Indiana, and Ohio, suits have been brought against that organization not only for failing to inform parents when an abortion was performed on a minor, but also for failing to hold an "informed consent" meeting with the client prior to an abortion.[24] For example, Ohio Planned Parenthood recently settled out of court in a suit brought against them for emotional and psychological distress suffered by a fourteen-year-old girl upon whom they had performed an abortion. Although she was a minor at the time, the abortion agency did not inform her parents of the abortion, or the legal authorities that she was in an illegal and criminal sexual relationship with an adult, her 21-year-old soccer coach. Neither the abortionist nor any other agent of Planned Parenthood obtained the informed and voluntary consent of the girl before providing these medical "services". In a highly significant ruling, the Common Pleas Court judge found that the Planned Parenthood doctor breached a legal duty by not holding an "informed consent" meeting with the girl before the abortion.[25] The case dragged on for seven years, 2005 to 2012, when it was finally

---

23   Bill C-510: *An act to amend the criminal code (coercion)*. 1st Reading, April 14th, 2010, 40th Parliament, 3rd Session, 2010. http://www.parl.gc.ca/HousePublications/Publication.aspx?Language=E&Mode=1&DocId=4427296&File=24#1.
24   Bronson P. It's easier to get an abortion than an aspirin. *Cincinnati Enquirer*, Sept. 27, 2005: p. B7.
25   Perry K. Abortion provider loses ruling. Cincinnati Enquirer, Dec. 9, 2010: p. C1.

resolved to the satisfaction of the plaintiffs.[26] In short, abortion providers are now increasingly vulnerable to suits from women who believe they were not adequately informed of the risks entailed by the procedure, and by parents of minors who were informed neither of the abortion, nor that their underage daughters were the victims of rape. In addition there have been at least three recent cases of women who sued their abortion providers for failing to inform them of the link between abortion and breast cancer. None of the women had actually developed breast cancer when they brought their abortion providers to court, but they won damages merely because the courts recognized that their induced abortions had significantly increased their chances of developing breast cancer before the age of 45.[27]

This handful of cases may well open the floodgates to scores of other cases in the future. Strengthened by these recently established legal precedents, the victims of abortion will certainly prove less and less willing to accept any failure on the part of abortion providers to inform them of the risks of the procedure before they perform it.

---

26   Jamie and Brenda Wallace, parents of Jane Roe, a minor v. Planned Parenthood Southwest Ohio region, et al. Court of Common Pleas, Civil Division, Hamilton County, Ohio. Case No. A0502691 (2007). We are grateful to Brian Hurley, one of the prosecuting attorneys, for providing details and court documents related to the case.
27   The three cases occurred in Pennsylvania, Oregon and Ohio: Stephanie Carter v. Charles D. Benjamin, D.O., et al., Court of Common Pleas, Philadelphia., April Term, 2000, No.: 3890 (settled Oct. 2003);   Felicia. Bautista. v. All Women's Health Services, Multnomah County, Oregon Circuit Court Case # 0307-07422, 7 July 2003 (settled 24 January 2005);   Chelsey Wallace v. Planned Parenthood, Southwest Ohio region et al. Court of Common Pleas, Civil Division, Hamilton County, Ohio Case No A0502691(2007).

Section II: The Medical Impact

Abstract

The immediate complications of induced abortion include bleeding (hemorrhage), retained tissue, infection, uterine perforation, cervical laceration, and immediate psychiatric morbidity, or depression. Depending on the jurisdiction, these reported complications occur in 3.4 per cent to eleven per cent of all surgically-induced abortions. The immediate complication rate for "medical", or drug-induced, abortions is up to four times higher—twelve per cent to 44 per cent. Since abortion clinics do not follow up with their patients, the true immediate complication rate may well exceed the figures quoted in various studies.

Chapter 7 presents the overwhelmingly strong evidence, both biological and epidemiological, for the link between induced abortion and breast cancer. A woman who carries her pregnancy to term decreases her risk of breast cancer. On the other hand, aborting a first pregnancy significantly increases the risk of later developing breast cancer. Recent research on the physiology of the breast explains why this is so. When a woman becomes pregnant for the first time her immature and cancer-vulnerable breast tissue matures into cancer-resistant tissue. Approximately 85 per cent of her breast turns into fully mature, cancer resistant Type 4 lobules, which contain the first milk, colostrum. After weaning, these lobules regress to Type 3 lobules, which are also cancer-resistant. This biological change accounts for the recognized fact that never having a full-term pregnancy (nulliparity) increases a woman's risk of breast cancer. After a full-term pregnancy, only fifteen per cent of her breast tissue remains susceptible to forming cancer. It is the genetic changes that occur in the breast lobules during a full-term pregnancy that give lifelong protection. Molecular biologists have also determined that progenitor or stem cells in the breast do not become terminally differentiated (reach their full potential growth or maturity) until they have undergone the environment

Chapter 7:

Biology and epidemiology confirm the abortion-breast cancer link

of pregnancy and have lactated. A woman who aborts an early pregnancy denies herself this protection against breast cancer.

As for the epidemiological evidence, most scientists worldwide, except in the US, agree that induced abortion is a known risk for breast cancer. This agreement is based on 56 studies (35 of them statistically significant) from many countries. Studies that compare countries have demonstrated that those with high rates of induced abortion also experience significantly higher rates of breast cancer. Racial comparisons are also instructive. African Americans have a much higher rate of induced abortion than Caucasian Americans. Their rate of breast cancer is also much higher. Yet in the face of all this multi-faceted evidence, the National Cancer Institute in the US continues to deny the abortion-breast cancer link, even though one of its own researchers has published a study demonstrating the link. As with this Institute's previous refusal to recognize the link between cigarette smoking and lung cancer, the explanation now appears to be mainly political.

Chapter 8:

Prenatal testing and abortion for fetal anomaly

Prenatal testing, through the technologies of amniocentesis, ultrasound imaging, and chorionic villi sampling are the subject of Chapter 8. Now that prenatal diagnosis has become standard medical practice, there is widespread disapproval of women who decline to undergo the tests. They are accused of not doing their duty to ensure the birth of healthy children. Overwhelmingly, medical professionals stress the negative aspects of bearing a child with disabilities, and convey the expectation that a diagnosis of physical or mental disabilities should be followed by a decision to abort.

Prenatal diagnosis programs are markedly decreasing the number of children born with certain conditions. Unfortunately, there is no sign that any increased support is being given to pregnant mothers or children with genetic disorders, still less that testing is being used to prevent or treat illness and disability in unborn children. The resort to prenatal testing to weed out the "unfit" is reminiscent of the discredited science of eugenics. Encouragingly, when the option of perinatal palliative care—a supportive option for parents whose child has been diagnosed with a life-limiting anomaly—is offered, between 40 and 80 percent of parents request this care and choose to continue their pregnancy.

Prenatal diagnosis is a far from perfect science. Unborn children diagnosed as suffering from serious conditions such as Down Syndrome have occasionally been born perfectly normal. It is impossible to know how many unaffected babies have been aborted because of a faulty diagnosis.

Forty per cent of women who abort for fetal abnormality suffer long-term emotional distress. Nor does the distress diminish over time.

Chapter 9 concerns infection and infertility after abortion. Women who undergo an induced abortion later suffer a higher rate of Pelvic Inflammatory Disease (PID) than the general population. The sequelae of PID include chronic pelvic pain, subfertility, infertility, ectopic pregnancy, intra-amniotic infection, neonatal sepsis, and stillbirth.

Chapter 9:

Physical complications: Infection and infertility

Although research on induced abortion and infertility is limited, there is recent evidence that abortion increases the risk of infertility. An English study documents a 620 per cent increase in subfecundity among women who terminated their pregnancies. The evidence linking ectopic pregnancy to previous induced abortion is overwhelming.

Chapter 10 examines the serious physical injuries arising from induced abortion. The rate of perforation of the uterus during induced abortion is higher than often recognized, because most post-abortion perforations appear to go undetected. Perforation of the uterus can result in scarring and lead to infertility from Asherman's Syndrome (intrauterine adhesions). Dilation of the cervix during a surgical abortion can render the cervix

Chapter 10:

Physical complications: Injury, miscarriage, placenta previa

incompetent, resulting in miscarriage or preterm births in subsequent pregnancies. The risk of placenta previa also rises after one or more induced abortions. The complications of induced abortion can on rare occasions necessitate a hysterectomy.

The incidence of hysterotomies after abortion may well be underestimated in the literature. The risk of cervical trauma after surgical abortion may be as high as one in 100. A prior induced abortion also increases the risk of placenta previa in a subsequent pregnancy. This occurs when the placenta implants itself near or covering the cervix. Why does this happen? For the simple reason that "vacuum aspiration or dilation and curettage may cause scarring and adhesions in the uterus that impede proper placentation in subsequent pregnancies."[1]

Chapter 11:

Physical complications: Autoimmune diseases

The disturbing rise in autoimmune diseases among women over the past four decades is the subject of Chapter 11. It appears to be attributable, at least in part, to the increased incidence of induced abortion during the same period. An astonishing discovery is that women who undergo an induced abortion have a significant fetal-maternal transfusion of cells, at a much greater volume than during a normal, completed pregnancy.

Chapter 12:

Physical complications: Maternal mortality from abortion

Chapter 12 weighs a recent study claiming that abortion is much safer for women than giving birth, and finds it wanting. This study's erroneous conclusions are based on incomplete data, stemming from the continuing failure in both the US and Canada to maintain accurate and comprehensive records on maternal deaths from abortion.

Contradicting that study are four large-scale data linkage studies from the US, Britain, Denmark and Finland. All four show that women who have induced abortions have a sharply higher death rate than women

---

1 Hung TH, Hsieh CC, Hsu JJ, Chiu TH, Lo LM and Hsieh TT. Risk factors placenta previa in an Asian population. International Journal of Gynecology and Obstetrics 2007 April; 97(1): 26-30.

who give birth. These international studies shatter the myth that abortion is safer for women than childbirth.

"Medical", that is drug-induced, abortion has been acclaimed as a more efficient, less traumatic means of terminating a pregnancy than surgical abortion. Yet, as Chapter 13 points out, it has two serious drawbacks. First, it is significantly less successful in achieving the intended result of terminating a pregnancy. Second, reported complication rates are much higher than for surgical abortion.

Chapter 14 explores the dilemma faced by many infertile couples who use *in vitro* fertilization and are then pressured to undergo multi-fetal pregnancy reduction (MFPR), a form of selective abortion in which one or more fetuses are terminated.

The great majority of women who have had an induced abortion wish to get pregnant again. That is why it is of the utmost importance that women contemplating an abortion should be aware of the possible consequences of that abortion for a subsequent pregnancy. The link between induced abortion and the risk of later preterm births is the subject of Chapter 15.

Two recently-published systematic reviews have now clarified why women who have had one or more induced abortions significantly increase their chances of later giving birth to a preterm or low birth weight child. Children who are born prematurely, or with low, or very low birth weights, suffer from significantly higher rates of:

- Infant mortality
- Cerebral palsy
- Intellectual Handicap
- Autism
- Epilepsy
- Blindness

Chapter 13:

Medical or drug-induced abortion: How safe?

Chapter 14:

Multi-fetal pregnancy reduction (MFPR)

Chapter 15:

Premature or preterm births after abortion

Chapter 16:

Pain during and after abortion

The practice of induced abortion is thus responsible for significantly higher social and health costs by causing a higher percentage of children to be born preterm, or with low birth weight. In the light of these findings, it is difficult to exaggerate the personal and social catastrophe caused by the widespread practice of induced abortion.

Lastly, in this Section we consider how physically painful the abortion procedure is for the woman undergoing it. Doctors and abortion providers commonly underestimate the amount of pain that women experience. Despite advances in pain control, the great majority of women say that they experience at least moderate pain during a surgical abortion. General anaesthetic is most effective in controlling pain, but only hospitals are authorized to administer it. Abortion clinics must rely on sedation and local anaesthetic. In their publicity, abortion providers downplay abortion pain, or do not mention it at all.

Chapter 6

Immediate physical complications of abortion: An overview

KEY POINTS

- The immediate complications of induced abortion include hemorrhage, retained tissue, infection, uterine perforation, cervical laceration, and immediate psychiatric morbidity.

- The longer-term complications include infertility, premature birth, ectopic pregnancy, placenta previa and breast cancer.

- Immediate complications occur in 3.4 to eleven per cent of surgically-induced abortions, depending on the jurisdiction.

- The rate of complications following medical (drug-induced) abortion is up to four times higher than for surgically-induced abortions.

- Another complication is unsuccessful (or failed) abortion, which means either that the procedure has to be repeated, or the child carried to term is often damaged.

Defining Physical Complications

What are the physical complications of induced abortion? Complications are classed as immediate or late. An immediate complication is an outcome that occurs very close to the time of the induced abortion, for up to six weeks afterwards. These include hemorrhage, retained tissue, infection, uterine perforation, cervical laceration, and immediate psychiatric morbidity. A late complication may occur weeks, months or even many years following the induced abortion. These include infertility, premature birth, ectopic pregnancy, placenta previa and breast cancer.

Complication Rates

The rates of immediate complication following an induced abortion vary among places and studies. The growing number of women who abort, particularly those who are having a second abortion, also changes the complication numbers considerably.

In Canada, the number of known abortions performed in 1970, the first year after abortion was partially decriminalized, was 11,200.[1] Between 1970 and 2005 Statistics Canada recorded over 2.8 million induced abortions[2]— an increase from 1970 to 2005 of 768 per cent, while the total population of Canada grew by only 60 per cent between 1970 and 2012[3]. There was a sharp rise in the number of women of child-bearing years after 1969, but this rise would not nearly account for the massive increase in abortion.

Abortion statistics in Canada are currently collected by the Canadian Institute for Health Information (CIHI). In 2009 CIHI reported 41,640 induced abortions performed in hospitals, and at least 52,115 performed in clinics (clinic data from BC were incomplete), for a total of over 93,755

---

1   Induced abortions in hospitals and clinics, by area of report and type of facility performing the abortion Canada, provinces and territories, annual (Number) *Terminated*, 1970 to 2006. 13 June 2012. http://www5.statcan.gc.ca/cansim/a26?lang =eng&retrLang=eng&id=1069005&pattern=abortion&tabMode=dataTable&srchLan=-1&p1=1&p2=1.
2   Ibid.
3   This percentage is derived from the population numbers found in: Statistics Canada. Estimated Population of Canada, 1605 to present. Table 75-001, www.statcan.gc.ca; Statistics Canada, Estimates of Population, Canada, provinces and territories, Table 051-005. 26 September 2012.

induced abortions in Canada.[4] The true number of abortions is unknown, as only hospitals are required to report them. Clinics report abortions on a voluntary basis only, and some provinces do not record any clinic data. However, abortion complication rates reported by clinics are consistently higher than the rates reported by hospitals. Additionally, "Quebec hospitals report only induced abortions covered by the provincial health insurance plan."[5]

A 2011 study by the Project for an Ontario Women's Health Evidenced-Based Report (POWER) is more comprehensive. In addition to statistics from the Ministry of Health and Long Term Care, they used data from insurance billing (OHIP), and determined an annual abortion rate of 1.5 for every 100 women, or 37 abortions for every 100 live births. Of these, 40 per cent of women having a hospital-induced abortion reported having had a previous induced abortion. The true percentage may be a shade higher owing to a slight tendency by women to underreport their abortion history.[6]

The same report tells us that "Overall in Ontario, emergency department/same-day surgery visits or hospitalizations within fourteen days and for any reason were observed after 4.5 per cent of abortions, [while] 0.4 per cent of abortions resulted in hospitalization."[7] While 4.5 per cent was the average complication rate, the range of complication rates given was 5.2 per cent for women aged fifteen to nineteen years, and 3.5 per cent for women aged 40 to 49 years. These rates do not include complications handled by attending physicians, community health clinics or nurse practitioners in a community practice.

Given a complication rate of 4.5 per cent and Canada's abortion statistics, at least 126,000 women from 1970 to 2005 alone have suffered from physical consequences of induced abortion. With the United States' one million abortions a year, at least 45,000 women a year experience physical complications. As the authors of a Scandinavian study put it, "although the occurrence of immediate complications is not expected to be high, even

---

4   Canadian Institute for Health Information. Induced abortions performed in Canada in 2009: p. 1. http://www.cihi.ca/CIHI-ext-portal/pdf/internet/TA_09_ALLDATATABLES20111028_EN.
5   Ibid.
6   Dunn S, Wise MR, Johnson LM, et al. Reproductive and gynaecological health. In Bierman AS, ed. *Project for an Ontario women's health evidence-based report (POWER): volume 2*: Toronto; 2011: p. 87.
7   Ibid., p. 89.

a small excess risk has public health importance because the procedure is frequent."[8]

Other studies have reported complication rates after induced abortion as low as 3.4 per cent and as high as 9.2 per cent, depending on follow-up time. A register-based study of 56,117 abortions in Denmark found a complication rate of five per cent in the two weeks following the induced abortion, with the most frequent complications being bleeding and infections.[9]

In a study sponsored by the College of Physicians and Surgeons of Ontario, 41,039 women who had induced abortions were compared with a similar number who did not undergo induced abortions. The study only concerned itself with short-term consequences, but in the three-month period after the abortion, the women who obtained induced abortions had a more than four-times higher rate of hospitalizations for infections (6.3 vs. 1.4 per 1000), a five-times higher rate of "surgical events" (8.2 vs. 1.6 per 1000), and a nearly five-times higher rate of hospitalization for psychiatric problems (5.2 vs. 1.1 per 1000), than the matching group of women who had not had abortions. The community clinic patients fared somewhat better, but the authors cautioned that the clinics "cannot easily follow the medium-term outcomes subsequent to the services they provide."[10]

Sykes studied 2879 cases of abortion performed at Christchurch Women's Hospital in New Zealand and found a complication readmission rate of 5.8 per cent, including two patients who presented with immediately life-threatening conditions: a uterine hemorrhage due to perforation and a severe sepsis.[11] Although Sykes had all admissions for complications

---

8 Zhou W, Nielsen GL, Moller M and Olsen J. Short-term complications after surgically induced abortion: a register-based study of 56 117 abortions. Acta Obstetricia et Gynecologica Scandinavica 2002; 81(4): p. 332.
9 Ibid., pp. 331-36. Other studies found complication rates of 3.4 per cent at a family planning centre in Paris: Thonneau P, Fougeyrollas B, Ducot B, et al. Complications of abortion performed under local anesthesia. European Journal of Obstetrics and Gynecology and Reproductive Biology 1998; 81(1): pp. 59-63; 7.1 per cent in a study that included more side effects: Nesheim BI. Induced abortion by the suction method. An analysis of complication rates. Acta Obstetricia et Gynecologica Scandinavica 1984; 63(7): pp. 591-5.
10 Østbye T, Wenghofer EF, Woodward CA, Gold G and Craighead J. Health services utilization after induced abortions in Ontario: a comparison between community clinics and hospitals. American Journal of Medical Quality 2001; 16(3): 99-106, p. 105.
11 Sykes P. Complications of termination of pregnancy: a retrospective study of admissions to Christchurch Women's Hospital 1989 and 1990. New Zealand Medical Journal 1993; 106(951): pp. 83-5.

registered, he recognized that the actual complication rate may be much higher than their data showed because some complications might be presented to hospitals other than Christchurch, while other patients could also be lost to follow up as a consequence of being treated privately. One statistic that points to this conclusion is that women who lived outside the region accounted for about nine per cent of the abortions but only six per cent of the complications.

An American study of the psychological responses of women after abortion also discovered that seventeen per cent of these women reported physical complications such as bleeding or pelvic infection after their first-trimester abortion, suggesting that the true complication rate is not reflected by hospital records.[12]

In Britain, the Royal College of Obstetricians and Gynaecologists in 2000 gave an immediate physical complication rate of induced abortion of over eleven per cent,[13] but they did not report an overall complication rate for abortion in their 2004 or revised 2011 guidelines.

COMPLICATION RATES OF MEDICAL ABORTION

The rate of complications following medical (drug-induced) abortion and surgical abortion have been compared, revealing that drug-induced abortion carries a higher risk of side effects and adverse events, especially bleeding.[14] A recent register-based study of 42,619 first-trimester abortions in Finland showed that in the six weeks following abortion, the incidence of adverse events was four times greater with medical abortion than with surgical abortion.[15] The percentage of women with adverse events (complications) after medical abortion was twenty per cent, but only 5.6 per cent after surgical abortion.[16]

---

12 Major B, Cozzarelli C, Cooper ML, et al. Psychological responses of women after first-trimester abortion. Archives of General Psychiatry 2000; 57(8): 777-84.
13 Royal College of Obstetricians and Gynaecologists. *The care of women requesting induced abortion:* 4. Information for women. 2000.
14 Winikoff B, Sivin I, Coyaji KJ, et al. Safety, efficacy, and acceptability of medical abortion in China, Cuba, and India: a comparative trial of mifepristone-misoprostol versus surgical abortion. AJOG 1997; 176(2): pp. 431-7.
15 Niinimäki M, Pouta A, Bloigu A, et al. Immediate complications after medical compared with surgical termination of pregnancy. Obstetrics & Gynecology 2009 October; 114(4): 795-804.
16 Ibid. $p<0.001$ OR 4.23, 95 per cent CI 3.94-4.54.

A smaller prospective study done in the United States revealed that the rate of complication requiring suction curettage (for incomplete abortion, ongoing pregnancy, or acute or persistent bleeding) was 18.3 per cent after medical abortion and 4.7 per cent after surgical abortion.[17]

Overall, the complication rates reported in North America are notably lower than those reported in other Western countries with advanced medical systems. Is this because abortion services in Canada and the United States are safer and more efficient? Or is it because the North-American research methodology misses many complications owing to short-term follow up, incomplete coding, and political bias?

Risk Factors

Many risk factors have been identified that increase the likelihood of complications following abortion. Zhou identified a higher risk of complications among women younger than twenty years old (seventeen per cent) and women living in rural areas (43 per cent).[18] For Niinimaki, the most important risk factor for complications was the method of abortion, with medical abortion being significantly riskier. He also noted parity (number of pregnancies) and previous induced abortions as risk factors.[19]

Researchers agree that advanced gestational age is an important risk factor for complications following abortion,[20] citing a 28 per cent higher risk when gestational age was greater than twelve weeks,[21] and that the risk of complications after abortion increases exponentially with gestational age.[22] Advanced gestational age is a concern, as eleven per cent of abortions performed each year in the United States are done in the second trimester. Of these, 97 per cent are done by D&E (dilation and evacuation), which carries a significant risk of cervical laceration (0.9 per cent) and of uterine perforation (0.2 to 0.4 per cent).[23] This risk is minimized by the

---

17   RR 3.93, 95 per cent CI 1.87-8.29 (n=178); Jensen JT, Astley SJ, Morgan E and Nichols MD. Outcomes of suction curettage and mifepristone abortion in the United States: a prospective comparison study. Contraception 1999; 59(3): 153-9.
18   Zhou, Nielsen, Moller and Olsen. See n. 8, 331-6.
19   Niinimäki et al. See n. 15.
20   Ibid.
21   Zhou, Nielsen, Moller and Olsen. See n. 8, 331-6.
22   Diedrich J and Steinauer J. Complications of surgical abortion. Clinical Obstetrics and Gynecology 2009; 52(2): 205-12.
23   Hayes JL and Fox MC. Cervical dilation in second-trimester abortion. Clinical Obstetrics and Gynecology 2009; 52(2): 171-8.

use of preoperative cervical preparatory agents, such as laminaria, but not eliminated. Other risks include incomplete abortion, infection, and hemorrhage.

FAILED OR INCOMPLETE ABORTION:

> "Started to hemorrhage hours after abortion: in ER was told I had an incomplete abortion so had to have repeat abortion."
>
> "I collapsed a few days later in the hall of high school. They took me to the ER only to discover I needed a second D&C because they left some of the placenta in and it had started to rot. The only thing worse than the pain the first time was reliving it a second time."

An incomplete or failed abortion is one in which the fetus continues to survive or is not fully expelled, requiring a second procedure. However, as Creinin notes, there is a difficulty in defining incomplete abortion in the literature: "Comparing abortion failure rates between medical and surgical abortion is difficult because the definition of a "failure" is inherently biased by the procedure itself. Since the goal of a medical abortion is to achieve complete expulsion without requiring a surgical procedure, a suction aspiration performed for any reason (including incomplete abortion, hemorrhage, continuing [viable] pregnancy, or patient consent) is considered a failure of the method. However, with surgical abortion, a repeat aspiration for an incomplete abortion, hemorrhage, or hematometra is considered a "complication," but not a "failure." After a surgical abortion, the procedure is considered to be a failure only if there is a continuing pregnancy."[24]

In his study, Creinin used the definition of medical abortion failure, that is, any instance where repeat suction aspiration was performed, and found a failure rate of eight per cent following medical abortion and four per cent following surgical abortion in a small study.[25]

---

24   Creinin MD. Randomized comparison of efficacy, acceptability and cost of medical versus surgical abortion. Contraception 2000; 62(3): 117-24, p. 117.
25   Ibid., pp. 117-24.

Surgical Abortion

Very early abortions are seen as an important risk factor for failed surgical abortion. One study reported a failure rate of 0.23 per cent for abortions under twelve weeks gestation.[26] Another study of surgical abortions at three to six weeks gestation at a Planned Parenthood clinic in Massachusetts reported a failure rate of 2.3 per cent[27] and a total complication rate of 4.0 per cent including failed abortion.[28] Because the follow-up rate for this study was only 66 per cent, many more women could have experienced complications or incomplete abortion but gone to a hospital or different clinic for medical follow up.[29]

In 2002 Zhou reported a failure rate of 0.53 per cent after surgical abortion, while Kaunitz reported a failure rate of 0.23 per cent for surgical abortions at twelve weeks gestation or less. Medical abortion failure rates are reported at 1.4 per cent to 2.9 per cent.[30]

Niinimaki's large registry-based study in Finland revealed an incidence of incomplete abortion of 6.7 per cent for medical abortion, and 1.6 per cent for surgical abortion.[31] He also noted that 5.9 per cent of women required surgical evacuation after medical abortion, and 1.8 per cent required surgical re-evacuation after surgical abortion.[32] However, some instances of surgical (re-)evacuation were due to bleeding and other reasons, aside from incomplete or failed abortions.

Medical Abortion

Drug-induced or medical abortion has a higher failure rate than surgical abortion. When abortion is induced by the use of chemical prostaglandins or prostaglandin analogues, two possible scenarios may lead to an incomplete abortion.

---

26   Flett GMM and Templeton A. Surgical abortion: best practice & research. Clinical Obstetrics and Gynaecology 2002; 16(2): 247-61.
27   95 per cent CI 1.3 per cent-3.7 per cent.
28   95 per cent CI 2.8 per cent-5.7 per cent.
29   Paul ME, Mitchell CM, Rogers AJ, Fox MC and Lackie EG. Early surgical abortion: efficacy and safety. AJOG 2002; 187(2): 407-11.
30   Royal College of Obstetricians and Gynaecologists. See n. 13.
31   Niinimaki et al. See n. 15. p<0.001, OR 5.37, 95 per cent CI 4.49-6.28 (n=42,619).
32   Ibid. p<0.001, (OR 3.58, 95 per cent CI 3.18-4.03).

The first is the actual failure of the drugs to complete the abortion. Grimes reports the overall complete abortion rate from his meta-analysis of seven chemical (drug-induced) abortion studies from 1991 to 1994 as 93.9 per cent. He goes on to say, "failed abortion is an infrequent but important complication of medical abortion. These women should undergo suction curettage as soon as the diagnosis is made."[33] Similarly, Collins and Mahoney noted that "...prostaglandins and their analogues must be given in doses yielding unacceptably high levels of side effects... [With a] lower dose... some failures will occur and these women will then need abortion by other methods."[34] Women may even be unaware that the abortion is incomplete and may only later seek medical help when infection develops.

The second scenario is the woman's own decision-making process: Drug-induced abortion requires at least two infusions of drugs at two separate office visits and may require up to two weeks to complete. During this time, a woman may change her mind and decide to continue with the pregnancy. Holmes and Fonseca and colleagues have found that "exposure during the first trimester to the synthetic prostaglandin misoprostol also has been associated with the occurrence of terminal transverse limb defects and scalp defects."[35] Likewise, Gonzalez identified Brazilian children suffering from limb deficiencies as a result of exposure to misoprostol in early pregnancy.[36]

On the other hand, Grimes records that "... some women with a failed abortion choose to continue the pregnancy and a small number of normal infants have been born after exposure to mifepristone in early pregnancy."[37]

Another recent study showed a ten per cent rate of retained placenta (and possibly also fetus) after medical abortion, as opposed to a one per cent rate of retained products after surgical abortion in the second trimester.[38]

---

33   Grimes D. Medical abortion in early pregnancy: a review of the evidence. [Review]. Obstetrics & Gynecology 1997; 89(5:2): 790-96: p. 793.
34   Collins FS and Mahoney MJ. Hydrocephalus and abnormal digits after failed first-trimester prostaglandin abortion attempt. Journal of Pediatrics 1983; 102(4): p. 621.
35   Holmes LB. Possible fetal effects of cervical dilation and uterine curettage during the first trimester of pregnancy. Journal of Pediatrics 1995; 126(1): p. 132.
36   Gonzalez CH, Vargas FR, Perez AB, et al. Limb deficiency with or without mobius sequence in seven Brazilian children associated with misoprostol use in the first trimester of pregnancy. American Journal of Medical Genetics 1993; 47(1): pp. 59-64.
37   Grimes. See n. 33.
38   Mauelshagen A, Sadler LC, Roberts H, Harilall M and Farquhar CM. Audit of short term outcomes of surgical and medical second trimester termination of pregnancy. Reproductive Health 2009; 30(6:16): 1-6.

A multi-centre study in three developing countries, China, Cuba and India (n=1373), comparing mifepristone-misoprostol medical abortion to surgical abortion found that medical abortion had a consistently higher failure rate than surgical—8.6 per cent vs. 0.4 per cent in China, sixteen per cent vs. four per cent in Cuba, and 5.2 per cent vs. zero per cent in India. The authors of this study identified three types of medical abortion failures: "acceptability failures" where the woman or physician felt the need for surgical intervention before the end of the study period; medical failure, where an adverse event or an incomplete abortion after seventeen days required surgical intervention; or erroneous diagnoses of incomplete abortion. They reported an overall failure rate of seven per cent,[39] but as we have seen previously, there is difficulty in comparing failure rates across studies as the definition of failure or incomplete abortion varies greatly.

CONSEQUENCES OF FAILED ABORTION

A 1996 Canadian literature review found that when abortion fails and women choose not to undergo a second procedure, the children born may have "limb or digit abnormalities and congenital contractures." The review goes on to note, "However, it is likely there has been bias leading to the reporting of abnormal cases."[40] Given that only seven studies in the past 45 years have addressed failed abortion, there may be systematic underreporting as well.

Holt and colleagues noted that for 3.4 per cent of women in the study of ectopic pregnancy, the original abortion procedure did not succeed and a D&C was performed. In these cases the abortion failed because the clinic did not test for ectopic pregnancy.[41] This failure to test for ectopic pregnancy can be life threatening.

Infants are also known to survive late-term abortions.[42] This outcome is now less frequent owing to the use of KCL injections (potassium chloride) in late-term abortion, to ensure that a viable fetus does in fact die. As Ferguson and colleagues state, "We use urea to be certain that we effect

---

39   Winikoff et al. See n. 14, 431-37.
40   Hall JG. Arthrogryposis associated with unsuccessful attempts at termination of pregnancy. American Journal of Medical Genetics 1996; 63(1): 293-300, p. 293.
41   Holt VL, Daling JR, Voigt LF, et al. Induced abortion and the risk of subsequent ectopic pregnancy. American Journal of Public Health 1989; 79(9): 1234-8.
42   Shaver J. *Gianna: aborted...and lived to tell about it*. Colorado Springs, CO: Focus on the Family Publishing, 1995; p. 174.

fetal death. It is unsettling to all personnel to deliver these fetuses when they are not stillborn."[43] In the Ferguson study, 34 per cent of the abortions were on fetuses over 22 weeks gestation. (Fetal viability in premature birth currently begins at 23 to 24 weeks, and babies born at 21 to 22 weeks have occasionally been resuscitated).

A recent Canadian court case has drawn attention to the plight of a child who suffered cerebral palsy as an abortion survivor. The child was born alive and left without oxygen or medical treatment for 40 minutes until a nurse took her to the neonatal intensive care unit. The hospital involved was found negligent and thus responsible for her disabilities, and was ordered to pay the plaintiff $8.7 million.[44] Holmes has also reported two cases of infant malformation following prenatal exposure to cervical dilation and uterine curettage.[45]

Abortion can also fail in cases where multiple pregnancies are reduced to one or two desired fetuses. "Selective reduction" is now a common practice in large teaching hospitals. Hall has documented cases where the procedure kills the intended fetus but "puts the remaining fetus(es) at risk for vascular compromise" and elevates the risk of miscarriage.[46] (See also Chapter 14 on "Multifetal Pregnancy Reduction").

The woman who seeks abortion is often promised a relatively painless and simple procedure to eliminate a pregnancy that she does not wish to carry to term. Failed abortion may involve her in a number of unanticipated outcomes. If she changes her mind about "medical" abortion and a child is born with anomalies, maternal grief and guilt may be anticipated and counselling may be necessary. If a second abortion procedure is successful at a late stage of fetal development, where the woman knows that procedures are chosen to ensure that an anticipated live birth cannot occur, grief and guilt may likewise ensue.

Women who choose to proceed with the pregnancy after a failed abortion are at a higher risk for miscarriage, premature rupture of

---

[43] Ferguson JE 2d, Burkett BJ, Pinkerton JV, et al. Intraamniotic 15(s)-15-methyl prostaglandin F2 alpha and termination of middle and late second-trimester pregnancy for genetic indications: a contemporary approach. AJOG 1993; 169(2:1): 332-40; p. 340.
[44] Hospital pays $8.7M settlement: premature baby was abandoned with dead foetuses. National Post, 31 July 1999; A:1.
[45] Holmes. See n. 35, pp. 131-4.
[46] Hall. See n. 40.

membranes, chorioamnionitis, intra-uterine growth retardation, and fetal malformations. There are limited data on these women, but normal births have also been reported.[47]

Hemorrhage

> "Hemorrhaged after second abortion. Had excessive bleeding with births of children. Three miscarriages and excessive bleeding. Had life-threatening hemorrhage with fifth birth (as well as uterine infection)."

Hemorrhage may be caused by the failure of the uterus to contract after the abortion (uterine atony), cervical laceration, retained tissue, uterine perforation, abnormal placentation, coagulopathy, or other etiologies. The definition of hemorrhage varies from study to study. Sometimes reports of bleeding or hemorrhage after abortion include all instances of blood loss that led to a consultation with a physician, other reports include estimated blood loss of greater than 250 ml or greater than 500 ml based on the physician's subjective estimate, while still others only include post-abortion hemorrhages that required a blood transfusion.

According to the Royal College of Obstetricians and Gynaecologists, the risk of hemorrhage after abortion is 0.88 per 1000 at less than thirteen weeks gestation, and 4.0 per 1000 at over twenty weeks gestation.[48] In their 2004 guidelines they also reported Zhou's Danish record linkage study findings that the risk of hemorrhage is 4.4 per 1000 abortions.[49] The discrepancies in reported rates can be attributed to ill-defined criteria in reporting hemorrhage.

Niinimaki's study documented the much higher rate of consultation for hemorrhage after medical abortion (15.6 per cent) compared with surgical abortion (2.1 per cent).[50] Because this was a record-linkage study, all cases of women returning to their physician for bleeding were documented, whereas other studies that do not use record linkage show a lower rate of

---

47 Flett and Templeton. See n. 26.
48 Royal College of Obstetricians and Gynaecologists. See n. 13.
49 Zhou, Nielsen, Moller and Olsen. See n. 8, pp. 331-336.
50 Niinimaki et al. See n. 15. $p<0.001$, OR 7.93, 95 per cent CI 7.15-8.81.

hemorrhage after abortion. In any case, the risk of bleeding is known to be much higher after medical abortion. The transfusion rate will therefore be correspondingly higher. Every transfusion carries the risk of HIV and hepatitis, which can have life-long morbidity, including death.

A small prospective study done in the United States confirms this, noting that of the 18.6 per cent of women requiring suction curettage after medical abortion, more than half were treated for acute or persistent bleeding. All the 4.7 per cent of women requiring suction curettage following surgical abortion did so for persistent bleeding.[51]

Sepsis

In rare cases, there have been reports of sepsis subsequent to the placement of intracervical laminaria (a form of seaweed used to dilate the cervix) during surgical abortion, which might carry infection from cervix to uterus. There are also case studies of bacteremia and toxic shock syndrome reported[52] and a fatality from Clostridium, perfringens and Escherichia coli sepsis after laminaria placement.[53] One woman developed sacroiliitis, endocarditis and septic pulmonary emboli from a Group B streptococcus infection following a second trimester D&E.[54] After medical abortion, a case of necrotizing fasciitis and toxic shock syndrome was reported in a woman who was positive for Group A streptococcus.[55] Between 2000 and 2009 eight deaths from Clostridium sordellii infections after medical abortions were reported in the US by the Centers for Disease Control and Prevention.[56]

---

51   Jensen, Astley, Morgan and Nichols. See n. 17.
52   Acharya PS and Gluckman SJ. Bacteremia following placement of intracervical laminaria tents. Clinical Infectious Diseases 1999; 29(3): 695-7; Sutkin G, Capelle SD, Schlievert PM and Creinin MD. Toxic shock syndrome after laminaria insertion. Obstetrics and Gynecology 2001; 98(5): pp. 959-61.
53   Jasnosz KM, Shakir AM and Perper JA. Fatal clostridium perfringens and Escherichia coli sepsis following urea-instillation abortion. American Journal of Forensic Medicine and Pathology 1993; 14(2): pp. 151-4.
54   McKenna T and O'Brien K. Case report: group B streptococcal bacteremia and sacroiliitis after mid-trimester dilation and evacuation. Journal of Perinatology 2009; 29(9): pp. 643-5.
55   Daif JL, Levie M, Chudnoff S, Kaiser B and Shahabi S. Group a streptococcus causing necrotizing fasciitis and toxic shock syndrome after medical termination of pregnancy. Obstetrics and Gynecology 2009; 113(2): pp. 504-6.
56   Meites E, Zane S and Gould C. Letter to the NEJM, 30 September 2010; 363(14): pp. 1382-3. This brought the infection rate from Clostridium sordelli and C. perifringens to 0.58 per 100,000 medical abortions.

It should be borne in mind that 30 per cent of abortion-related deaths are attributable to infection.[57]

Conclusion

Absolute certainty about the rates of physical complication after abortion is impossible. Statistics are usually drawn from clinic or hospital records that may under-represent the true rate if women experiencing complications follow up elsewhere. Even if the complication rates immediately following induced abortion are as low as sometimes reported, there are so many women who undergo the procedure that many thousands of them have, and will continue to have, such complications as failed abortion, hemorrhage, and sepsis. The later in gestation that an abortion is performed, the more likely the woman will experience complications. Medical abortions have a much higher rate of physical complications—bleeding in particular—than surgical abortions. Women deserve to be informed of these risks.

---

57   Achilles SL and Reeves MF. Prevention of infection after induced abortion: release date October 2010 SFP Guideline 2012. Contraception 2012; 83(4): 295-309.

Chapter 7

Biology and epidemiology confirm the abortion-breast cancer link

KEY POINTS

- Once pregnant, if a woman chooses to maintain her pregnancy and achieves a full-term pregnancy, she will *decrease* her risk of breast cancer.

- Never becoming pregnant *increases* breast cancer risk. If a woman undergoes an induced abortion she may remain childless, a condition that also *increases* her breast cancer risk.

- Delaying pregnancy after age twenty increases breast cancer risk. If a woman undergoes an induced abortion and brings a subsequent pregnancy to term, she has effectively delayed that full-term pregnancy, thereby *increasing* her risk of breast cancer.

- Every full-term pregnancy after the first further *decreases* the risk of breast cancer. If a woman has already had a full-term pregnancy and then chooses to abort a subsequent pregnancy she loses the risk reduction that an additional full-term pregnancy would have afforded her, thereby *increasing* her risk.

- The use of instruments such as dilators during an abortion increases a woman's risk of having a premature delivery in future births. If that premature delivery occurs before 32 weeks gestation, she will have an *increased* risk of breast cancer.

INTRODUCTION

Breast cancer is the leading cause of cancer death of women worldwide. One in ten of all new cancers in the world are female breast cancers. North America has the highest incidence of breast cancer in the world. The age-adjusted rate for non-invasive breast cancer, ductal carcinoma *in-situ* (DCIS), increased 660 per cent between 1973 and 2000, while the rate for invasive breast cancer increased 36 per cent. Ductal carcinoma *in-situ* differs from invasive cancer by the location of all the cancer cells that remain within the milk duct. By definition the *in-situ* cancer cells have not penetrated or invaded the wall of the milk duct (the basement membrane). Should these cells invade the basement membrane, the cancer would be classified as invasive breast cancer, which is able to spread throughout a woman's body. DCIS is the earliest detectable form of breast cancer, which is highly curable (97-99 per cent). Invasive breast cancers commonly arise in *in-situ* cancers. Breast cancer is the leading cause of cancer deaths of women between twenty and 59 years old.

For centuries it was known that remaining childless increased a woman's risk for breast cancer. Conversely, it was also known that pregnancy was protective. In 1743, Ramazzini of Padua observed that there was an increased amount of breast cancer among nuns. In 1842, a hundred years later, Rigioni-Stern noted a threefold increase risk of breast cancer among nuns. Nuns were largely childless whereas the rest of the population had pregnancies early on in their reproductive lives. Yet it was not until the 1980s that the normal physiology of breast development and maturation during pregnancy, which accounts for those reproductive risks, became clear. In the first decade of the 2000s, with advances in technology, scientists learned the genetic changes that occur in breast cells that explain why pregnancy affords protection from cancer.

It is well known that different pregnancy outcomes lead to changes in the rates of breast cancer among women. There are various long-established insights on the relation between pregnancy and breast cancer.

Delayed First Pregnancy

The longer a woman waits to have her first full-term pregnancy (FFTP), the higher her risk of breast cancer as her immature, cancer-vulnerable breast tissue is exposed to carcinogens for a longer duration. *A woman who remains childless or has her FFTP when she is more than 30 years of age has a 90 per cent higher* risk of breast cancer than a woman who has her first child before the age of twenty.[1]

For each year a woman delays pregnancy after age twenty, she has a *five per cent increase in risk* for pre-menopausal breast cancer and a *three per cent increase in risk* for postmenopausal breast cancer.[2] For example, having an induced abortion at age twenty followed by a full-term pregnancy at age thirty would increase her risk of pre-menopausal breast cancer by 50 per cent. Other studies have shown that breast cancer risk increases 0.7 per cent for each year that subsequent births are delayed after her first birth.[3] Yet another study has shown that if a woman has a pregnancy and lactates within five years after an abortion, her risk will be twenty per cent less than if she waits ten or more years to lactate for the first time.[4]

Increased Number of Pregnancies

For each pregnancy that the woman has subsequent to her first, her risk of breast cancer will decrease another ten per cent.[5]

Abortion and Subsequent Premature Births

Two large meta-analyses show that induced abortion increases a woman's risk of premature delivery.[6] Also, the more induced abortions a woman has, the higher her risk of subsequent premature births.[7] In 2006, the Institutes of

---

1   Bland K and Copeland E, eds. *The Breast: Comprehensive Management of Benign and Malignant Diseases*. Philadelphia: Saunders El Sevier, 4th edition, 2 vols, 2009, vol 1, chap. 19: p. 335, Table 19-1.
2   Clavel-Chapelon F and Gerber M. Reproductive factors and breast cancer risk: do they differ according to age at diagnosis? Breast Cancer Research and Treatment 2002 March; 72(2): 107-15.
3   Decarli A, La Vecchia C, Negri E and Franceschi S. Age at any birth and breast cancer in Italy. International Journal of Cancer 1996 July; 67(2): 187-9.
4   Daling JR, Malone KE, Voigt LF, White E and Weiss NS. Risk of breast cancer among young women: relationship to induced abortions. Journal of the National Cancer Institute Cancer Spectrum 1994 November; 86(21): 1584-92.
5   Lambe M, Hsieh C, Chan H, Ekbom A, Trichopoulos D and Adami H. Parity, age at first and last birth, and risk of breast cancer: a population study in Sweden. Breast Cancer Research and Treatment 1996 January; 38(3): 305-11.
6   Shah PS and Zao J. Induced termination of pregnancy and low birth weight and preterm birth: a systematic review and meta-analyses. BJOG 2009 October; 116(11): 1425-42; Swingle HM, Colaizy TT, Zimmerman MB and Morriss FH. Abortion and the risk of subsequent preterm birth: a systematic review with meta-analyses. Journal of Reproductive Medicine 2009 February; 54: 95-108.
7   Rooney B and Calhoun BC. Induced abortion and risk of later preterm births. Journal of the American Physicians and Surgeons 2003 Summer; 8(2): 46-9.

Medicine listed induced abortion as an immutable cause of premature birth.[8]

Except for those that end in spontaneous abortion, whatever the length of her pregnancy, in the first 32 weeks she will have changes in her breast tissue that will increase her risk of breast cancer. When a woman gives birth naturally, it takes many hours to dilate the cervix for birth. During an abortion the cervix is forcibly dilated and subjected to injury. Owing to the use of instruments such as dilators during an abortion she may deliver a subsequent pregnancy prematurely. If the premature delivery is before 32 weeks, she will have an increased risk of breast cancer. Approximately three per cent of all premature deliveries occur before 32 weeks.[9] Approximately 12.5 per cent of all births are before 37 weeks and are considered premature.[10]

Breast Tissue Changes in First Pregnancy

When a woman becomes pregnant for the first time, her immature and cancer-vulnerable breast tissue matures into cancer-resistant tissue. Approximately 85 per cent of her breast will become fully mature Type 4 lobules, which contain the first milk, colostrum. After weaning, theses lobules regress to Type 3 lobules, which are also cancer-resistant. This biological change accounts for the recognized fact that never having a full-term pregnancy (nulliparity) increases a woman's risk of breast cancer (as the experience of nuns demonstrates). After a full-term pregnancy, only fifteen per cent of her breast tissue remains susceptible to forming cancer.[11] It is the genetic changes that occur in the breast lobules during a full term pregnancy that give lifelong protection.[12] Molecular biologists have also determined that progenitor or stem cells in the breast do not become terminally differentiated (reach their full potential growth or maturity) until they have undergone

---

8   Alexander GR. Appendix B: prematurity at birth: determinants, consequences, and geographic variation. In *Preterm Birth: Causes, Consequences and Prevention.* Ed. Behrman RE and Butler AS. Washington, DC: National Academies Press (US), 2007: p. 625.
9   Ibid., p. 616.
10   Ibid.
11   Russo J, Rivera R and Russo IH. Influence of age and parity on development of the human breast. Breast Cancer Research and Treatment 1992; 23: 211-8; Russo H, Yang, Russo. Chapter 1: developmental, cellular, and molecular basis of human breast cancer. Journal of the National Cancer Institute Monograph 2000; 27: 17-37.
12   Russo J, Balogh GA and Russo IH. Full-term pregnancy induces a specific genomic signature in the human breast. Cancer Epidemiology, Biomarkers, and Prevention 2008 January; 17: 51-66; Verlinden I, Gungor N, Wouters K, Janssens J, Raus J and Michiels L. Parity-induced changes in global gene expression in the human mammary gland. European Journal of Cancer Prevention 2005 April; 14(2): 129-37.

the environment of pregnancy and have lactated.[13] A group of international researchers has found the numbers of these stem cells are lowest in women who have give birth in their early twenties while they are highest in women with high risk for breast cancer, such as those who have inherited a mutated BRCA gene.[14]

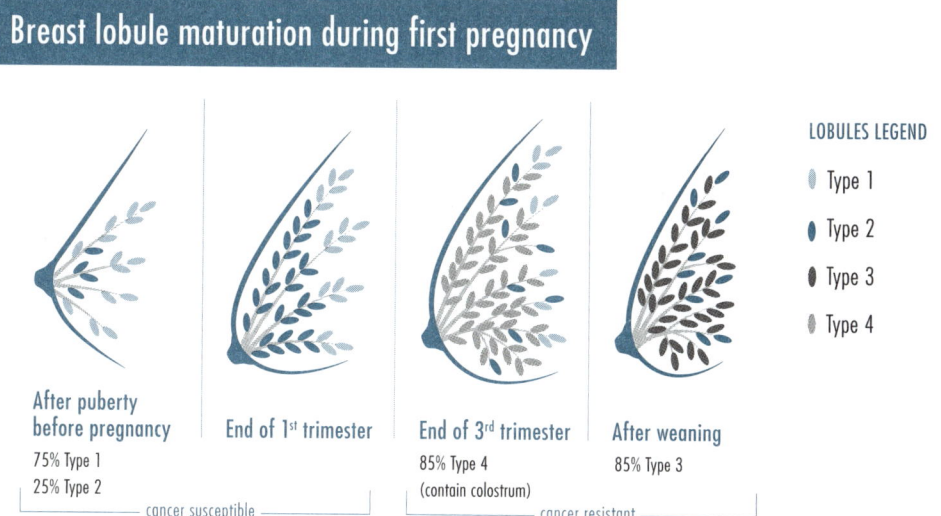

Early Termination of Pregnancy (through Prematurity or Abortion) and Increased Risk of Breast Cancer

Several studies have shown that prematurity before 32 weeks gestation increased breast cancer risk.[15] In fact, the biologic mechanism for premature delivery, induced abortion and second-trimester miscarriage as causes for increased risk of breast cancer is the same mechanism for all three: Abortion, premature delivery and second-trimester miscarriage all leave the breast with more places for cancers to start when the pregnancy ends. The woman's breasts have been exposed to the same pregnancy hormones (estrogen, progesterone, human chorionic gonadotropin (hCG)

---

13 Boecker W, Weigel S, Heindel W and Stute P. The normal breast. In *Preneoplasia of the Breast: A New Conceptual Approach to Proliferative Breast Disease.* Ed. Werner Boecker. Munich: Elsevier Saunders, 2006: 1-28.
14 Choudhury, S et al. Molecular Profiling of Human Mammary Gland Links Breast Cancer Risk to a p27+ Cell Population with Progenitor Characteristics. Cell Stem Cell 2013 July; 13, 117-130.
15 Melbye M, Wohlfahrt J, Andersen AMN, Westergaard T and Andersen PK. Premature delivery and breast cancer risk. British Journal of Cancer 1999 April; 80: 609-13; Vatten LJ, Romundstad PR, Trichopoulos D and Skjaerven R. Pregnancy related protection against breast cancer depends on length of gestation. British Journal of Cancer 2002 July; 87: 289-90.

and human placental lactogen hPL) all of which lead to the same breast changes. Elevated levels of estrogen and progesterone, stimulated by hCG, cause more cancer-vulnerable breast tissue to form. It is only *after* 32 weeks of gestation that the elevated levels of hPL, in concert with other pregnancy hormones, allow the full maturation to cancer-resistant breast tissue to occur. Therefore, whether the pregnancy ends before 32 weeks with a premature birth, a second-trimester miscarriage (which generally will have normal hormonal levels) or an induced abortion, breast cancer risk is increased.

THE INDEPENDENT LINK BETWEEN BREAST CANCER AND INDUCED ABORTION

There is evidence that induced abortion before 32 weeks gestation in and of itself increases breast cancer risk when other factors such as age at first birth are controlled for in the studies. The various types of evidence supporting an independent link will be addressed in this section.

For a study concerning breast cancer risk to be accurate, all known risks must be controlled for in the case group or cancer group, and the control group or non-cancer group, which is used for comparison. This is the basis for case-controlled studies. For instance, if a study was to look at whether candy increased breast cancer risk or not, the case group and the control group would have to be similar in all other known cancer risks. Thus if the case group had more women in it with a family history of breast cancer than the control group, the study would come under merited criticism if it found that candy increased breast cancer risk. In other words, the case group and control group would have to be comparable in all known risks for the study to be valid.

There have been several recent studies from groups of scientists all over the world that have controlled for induced abortion as a risk factor for breast cancer. For example, an American study looking at oral contraceptives as a risk for subtypes of breast cancer also controlled for induced abortion.[16] In the discussion section of the study, it reported that as in "previous studies, induced abortion was found to be a risk for breast cancer." The researchers included the chief of the Hormonal and Reproductive Section in the Division of Epidemiology at the National Cancer Institute. Another

---

16 Dolle JM, Daling JR, White E, et al. Risk factors for triple-negative breast cancer in women under the age of 45 years. Cancer Epidemiology, Biomarkers and Prevention 2009 April; 18(4): 1157-66.

recent study, this one from Iran, found that induced abortion carried a 62 per cent increased risk of breast cancer.[17] A paper from China looking into risk factors associated with sub-types of breast cancer found that induced abortion increased breast cancer risk by 26 per cent[18]. A recent Turkish study has also found induced abortion to be a risk for breast cancer, with an increased risk of 66 per cent.[19] In the discussion section of this paper the authors noted that their finding was consistent with previous findings in the world's literature concerning induced abortion. Another recent study, this time in Armenia, found an increased risk of breast cancer of 77 per cent for women who had had one to three induced abortions and 95 per cent for women who had had four to ten abortions.[20] A study in China found an increased risk of 52 per cent among post-abortive women, even when adjusting for other relevant reproductive factors. It too supports the existence of an independent link. The authors also studied pre- and post-menopausal women separately and found that the increase in risk for post-menopausal women was 82 per cent.[21] The study, like many others, also demonstrated a dose-response relationship regarding increase in risk (with an increased risk of 150 per cent for three or more abortions), which, as will be discussed later, is one of the Bradford-Hill criteria for establishing causality.

This year the authors of a Danish cohort study[22] reported that they "did

---

17   Naieni KH, Ardalan A, Mahmoodi M, Motevalian A, Yahyapoor Y and Yazdizadeh B. Risk factors of breast cancer in north of Iran: a case-control in Mazandaran province. Asian Pacific Journal of Cancer Prevention 2007; 8(3): 395-8. The finding was statistically significant.
18   Xing P, Li J and Jin F. A case-control study of reproductive factors associated with subtypes of breast cancer in Northeast China. Medical Oncology 2010 September; 27(3): 926-31. Another separate Chinese study, that unfortunately did not distinguish between spontaneous and induced abortions, nevertheless showed an increased risk of 120 per cent for one to two abortions and 662 per cent for three or more abortions: Zeng Y, Xu M, Tan S and Yin L. Analysis of the risk factors of breast cancer. Journal of Southern Medical University 2010; 30(3): 622-3.
19   Ozmen V, Ozcinar B, Karanlik H, et al. Breast cancer risk factors in Turkish women - a university hospital based nested case control study. World Journal of Surgical Oncology 2009 April; 7(37): 37-44. The finding was statistically significant.
20   Khachatryan L, Scharpf R and Kaan S. Influence of diabetes mellitus Type 2 and prolonged estrogen exposure among women in Armenia. Health Care for Women International 2011 October; 32(11): 953-71.
21   Jiang AR, Gao CM, Ding JH, et al. Abortions and breast cancer risk in premenopausal and postmenopausal women in Jiangsu province of China. Asian Pacific Journal of Cancer Prevention 2012; 13: 33-5. http://www.apjcpcontrol.org/page/popup_paper_file_view.php?pno=MzMtMzZUgMTIuMiZrY29kZT0yNzAxJmZubz0w&pgubun=i . The finding was statistically significant.
22   Brauner C, Overvad K, Tjonneland A and Attermann J. Induced abortion and breast cancer risk among parous women: a Danish cohort study. Acta Obstetricia et Gynecologica Scandinavica 2013. http://onlinelibrary.wiley.com/doi/10.1111/aogs.12107/abstract.

not find evidence of an adverse effect of induced abortion on breast cancer risk in parous women overall..." However, their study is seriously flawed, since they only looked at women between 50 and 65 years of age, whom they followed for "approximately 12 years." Given that the average age at abortion in Denmark is 27, and the average age of the women recruited was 57, and that the study design excluded all women with previous cancers, all of the post-abortive women who developed cancer within 25 to 30 years of their abortion were excluded. We also know that parous women are less likely to get cancer, especially if they have children soon after an abortion. Another study this year, from India,[23] shows induced abortion as its strongest risk factor. Finally, just as we go to press, a statistically-significant study from Bangladesh reports a more than twenty times increased risk of breast cancer after induced abortion.[24]

If scientists worldwide did not know and agree that induced abortion is a known risk for breast cancer, they would not refer to it as commonly accepted in their studies and analyses. Induced abortion is specifically acknowledged as a known risk factor in the performance of such studies, as well as in the methodology and discussion sections of the published papers. This is because induced abortion is now a commonly-accepted risk factor for breast cancer—except in North America, where it is denied chiefly for political reasons.

The Biological Evidence

An abortion does not turn back the clock and make a pregnant woman "unpregnant". As soon as conception occurred and before implantation, the embryo released the hormone hCG (human chorionic gonadotropin), which immediately caused the mother's ovaries to produce higher levels of estrogen and progesterone and change her breasts. That earliest sign of pregnancy, sore and tender breasts, is the result of the multiplication of breast cells to produce more breast tissue in preparation for breastfeeding. Abortion cannot remove those newly made cells that will remain cancer-vulnerable for her lifetime or until she completes a pregnancy past 32 weeks. If that same pregnant woman chooses to carry her pregnancy to term, she will have the lifelong benefit of a lower breast cancer risk. These are the undisputed biological facts that cause abortion to be a risk for breast cancer.

There are well-documented, physiological changes that occur in the

---

23 Kamath R, Mahajan KS, Ashok L and Sanai TS. A study on risk factors of breast cancer among patients attending the tertiary care hospital, in Udupi district. Indian Journal of Community Medicine, 2013; 38(2): 95-99.
24 Jabeen S, Haque M, Islam J, Hossain MZ, Begum A, Kashem MA. Breast cancer and some epidemiological risk factors: A hospital based study, J Dhaka Med Coll 2013; 22(1): 61-6.

mother's breast with a normal pregnancy and result in a lowering of her breast cancer risk if the pregnancy goes past 32 weeks.[25] This reduction is due to the maturing hormones produced by the fetus and placenta (after birth) in preparation for breastfeeding.

An overview of breast physiology during pregnancy is necessary to facilitate understanding of the physiological evidence supporting the abortion-breast cancer link. A lobule is a unit of breast tissue consisting of milk glands and ducts that carry the milk toward the nipple. Prior to a first full-term pregnancy, the breast is about 75 per cent Type 1 and 25 per cent Type 2 lobules where ductal and lobular breast cancers form respectively. By the end of the pregnancy, the breast is about 85 per cent fully matured to cancer-resistant Type 4 lobules and only fifteen per cent immature, cancer-vulnerable lobules, thereby reducing the mother's future risk of breast cancer.

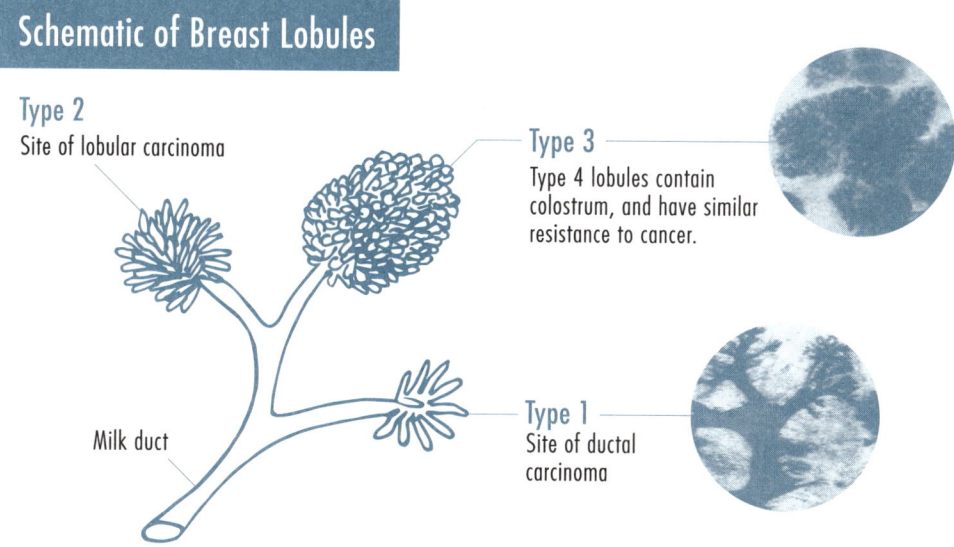

Reproduced with permission of Dr. José Russo, Fox Chase Cancer Center, Philadelphia.

During a pregnancy, the absolute numbers of these lobules also increase as the breast doubles in volume with an increase in number of lobules and

---

25 Hsieh CC, Wuu J, Lambe M, Trichopoulous D, Adami HO and Ekbom A. Delivery of premature newborns and maternal breast cancer risk. The Lancet 1999 April; 353(9160): p. 1239.

a decrease in stroma (the surrounding connective tissue).[26] A premature delivery before 32 weeks *for any reason*, whether physician-induced or because of an incompetent cervix (which is commonly due to previous abortions) or any other natural cause, *increases breast cancer risk*, because the breast has already responded to the hormones estrogen and progesterone, which are produced by the ovaries, fetus or placenta in response to fetal-placental secretion of human chorionic gonadotropin (hCG)[27]. These hormones cause an increase in breast tissue, Type 1 and 2 lobules, where cancers start. Only after 32 weeks' gestation does the fetal-placental hormone human placental lactogen (hPL) and other hormones enable the breast to fully mature its breast lobules into Type 4, making them cancer-resistant. This cancer resistance is the result of known permanent genetic changes that occur within the breast cells' genome, providing the molecular basis for the protective effect of a full-term pregnancy.[28] *An induced abortion before 32 weeks has the same physiological effect on the breast. Its only difference from premature delivery is that the fetus is delivered dead rather than alive.*

The breast physiology described above explains the independent breast cancer risk that induced abortions cause in addition to losing the protective effect the mother could have gained by carrying her pregnancy to term. The longer the gestation up to 32 weeks before the induced abortion, the higher the mother's breast cancer risk because she has developed more places for cancers to start.[29]

Another reason why induced abortion causes an increased risk of breast cancer is its secondary effect of increasing the rate of premature birth in the mother's subsequent pregnancies. Any premature delivery before 32 weeks will increase breast cancer risk through the same biological mechanism that causes induced abortion to increase breast cancer risk. With the stimulation by the pregnancy hormones of estrogen and progesterone, the numbers of cells that are immature and cancer vulnerable are markedly increased in number. In other words, there are more places (cells) for cancers to start. It is only in the hormonal environment that occurs *after* the first 32 weeks of pregnancy—during which time hPL (human placental lactogen) has been very elevated—that these cells mature through specific genetic changes, which cause them to become cancer resistant. There have been two large

---

26   Russo J, Lynch H and Russo IH. Mammary gland architecture as a determining factor in the susceptibility of the human breast to cancer. Breast Journal 2001 September; 7(5): 278-91.
27   Vatten, Romundstad, Trichopoulos and Skjaerven. See n. 15; Melbye et al. 1999. See n. 15.
28   Russo, Balogh and Russo. See n. 12.
29   Melbye M, Wohlfahrt J, Olsen JH, et al. Induced abortion and the risk of breast cancer. NEJM 1997 January; 336: 81-5.

meta-analyses confirming that induced abortion increases a woman's risk for premature delivery.[30]

Even pregnancies ending after 32 weeks but before 40 weeks gestation do not offer the maximum protection afforded by a full-term pregnancy.[31] Women who remain childless (nulliparous) have an increased risk for breast cancer because they have lifelong, immature, cancer-susceptible lobules, Types 1 and 2.

Without the maturing effects of hPL to form cancer-resistant Type 4 lobules, any mutated or clinically dormant cancer cells present in the mother's breasts before her pregnancy may become cancerous or start to grow under the influence of elevated levels of estrogen and progesterone, causing proliferation and the genotoxic estrogen metabolite 4 hydroxy catechol estrogen quinone. Estrogen levels increase 2000 per cent by the end of the first trimester. This explains why women who have their first child late in life will also have a higher risk of breast cancer. It is because of the additional time that has elapsed for mutations to have formed before pregnancy. This also explains the transient increase in the risk of breast cancer in women who have their first children late in their reproductive life.

The more menstrual cycles a woman has (whether owing to an early age at menarche [first period] or a late menopause), the longer her exposure to estrogen and progesterone during her menstrual cycles and, therefore, the higher her risk of developing breast cancer. Irregular periods during the first five years after menarche lower risk as there are fewer cycles and many are anovulatory (no egg produced), thus exposing a women to less estrogen and progesterone. Breastfeeding lowers a woman's risk for breast cancer because she will often stop menstruating and her cycles can be anovulatory (no ovulation).

Most spontaneous abortions (miscarriages) do not carry the same risk as induced abortions because most spontaneous abortions occur before three months gestation and are therefore associated with low levels of the pregnancy hormones needed for breast development. This in turn is due to an abnormality in the fetal-placental unit or the mother's ovaries, which then results in a spontaneous abortion (miscarriage).[32] Women who miscarry often

---

30   Swingle, Colaizy, Zimmerman and Morriss. See n. 6; Shah and Zao. See n. 6.
31   Vatten, Romundstad, Trichopoulos and Skjaerven. See n. 15; Melbye et al. 1999. See n. 15.
32   Kunz J and Keller PJ. HCG, HPL, oestradiol, progesterone and AFP in serum in patients with threatened abortion. BJOG 1976 August; 83: 640-4.

report having "not felt pregnant" owing to these low hormonal levels.

Epidemiological Studies

There were seventeen studies that showed a statistically significant increased risk of breast cancer before 1996, when Brind published a quantitative meta-analysis of them in the *British Journal of Epidemiology and Community Health*.[33] The meta-analysis excluded studies that did not differentiate between induced and spontaneous abortion and showed that seventeen of the 23 studies indicated a positive association, ten of which were statistically significant, meaning that there was a 95 per cent certainty that those studies did not show the association by chance. Since that time, many other studies have been published that show a statistically significant risk.[34]

---

[33] Brind J, Chinchilli VM, Severs WB and Summy-Long J. Induced abortion as an independent risk factor for breast cancer: a comprehensive review and meta-analysis. Journal of Epidemiology and Community Health 1996 October; 50(5): 481-96.

[34] Those studies that show a statistically significant link between abortion and breast cancer are as follows: Segi M, Fukushima I, Fujisaku S, et al. An epidemiological study of cancer in Japan. GANN 1957; 48(Supplement): 1-43; Rosenberg L, Palmer JR, Laufman DW, Strom BL, Schottenfeld D and Shapiro S. Breast cancer in relation to the occurrence and time of induced and spontaneous abortion. American Journal of Epidemiology 1988 May; 127(5): 981-9; Howe HL, Senie RT, Bzduch H and Herzfeld P. Early abortion and breast cancer risk among women under age 40. International Journal of Epidemiology 1989 June; 18(2): 300-4; Laing AE, Demenais FM, Williams R, Kissling G, Chen VW and Bonney GE. Breast cancer risk factors in African-American women: the Howard University Tumor Registry experience. Journal of the National Medical Association 1993 December; 85(2): 931-9; Laing AE, Bonney GE, Adams-Campbell L, et al. Reproductive and lifestyle factors for breast cancer in African-American women. Genetic Epidemiology 1994; 11: 285-310; Daling et al. 1994. See n. 4; Daling JR, Brinton LA, Voigt LF, et al. Risk of breast cancer among white women following induced abortion. American Journal of Epidemiology 1996 August; 144(4): 373-80; Newcomb PA, Storer BE, Longnecker MP, Mittendorf R, Greenberg ER and Willett WC. Pregnancy termination in relation to risk of breast cancer. JAMA 1996 January; 275(4): 283-7; Palmer JR, Rosenberg L, Rao RS, et al. Induced abortion in relation to risk of breast cancer (United States). Cancer Causes and Control 1997 November; 8(6): 841-9; Nishiyama F. The epidemiology of breast cancer in Tokushima prefecture. shikoku Ichi 1982; 38: 333-43 (in Japanese); Le MG, Bachelot A, Doyon F, Kramar A and Hill C. Oral contraceptive use and breast or cervical cancer: preliminary results of a French case-control study. *Hormones and sexual factors in human cancer aetiology*. EdS. Wolff JP and Scott JS. Amsterdam: Elsevier, 1984: 139-47; Lipworth L, Katsouyanni K, Ekbom A, Michels KB and Trichopoulos D. Abortion and the risk of breast cancer: a case-control study in Greece. International Journal of Cancer 1995 April; 61(2): 181-4; Rookus MA and van Leeuwen FE. Induced abortion and risk for breast cancer: reporting (recall) bias in a Dutch case-control study. Journal of the National Cancer Institute 1996 December; 88(23): 1759-64; Bu L, Voigt L, Yu Z, Malone K and Daling J. Risk of breast cancer associated with induced abortion in a population at low risk of breast cancer. American Journal of Epidemiology 1995; 141: S85 (abstract 337); Talamini R, Franceschi S, La Vecchia C, et al. The role of reproductive and menstrual factors in cancer of the breast before and after menopause. European Journal of Cancer 1996 February; 32(2): 303-10; Luporsi E. Breast cancer and alcohol. PhD dissertation, University of Paris-Sud, 1988. In Andrieu N, Duffy SW, Rohan TE, et al. Familial risk, abortion and their interactive effect on the risk of breast cancer—a combined analysis of six case-control studies. British Journal of Cancer 1995 September; 72(3): 744-51; Rohan TE, McMichael AJ and Baghurst PA. A population-based case-control study of diet and breast cancer in Australia. American Journal of Epidemiology 1988 September; 128(3): 478-89; Dolle et al. See n. 15; It was significant 1.4(1.1-2.52); Jabeen S, Haque M, Islam J, Hossain MZ, Begum A, Kashem MA. Breast cancer and some epidemiological risk factors: A hospital based study, J Dhaka Med Coll 2013; 22(1): 61-6; Xing, Li and Jin. See n. 17; Ozmen et al. See n. 18; Khachatryan, Scharpf and Kaan. See n. 19; Jiang et al. See n. 20; Lecarpentier J, et al. Variation in breast cancer risk associated with factors related to pregnancies according to truncating mutation location, in the French National BRCA1 and BRCA2 mutations carrier cohort (GENEPSO). Breast cancer research 2012; 14: R99; Yanhua C, et al. Reproductive variables and risk of breast malignant and benign turmours in Yunnan Province, China. Asian Pacific Journal of Cancer Prevention 2012; 13: 2179-218.

There are now 56 studies that show a positive association between abortion and breast cancer, of which 35 are statistically significant. The first was published in Japan and showed a three-fold increase in the risk of breast cancer in women with a history of induced abortion.[35] In 2012, three studies were published, two from China and one from France. All three were statistically significant, and all three supported the ABC (abortion-breast cancer) link.[36] In one Chinese study it was found that women who had a previous induced abortion experienced a 58 per cent increased risk of breast cancer even when factors such as number of full-term pregnancies and age at first birth had been controlled. The study also showed a dose-response relationship between abortion and breast cancer risk (with an increased risk of 33 per cent for one abortion, 76 per cent for two abortions and 165 per cent for three or more abortions), and did not show any significant increase in risk with spontaneous abortion. In the other Chinese study,[37] one abortion increased breast cancer risk by 150 per cent. The French study showed that an abortion before a full-term pregnancy increased risk by 70 per cent.

Ecological Epidemiological Studies

Ecological epidemiological studies examine trends in large populations based upon comparisons using statistical records kept by governmental agencies.

In 2007 an actuary, Patrick Carroll, published "The breast cancer epidemic: modeling and forecast based on abortion and other risk factors" in the *Journal of American Physicians and Surgeons*. He found that abortion was the greatest predictor of breast cancer incidence in nine European countries: England, Wales, Scotland, Northern Ireland, the Irish Republic, Sweden, the Czech Republic, Finland and Denmark. Using computerized abortion and breast cancer registries, he found that the greatest predictor of future breast cancer incidence was a nation's abortion rates. Within the United Kingdom, the constituent nations that have the highest abortion

---

35   Segi et al. 1957. See n. 34: 1-63.
36   Jiang et al. See n. 21; Lecarpentier J, et al. Variation in breast cancer risk associated with factors related to pregnancies according to truncating mutation location, in the French National BRCA1 and BRCA2 mutations carrier cohort (GENEPSO). Breast Cancer Research 2012; 14: R99.http://www.apocpcontrol.org/paper_file/issue_abs/Volume13_No5/2179-84%204.17%20Che%20Yanhua.pdf Yanhua, C, et al. Reproductive variables and risk of breast malignant and benign tumours in Yunnan Province, China. Asian Pacific Journal of Cancer Prevention 2012; 13: 2179-84. http://www.apocpcontrol.org/paper_file/issue_abs/Volume13_No5/2179-84%204.17%20Che%20Yanhua.pdf
37   Yanhua et al. See n. 34.

rates also have the highest breast cancer rates.[38] Thus, England, with the highest abortion rates, has an incidence of breast cancer of 116 per 100,000, while Northern Ireland, where abortion is much less prevalent, has an incidence of 97 per 100,000. Scotland lies between England and Northern Ireland in both breast cancer and abortion rates. There has been a 70 per cent increase in the risk of breast cancer in the United Kingdom between 1971 and 2002.

A 1989 study of breast and cervical cancers in three republics of the USSR (Russia, Estonia and Soviet Georgia) found that their breast cancer rates increased from between 270 and 330 per cent as their abortion rates increased.[39] The author commented that in the USSR, the majority of women used abortion as the principal method of birth control, and that in every year since legalization in 1955, the number of abortions has exceeded the number of live births. In the discussion the author declared that, "all four abortion indicators used in the study ... appeared to be the most significant correlates of the incidence of both cancers."[40] The four independent variables ('indicators') she referred to were: frequency of induced abortion, abortions to live birth ratio, frequency of out-of-hospital abortions and frequency of the termination of the first pregnancy.

Romania had one of Europe's lowest breast cancer rates while abortion was illegal under Ceausescu. Since its legalization in 1989, breast cancer rates appear to have risen dramatically, based on an analysis of the experience in one major county. Breast cancer incidence there increased from 25 per 100,000 women in 1988 to 40 in 1996 and 51 in 2006.[41] The total number of abortions reported in Romania jumped from 193,084 in 1989 to 992, 265 in 1990.[42] In 1960 breast cancer comprised seven per cent of all malignant tumors; by 1996 it had risen to 23 per cent, ranking it first in cancers among women. Given the explosion in the abortion rate, we may expect the incidence of breast cancer to rise even higher in coming years.

---

38 Carroll P. The breast cancer epidemic: modeling and forecasts based on abortion and other risk factors. Journal of American Physicians and Surgeons 2007 September; 12(3): 72-8.
39 Remennick LI. Reproductive patterns and cancer incidence in women: a population based correlation study in the USSR. International Journal of Epidemiology 1989 September; 18(3): 498-510.
40 Ibid.
41 Lucaci L and Szucsik IA. Statistical study on the incidence and prevalence of breast cancer, in Arad County, between the years 1999-2009. Arad Medical Journal 2010 November; 13(4): 5-10.
42 Council of Europe. Romania, Table 2: births, deaths, and legal abortions. *Recent Demographic Developments in Europe: Demographic Yearbook 2003*, 2004 January. http://www.coe.int/t/e/social_cohesion/population/RTAB2.xls.

In China, the enforcement of a one-child policy, which included compulsory abortion, was followed by a substantial increase in breast cancer rates. Since 1983, there has been an increased incidence of breast cancer in China.[43] Over the last ten years, the incidence of breast cancer rose 31 per cent to 55 per 100,000 women per year in Shanghai, and 23 per cent to 45 per 100,000 women per year in Beijing.[44] Even more alarming, a study published in 2008 reported that China was on the "cusp of a breast cancer epidemic,"[45] forecasting an incidence of 100 new cases of breast cancer per 100,000 women aged between 55 and 69 by 2021.[46]

In the United States, subsequent to the legalization of abortion in 1973, there has been a marked increase in the risk of both non-invasive and invasive breast cancers from 1975 to 2000.[47] Invasive cancer incidence went from 105 to 136 per 100,000 women. Non-invasive cancer in pre menopausal women went from four to twelve per 100,000 women, a nearly 400 per cent increase in incidence. On a smaller scale, Washington State breast cancer rates in black women rose after abortions began being state-funded (which increased abortion availability to poor black women).[48]

The Bradford-Hill Criteria

Before any causal statements may be made that a risk factor is a *cause* of a disease, and not just merely associated with it, strict criteria must be met. Just because a study shows a positive association of a factor with a disease, does not necessarily mean that factor is the cause.

---

43   Ferlay J, Héry C, Autier P and Sankaranarayanan R. "Chapter 1: global burden of breast cancer." In *Breast Cancer Epidemiology*. Ed. Li C. New York: Springer, 2010: pp. 13-15.
44   Beijing Centers for Disease Control and Prevention. China says breast cancer on rise in Beijing, Shanghai. Reuters, 30 October 2007. http://in.reuters.com/article/2007/10/30/us-china-cancer-idINPEK20120020071030.
45   Linos E, Spanos D, Rosner BA, et al. Effects of reproductive and demographic changes on breast cancer incidence in China: a modeling analysis. Journal of the National Cancer Institute 2008 October; 100(19): 1352-60, p. 1352.
46   Ibid.
47   National Cancer Institute. Cancer prevalence. *SEER Cancer Statistics Review 1975-2005*, 2008. http://seer.cancer.gov/csr/1975_2005/results_merged/topic_prevalence.pdf; White E, Daling JR, Norsted TL and Chu J. Rising incidence of breast cancer among young women in Washington State. Journal of the National Cancer Institute 1987 August; 79: 239-43.
48   Krieger N. Exposure, susceptibility, and breast cancer risk: a hypothesis regarding exogenous carcinogens, breast tissue development, and social gradients, including black/white differences, in breast cancer incidence. Breast Cancer Research and Treatment 1990 January; 13(3): 205-23.

For example, large, statistically significant and reproducible studies might show that people who carry matches in their pockets have a higher risk of lung cancer. Without the additional criteria of a plausible biological theory of how the matches cause lung cancer, these studies, no matter how many are done, show only a positive association between matches and lung cancer. Knowing that matches were associated with lung cancer might lead scientists to the discovery that the matches were mostly used to light cigarettes. This in turn would uncover the true cause of lung cancer. It was the Bradford Hill criteria, published in 1964, that brought the United States Surgeon General to place warnings on cigarette packages to the effect that they increased the risk of lung cancer.

Epidemiological studies done concerning the abortion-breast cancer link do show that they meet the criteria for classifying abortion as a causal risk for breast cancer. The following nine criteria were established by Sir Austin Bradford Hill in 1964 and were used to show the causal link between cigarettes and lung cancer.

Criterion 1: Strength of Association

Studies should show a large relative risk (RR), greater than 3.0. An RR of 3.0 means there is a 200 per cent increase in risk. (1.0 is null. 0.5 is a 50 per cent decrease in risk.)

If there is only a ten per cent increase in risk, it is difficult to say the risk is causal. There are subsets of women that show a greater than 200 per cent increased risk in breast cancer with abortion. There have been many studies such as the one by Daling (1994) that showed risks in some sub-groups of women to be much more than 200 per cent.[49] For instance, abortions done on women under the age of 18, at between nine and 24 weeks' gestation, had a relative risk of 9.0, meaning an 800 per cent increase in risk. If a woman aged 30 or older had an abortion at between nine and 24 weeks' gestation, her risk of breast cancer increased by 230 per cent.

Studies must be statistically significant.

Scientists require 95 per cent certainty that the study results were not obtained by chance alone. There are now 35 statistically significant studies that show the abortion-breast cancer link.

---

49   Daling et al. 1994. See n. 4.

Criterion 2: Temporality

The exposure to the risk must occur before the disease is detected, meaning that the abortion must occur before the breast cancers form.

This may seem so obvious that it need not be mentioned. However, a well-known study, that by Melbye and colleagues (1997) violated this rule when it collected breast cancer cases from a registry starting in 1968, but abortions only from 1973.[50] The cancer cases between 1968 and 1972 had no place in the study. By including them the authors minimized the link between breast cancer and abortion.

Criterion 3: Consistency

The preponderance of studies must show a positive association.

One or two studies by themselves can never be thought to support a causal link. Out of 73 published world wide studies done to date, 56 show a positive association,[51] of which 35 are statistically significant, while a total of seventeen studies show no link.

There are many reasons why studies might not show a link. If the population studied had abortions followed shortly by a full-term pregnancy in many instances, a very small effect would be expected and might not be observed. If the abortions were used to limit enlarging a family with many children, a small effect would be expected as the mother's breast tissue would have largely matured in previous pregnancies. This circumstance occurs in countries such as Italy, where the effect of induced abortion on breast cancer risk has been found to be less than other European countries. There may be bias in selection of patients so that very few young women, who have the highest risk with abortion, are included. The study may not follow most of the patients long enough for cancers to form; breast cancers take at least eight or more years to be detected, based upon the average doubling time for breast cancer cells. The study may choose not to look at all breast cancers and consider only some, such as invasive breast cancers, thereby eliminating approximately 25 per cent of cancers. For instance, in the US there were 230,480 cases of invasive breast cancers and 57,650 non-

---

50   Melbye et al. 1997. See n. 29.
51   Breast Cancer Prevention Institute. Epidemiologic studies: induced abortion and breast cancer risk. Fact Sheet. 2012 September. .www.bcpinstitute.org.

invasive breast cancers in 2011.[52]

Criterion 4: Theoretical Plausibility

The biological mechanism that explains the reason for the risk association must be biologically plausible.

The breast physiology, which explains the risk of breast cancer with induced abortion, has been thoroughly explained in a previous section. Elevated levels of estrogen during pregnancy leave the breast with increased numbers of Type 1 and 2 lobules where breast cancers arise, and without the benefit of a full-term pregnancy maturing the breast into predominantly Type 3 lobules, which are cancer-resistant. This same physiology can account for other well-accepted reproductive risks such as nulliparity (no births) and premature delivery. It has been shown that the longer a woman is pregnant before an abortion (up to 32 weeks), the higher her risk of breast cancer.[53]

Criterion 5: Coherence

The hypothesis, when proven, does not do violence to related sets of scientific findings but, instead, fits in with them.

The biological hypothesis of the abortion-breast cancer link (abortion causes an increase in the number of cancer-susceptible lobules and cells and, therefore, risk) is consistent with all other reproductive risk factors concerning pregnancy, such as: the protective effect of a full-term pregnancy while nulliparity (no births) increases risk; early age at full-term pregnancy decreasing risk; late age at full-term pregnancy increasing risk; the transient increase in breast cancer risk in older women who have their first pregnancy late in their reproductive life; lower exposure to estrogen and therefore risk after a full-term pregnancy because of an increase in sHBG (serum hormone binding globulin); lower prolactin levels in parous women (who have given birth) decreases risk; lower risk with each full-term pregnancy, and higher risk with premature delivery before 32 weeks.

---

52 American Cancer Society (ACS). *Breast Cancer Facts and Figures 2011-2012*. Atlanta, GA: ACS, Table 1, p. 2. http://www.cancer.org/acs/groups/content/@epidemiologysurveilance/documents/document/acspc-030975.pdf.
53 Melbye et al. 1997. See n. 29. After 32 weeks of course, the risk of breast cancer declines sharply.

Lung cancer does not form the day after you smoke a pack of cigarettes; it takes many packs over many years. Similarly, breast cancer does not develop immediately after an abortion. Yet, the association of breast cancer and abortion is in accord with the known natural history and biology of breast cancer. It takes an average of eight to ten years for one breast cancer cell to keep doubling so that it forms a tumor of clinically detectable size — about one centimetre. Most studies show the increase in breast cancers occurring in the time frame appropriate for the development of breast cancer, namely, at least eight to ten years after exposure.

Criterion 6: Specificity of Cause

Factor X leads to outcome Y.

There are ecological epidemiological studies that show induced abortion is the best predictor of breast cancer rates in a country. Induced abortion was found to be the greatest predictor of breast cancer rates in nine European countries.[54] Another study done in the USSR also showed such a link.[55]

Criterion 7: A Dose Effect is Observed

Based on biological mechanisms, the more one is exposed to the risk, the higher the risk of the disease if a factor is causal.

For example, the more cigarettes one smokes, the higher the risk of lung cancer. The longer one is pregnant before an abortion, the more immature breast tissue would be formed up to 32 weeks, and the higher the risk of breast cancer. The Melbye study showed a three per cent increase in the risk of breast cancer with each week of gestation.[56] However, it lumped together all late-term abortions after eighteen weeks' gestation. There is also evidence that the more abortions a woman has, the greater will be her risk of breast cancer.[57] Yet it is also true that, just as one exposure to

---

54 Carroll. See n. 38.
55 Remennick. See n. 39.
56 Melbye et al. 1997. See n. 29; Goldacre MJ, Kurina LM, Seagroatt V and Yeates D. Abortion and breast cancer: a case control record linkage study. Journal of Epidemiology and Community Health 2001 May; 55(5): 336-7; Erlandsson G, Montgomery SM, Cnattingius S and Ekbom A. Abortions and breast cancer: record based case-control study. International Journal of Cancer 2003 February; 103(5): 676-9.
57 Jiang et al. See n. 21; Yanhua et al. See n. 34; Remennick. See n. 39.

asbestos can cause a mesothelioma to form, so only one abortion may be enough to induce breast cancer.

Criterion 8: Experimental Studies

Variables are experimentally controlled for and yield predicted results consistently, first in animal studies, later in human (if ethically permissible, which, of course, is not the case with abortion).

Two pathologists studied the effect of a breast carcinogen (DMBA) given to groups of rats. The rats were either virgin, had a litter of pups, or had been aborted. The aborting rats developed breast cancers at a much higher rate when given DMBA than the virgins. No cancers occurred in one group of rats that had had a full-term pregnancy.[58]

Criterion 9: Analogy

Similar exposures should result in similar effects; for example, cigarette smoking causes bladder, as well as lung, cancer.

By the same token, premature deliveries before 32 weeks also double breast cancer risk because the breasts are left with more lobules where breast cancers can start. An abortion can be thought of as premature delivery by an abortionist.[59]

US racial trends of abortions and breast cancer incidence

In the US, although the incidence of breast cancer is highest among the Caucasian population, African-Americans under the age of 35 have an even higher incidence. The phenomenon has been labeled "inexplicable" by a prominent breast surgeon.[60] However, it becomes both explicable and predictable when abortions and premature births are compared between these racial groups. Although African-Americans make up twelve per cent of the population, they account for 35 per cent of total abortions, even though they constitute barely 12 per cent of the population. Caucasians

---

58   Russo J and Russo IH. Susceptibility of the mammary gland to carcinogenesis. American Journal of Pathology 1980 August; 100(2): 497-512.
59   Melbye et al. 1999. See n. 15.
60   Bland K. William Hunter Herridge Lecture: Contemporary management of pre-invasive and early breast cancer. American Journal of Surgery 2011 March; 201(3): 278-89, p. 279.

account for 55 per cent of all abortions. African Americans are thus three times more likely to have an abortion than Caucasians.[61] According to the Institutes of Medicine, in the US the overall premature birth rate before 37 weeks is 12.5 per cent, but 17.8 per cent in African Americans. As we have seen, both abortion and preterm birth are risk factors for breast cancer.[62]

QUESTIONING THE ABORTION-BREAST CANCER LINK

Recall Bias

"Recall bias" is the most widely and oft-reported argument used against the ABC link. This is the hypothesis that women who have developed breast cancer will be more likely to admit that they have had abortions than women who are well. The theory is based on the assumption that healthy women are more likely to conceal what could be embarrassing behavior but are more likely to tell the truth should they become ill, seeking a reason for their illness. Recall bias thus supposes that many women who do not have cancer will not report their abortions while those who do have cancer will report them. Case control studies in which researchers rely on interviews for their data are thought to be those potentially susceptible to recall bias. This is because researchers assume interviewees will not admit in an interview to "socially unacceptable behavior," such as abortion—unless they are sick. However, recall bias has not posed any such problem in other areas of medical research where case control studies have been used to gather data of other socially unacceptable behavior. For instance, in case control studies testing for a link between alcohol consumption and liver damage, interviewees were assumed to report their alcohol consumption accurately. The same is true for interviews in which interviewees were asked how many sexual partners they had, when inquiring into connections with cervical cancer, and whether they were involved in anal intercourse, when inquiring into HIV. Abortion would not seem to be a more socially unacceptable act than any of these. Why then should recall bias be thought to taint research about abortion but not the others?

Often the "Swedish" study is cited when using the argument of recall

---

61   Elam-Evans LD, Strauss LT, Herndon J, Parker WY, Bowens SV, Zane S and Berg CJ. Abortion surveillance—United States, 2000. Centers for Disease Control and Prevention. 28 November 2003. www.cdc.gov/mmwr/preview/mmwrhtml/ss5212al.htm.
62   Institute of Medicine. Preterm birth: causes, consequences and prevention. 13 July 2006. www.iom.edu/Reports/2006/Preterm-Birth-Causes-Consequences-and-Prevention.aspx.

bias[63]; yet it was convincingly refuted in a subsequent letter to the editor.

Recall bias is a hypothesis worth testing. Yet, studies that have confirmed the ABC link internally controlled for recall bias in their study populations.[64] Moreover, a study conducted specifically to test for recall bias in abortion-breast-cancer research reported having found evidence of it; however, methodological problems with the study acknowledged after publication revealed that it actually failed to show that recall bias taints such research. Instead, the study's results supported what is true to clinical experience: almost equal numbers of women with cancer and without cancer concealed their abortions.[65] Researchers in the Lindefors-Harris study had before them both cancer and abortion computer registries in order to verify the responses of the women who were interviewed. Two groups of women were interviewed: those with cancer and those without. The researchers hypothesized that more of those without cancer would deny their abortions while more of those with cancer would admit to them. Such a result would be evidence of recall bias. Instead, they found no statistically significant difference between the responses of the two groups of women.[66] In short, most healthy women and sick women admitted to the abortions officially documented in the abortion registry while some healthy women and some sick women lied. There was a statistically insignificant difference of barely six per cent between the two groups, which even in large studies would not greatly affect the results. On the other hand, researchers did find women—both healthy and sick—who admitted to abortions that were not documented in the abortion computer registry. The researchers labeled this phenomenon "over reporting," claiming that women who told the researchers that they had had abortions that had not been reported in the computer registry were mistaken or lying. The researchers would have been better advised to assume a mistake in the registry or that the women had their abortions in another country. Only with this wrongheaded assumption of *over* reporting did the authors then conclude that they had significant evidence of recall bias. Over reporting, of course, does not exist. The researchers were forced to acknowledge their error in a subsequent

---

63   Lindefors-Harris BM, Eklund G, Adami HO and Meirik O. Response bias in a case-control study: analysis utilizing comparative data concerning legal abortions and two independent Swedish studies. American Journal of Epidemiology 1991 November; 134(9): 1003-8.

64   Daling et al. 1994. See n. 4; Lipworth, Katsouyanni, Ekbom, et al. 1995. See n. 34.

65   Lindefors-Harris, Eklund, Adami and Meirik. See n. 63.

66   Women with cancer and women without cancer both underreported their abortion in similar percentages (5 out of 24 women or 21 per cent, and 16 out of 59 or 27 per cent, respectively).

exchange of letters to the editor.[67] Unfortunately, since most doctors read only the abstract of a paper and do not follow letters to the editor, a false impression of the study's results remains.

Studies with Contrary Findings

It is widely reported that the reason that "early" studies showed an association between abortion and breast cancer was that they were small, "case controlled" studies, subject to recall bias.

There is a belief that record linkage studies, in which patients are not interviewed, are more reliable. One such study showed a 90 per cent increased risk of breast cancer in women under 40 who had undergone one or more abortions.[68] New York State fetal death certificates and breast cancer registries were used, ensuring that there could be no "recall bias", as patients were not interviewed. That study is ignored when web sites of cancer organizations state that there are no record linkage studies demonstrating an abortion-breast cancer link. Rather there are very well-publicized studies, often cited, that purport to show no link. When scrutinized, these studies are found to have major flaws.

Between 1996 and August 2005, ten epidemiological studies were published based on prospective data regarding induced abortion and breast cancer. Brind soon published an analysis of these studies.[69] In great detail, he uncovered egregious errors, too many to list here. However, we will now analyze five studies often cited to show no link between abortion and breast cancer. In the first, the Scottish Brewster study, we find the transparent use of selection bias.[70] That study selectively used a data base that was not representative of the Scottish population. Although 58 per cent of abortions in Scotland are done on young nulliparous (no

---

67 Meirik O, Adami HO and Eklund G. Letter re: relation between induced abortion and breast cancer. Journal of Epidemiology and Community Health 1998 March; 52(3): p. 209; Brind J, Chinchilli VM, Severs WB and Summy-Long J. Reply to letter re: relation between induced abortion and breast cancer. Journal of Epidemiology and Community Health 1998 March; 52(3): 209-11.
68 Howe, Senie, Bzduch and Herzfeld. See n. 34.
69 Brind J. Induced abortion as an independent risk factor for breast cancer: a critical review of recent studies based on prospective data. Journal of American Physicians and Surgeons; 2005 Winter; 10(4): 105-10.
70 Brewster DH, Stockton DL, Dobbie R, Bull D and Beral V. Risk of breast cancer after miscarriage or induced abortion: a Scottish record linkage case-control study. Journal of Epidemiology and Community Health 2005 April; 59(4): 283-7.

births) women who would be most affected by abortion, the group that was studied had only 5.6 per cent nulliparous women. Another often cited study, known as the California Teachers Study and which attempts to deny the abortion-breast cancer link, is an extreme example of selection bias.[71] Women were eliminated from this study if they were diagnosed with non-invasive breast cancer (ductal carcinoma *in-situ* or DCIS) while being followed. DCIS is a *precursor* of invasive ductal cancer, which may take years to form. So the women most *likely* to develop invasive breast cancer were eliminated from the study before that cancer could develop! Another large British study reportedly showed no association of breast cancer and abortion.[72] However, for the more than 28,000 patients, only 300 abortions were listed over a 30-year period, despite the fact that in the UK the recorded abortion rate was one per cent per year for the study period. This means that 90 per cent of the women listed as having no abortion, almost certainly did have one. In fact, the authors admitted that their "data on abortion are substantially incomplete."[73] Their data were incomplete because the authors only considered abortions performed in inpatient hospital facilities, while most abortions are done in outpatient facilities, not in hospitals. Yet this publication is commonly reported as a large study showing no abortion-breast cancer link.

Melbye (1997): 1.5 Million Danish women

When it was published, the Melbye study was hailed as the definitive answer to the question "Does abortion increase breast cancer risk"?[74] It was the first large study to be published after Dr. Brind's 1996 meta-analysis. In an editorial accompanying the publication, NCI epidemiologist Patricia Hartge proclaimed the 1997 Melbye to be a definitive study so that "In short, a woman need not worry about the risk of breast cancer when facing the difficult decision of whether to terminate a pregnancy."[75] However, it misclassified 60,000 women who had legal abortions as not having had abortions because the authors used abortion registries starting in 1973 instead of 1940. It also violated the Bradford Hill criterion of temporality

---

71   Henderson KD, Sullivan-Halley J, Reynolds P, et al. Incomplete pregnancy is not associated with breast cancer risk: the California Teachers Study. Contraception 2008 June; 77(6): 391-6.
72   Goldacre 2001. See n. 56.
73   Ibid., p. 337.
74   Melbye et al. 1997. See n. 29.
75   Hartge P. Editorial: abortion, breast cancer, and epidemiology. NEJM 1997; 336(2): 127-8.

by collecting breast cancer cases starting in 1968 while collecting data on abortions using records that started in 1973. Another factor that contributed to the study's methodological flaws relates to the biology of breast cancer. It takes an average of eight to ten years for a cancer cell to grow into a clinically detectable cancer of one cm. diameter, based on average doubling times for cancer cells (the time needed to undergo one mitosis or cell replication). If an abortion in an eighteen-year-old causes a breast cancer cell to form, it is not likely to be detectable until she is at least 26. Fully one-quarter of the patients in the Melbye study were under 25 when the study ended, accounting for only eight cases of breast cancer. Because of what is known about the time needed for the development of breast cancer, none of these young women should have been included in the study.[76]

Yet even with this and other major flaws, the study showed a statistically significant risk in women who have had abortions performed over eighteen weeks' gestation. This fact was not mentioned in the conclusion of the paper, which merely stated that there was no link at all between abortion and breast cancer. This paper is still cited as large and conclusive, as if a single study could be conclusive. It is often used in major textbooks to show there is no link between abortion and breast cancer (see below, pp. 136-7).

Beral Re-Analysis

In 2004, *The Lancet* published a study[77] hailed by its authors, Valerie Beral and colleagues, as the definitive analysis that puts to rest the claim that abortion increases breast cancer risk. Beral was quoted as saying, "Scientifically, this is really a full analysis of the current data."[78] However, a review of the study reveals that it is not a "full analysis". Indeed, serious methodological flaws—especially in the selection of studies to be included—render the Beral study unreliable. The authors were guilty of several errors in selecting the studies to include in their analysis. First, they eliminated eleven studies for unscientific reasons (e.g., "principal investigators could not be found," or "researchers declined to take part in collaboration"), and four other studies'

---

76   Gersho-Cohen J, et al. Roentgenography of Breast Cancer Moderating Concept of "Biologic Predeterminism". Cancer 1963 August; 16: 961-4.
77   Collaborative Group on Hormonal Factors in Breast Cancer. Breast cancer and abortion: collaborative reanalysis of data from 53 epidemiological studies, including 83,000 women with breast cancer from 16 countries. The Lancet 2004 March; 363(9414): 1007-16.
78   Wahlberg D. Study: breast cancer not tied to abortion. Atlanta Journal Constitution, 26 March 2004.

worth of data were simply not mentioned at all.[79] Thus, in the end they included only 24 of the 41 studies in existence at the time of the re-analysis that contained data on induced abortion and breast cancer. To supplement these 24 studies, the researchers added a further 28 unpublished studies. This means that the majority of the studies included in their analysis had not themselves stood the test of peer review, nor could they be consulted by other researchers.

A closer look reveals that many of the statistically significant studies that demonstrate a link between abortion and breast cancer have been excluded. To be precise, of the 41 studies published up to 1994, 29 actually showed increased risk of breast cancer among women who chose abortion (epidemiologists call this a "positive association"). Seventeen of these 29 studies were statistically significant. Yet ten of the seventeen significantly positive studies in the literature were excluded by Beral and her colleagues. If the results of the fifteen studies supposedly excluded for being unscientific are averaged, they show an increase in breast cancer risk of 80 per cent among women who had abortions.

Beral and colleagues also divided the studies into two separate categories: those that used retrospective methods of data collection (i.e., interviews of breast cancer patients versus control subjects), and those that used prospective methods (i.e., medical records taken long before the breast cancer diagnosis). The 39 studies that used retrospective methods showed a significant overall eleven per cent increase in risk with abortion. The thirteen studies that used prospective methodology showed a significant seven per cent decrease in risk with abortion. Instead of reporting the results of her findings accurately (that is, that the retrospective studies showed that abortion increases the risk of breast cancer), they simply declared that these studies were unreliable—because of "recall bias". Despite the theoretical possibility that recall bias exists, we have seen that tests for such bias have proven negative.

Finally, at least three of the prospective data-based studies merit

---

79   The four studies not mentioned in the Beral et al. analysis were: Laing, Demenais, Williams, Kissling, Chen and Bonney. See n. 34: A300; Bu, Voigt, Yu, Malone and Daling. See n. 34; Bu, et al. Risk of breast cancer associated with induced abortion in SER Abstracts S85 (abstract 337); Luporsi. See n. 34; Zaridze DG 1988, in Andrieu, Duffy, Rohan, et al. Familial risk, abortion and their interactive effect on the risk of breast cancer—a combined analysis of six case-control studies. British Journal of Cancer 1995; 72(3): 744-751.

exclusion from the Beral study because of vast gaps in their databases, and consequent misclassification of subjects.[80] The Melbye study, discussed above, is one such study that should have been excluded. Another major flaw was that an inappropriate comparison group was chosen. Beral compared apples and oranges when the effects of having had a pregnancy that ended in abortion were compared with the effect of "not having had that pregnancy." Once a woman has had a healthy pregnancy, however long, her breasts are different than before that pregnancy started. Pregnancy forever alters the breast and physiologically these women are as different as pre- and post-menopausal women. Just as the effect of hormone replacement for post-menopausal women is studied in relation to other post-menopausal women who have no exposure to hormones, pregnant women who undergo abortion need to be compared to pregnant women who do *not* undergo induced abortion.

The National Cancer Institute

In addition to denying the abortion-breast cancer link, flatly incorrect information regarding breast cancer risk is given to patients on the website of the National Cancer Institute (NCI) in Washington D.C. For example, under the section on protective factors and decreased exposure to estrogen, it is stated that the exposure to estrogen "is reduced in the following ways: Pregnancy: estrogen levels are lower during pregnancy."[81] In fact, *estrogen levels rise 2000 per cent by the end of the first trimester.* Either the scientists at the NCI are unaware of this, or they are avoiding the biological explanation of why an early first full-term pregnancy reduces breast cancer risk.

In 2003, the NCI conducted a "Workshop on Early Reproductive Events and Breast Cancer Risks". The opinion and conclusion arrived at by the 100 scientists who attended the workshop are often cited to justify disregarding the evidence for the abortion-breast cancer link. They asserted that induced abortion was not a risk factor for breast cancer and need not be studied any further. However, they did note that premature birth was a risk for breast cancer. Interestingly, they also declared premature delivery to be an "epidemiological gap" that should be studied further. The obvious analogy between induced abortion and premature delivery causing the same physiological changes in a woman's breasts, and thereby similar

---

80   Melbye et al. 1997. See n. 29; Goldacre 2001. See n. 56; Erlandsson, Montgomery, Cnattingius and Ekbom. See n. 56.
81   National Cancer Institute. Breast cancer prevention. 20 September 2011. http://www.cancer.gov/cancertopics/pdq/prevention/breast/Patient/page3.

breast cancer risks, was ignored. Researchers who had conducted studies that supported the abortion-breast cancer link were not asked to present on that topic. Scientists present were not permitted to see the data presented before they were published. More telling was an interview given the day the workshop ended by an epidemiologist and workshop leader, Leslie Bernstein. She stated that having a child was the surest way to reduce breast cancer risk, but added "I would never be a proponent of going around and telling them that having babies is the way to reduce your risk." More tellingly, she went on, "I don't want the issue relating induced abortion to breast cancer risk to be a part of the mix of the discussion of induced abortion, its legality, its continued availability."[82] A detailed report by a workshop participant who disagreed with the official conclusion and noted the irregularities in the conduct of the meeting was submitted as a "Minority Report."[83] In 2009, a more damning situation arose with the publication of a paper regarding oral contraceptives and breast cancer risk, which put the veracity of the "consensus" in doubt.[84] The fourth author, affiliated with the NCI, was Louise Brinton, who had also chaired their February 2003 Workshop. This was significant because the paper concluded that induced abortion was a 40 per cent statistically significant risk factor for breast cancer. When a journalist for the Toronto *Globe and Mail*, Gloria Galloway, tried to question Louise Brinton in January 2010 about her apparent change of view on induced abortion and breast cancer risk, Brinton refused to be interviewed.[85] It should be borne in mind that scientific truth is determined by the examination of evidence derived through study and experiment, not by voting or consensus, which are subject to political and personal pressures. After all, it was once the scientific consensus that the universe was composed of only four elements, and that the sun revolved around the earth. The NCI's directors are political appointees of the US President. As appointees, they are influenced by political forces and agendas.

---

82   Lanfranchi A. The federal government and academic texts as barriers to informed consent. Journal of American Physicians and Surgeons 2008 Spring; 13(1): 12-15.
83   Brind J. Early reproductive events and breast cancer: a minority report. 2003 March. Paper given at the NCI workshop "Early Reproductive Events and Breast Cancer," February 24—26, 2003, Bethesda, MD.
84   Dolle et al. See n. 16.
85   Galloway G. Was Maurice Vellacott right about abortion? The Globe and Mail, 8 January 2010. http://www.theglobeandmail.com/news/politics/ottawa-notebook/was-maurice-vellacott-right-about-abortion/article4351341/.

Political and Social Pressures

In 1860, Dr. Oliver Wendell Holmes, a physician, essayist, and father of the celebrated US jurist, in an address to the Massachusetts Medical Society, stated, "Theoretically, [medicine] ought to go on its own straightforward inductive path without regard to changes of government or to fluctuations of public opinion [...] The truth is that medicine, professionally founded on observation, is as sensitive to outside influences, societal, religious, philosophical, imaginative, as the barometer is to the changes of atmospheric pressure."[86] That powerful statement also reflects what has continued to be a part of the fabric of medicine today. Physicians are human and susceptible to the same pressures as other people. Although ideally physicians are trained to be inured to those pressures, sadly we are not. There is documented evidence of widespread fraud in connection with National Institute of Health (NIH) funded research. (The NCI is a part of the NIH.) A paper in the British journal, *Nature*, using anonymous questionnaires, revealed that a statistically significant 15.5 per cent of scientists admitted to "changing the design, methodology or results of a study in response to pressure from a funding source." That funding source was the NIH.[87]

There is extensive evidence for the existence of the bias, which continues to make the independent abortion-breast cancer link ignored or unknown.

i. Pressure to include public advocacy in epidemiology

It is recognized that there are two competing schools of thought regarding the field of epidemiology. Epidemiology is viewed as an objective science in one school and as a science that must include public advocacy in the other. Raj Bhopal, an eminent epidemiologist, has stated that the fundamental question is "...whether epidemiology is primarily an applied public health discipline...or primarily science in which methods and theory dominate over practice and application." In 1999, a commentary in the *American Journal of Public Health* succinctly put the question as whether epidemiology was a science or mission. Clearly a strong advocacy position can lead to bias in reporting the data that science has collected. Recent revelations in

---

86   Holmes OW. Address to annual meeting, Massachusetts Medical Society, 30 May 1860. Para. 7. In *Currents and Counter-currents in Medical with Other Addresses and Essays*. Boston: Ticknor and Fields, 1861.
87   Martinson BC, Anderson MS and deVries R. Scientists behaving badly. Nature 2005 June; 435: 737-8.

the media concerning the global warming controversy have shown that eminent scientists on either side are capable of suppressing or ignoring data that do not support their position. Imagine if an epidemiologist wants to advocate for zero population growth as a method to help reduce pollution and disease. Is it not doubtful that he or she would also favour widespread dissemination of data that support the abortion-breast cancer link when abortion is still used as the primary method of birth control in China and the countries that once constituted the USSR? For example, an epidemiologist financially supported by the NCI, Lynn Rosenberg, is on the record as a staunch abortion advocate who has also testified as an expert before governmental bodies making laws on abortion regulation.[88] Rosenberg also wrote an editorial in the Journal of the NCI dismissive of Janet Daling's 1994 landmark study, which appeared in the same issue and showed an overall 50 per cent increase in breast cancer risk with abortion.[89]

ii. Misleading academic texts

Bias is seen in academic breast cancer texts concerning prevention and risks. The preventive effects of child-bearing and the risk-increasing effects of induced abortion are misstated in major textbooks. In the 2000 edition of *Diseases of the Breast* by Jay Harris and colleagues, early full-term pregnancy is not listed in its table of methods of prevention because, according to the accompanying text, "unplanned early pregnancy and an average of more than two completed pregnancies per woman have undesirable social and ecologic consequences."[90] The fact that it takes a fertility of at least 2.1 children per woman just to maintain a given population is disregarded. The book's recommendations appear to be influenced by the notion that human beings are bad for the "ecology." Busy practising clinicians may rely on tables for a quick answer, rather than reading the whole text.

Although the 1991 and 1998 editions of *The Breast: Comprehensive Management of Benign and Malignant Disease* clearly stated that induced abortion was a risk factor for breast cancer in the chapter concerning

---

88   North Florida Women's Health and Counselling Services, Inc., et al., v. State of Florida, et al. Circuit Court, Second Judicial District, Leon County, FL, No. 99-3203, 1999.
89   Rosenburg L. Induced abortion and breast cancer: more scientific data are needed. Journal of the National Cancer Institute 1994 November 2; 86(21): 1569-70.
90   Harris J, Lippman ME, Morrow M and Osborne CK. *Diseases of the breast*, 2nd ed. Baltimore, MD.: Lippincott, Williams & Wilkins, 2000: 211-2. Editions are as follows: 1st Ed. (1996 Lippincott Raven); 2nd Ed. (2000 Lippincott Williams & Wilkins); 3rd Ed. (2004 Lippincott Williams & Wilkins); 4th Ed. (2010 Lippincott Williams & Wilkins).

molecular biology, the 2004 edition removed that information.[91] In its place was a misleading table of breast cancer risks. Induced abortion is listed in the table as having "no effect" on breast cancer risk. This statement is contradicted by the accompanying text, which states that abortion after 12 weeks carries a relative risk of 1.38, a 38 per cent increase.[92] By the 2009 edition, induced abortion was not listed in any of the tables that tabulated risk factors; yet, it had a similar paragraph of text as in the 1998 edition.

iii. Sociological pressures

It is very difficult for the public to believe that physicians who are thought to put their patients' health first, or scientists looking for scientific truth, could be involved in misinformation. It is difficult for breast surgeons to tell their patients that abortion increases breast cancer risk when the referring physician performs abortions. It may also be seen by their patient that they are being told that their own behavior has caused their cancer. Even patients who have had no abortions yet developed breast cancer may feel tainted by being perceived to have abortion as part of their medical history.

Knowing that approximately 40 per cent of women in the US will have had an abortion by the age of 40, there is the risk of telling a cancer patient that she may have contributed to the development of her own disease. It is much more comfortable not to risk offending professional colleagues who perform abortions, refer for abortions, or have had abortions as part of their personal history. Maintaining a cordial professional relationship ensures continued referrals and a pleasant practice environment.

iv. Political pressures

There are many historical examples of political pressures on governmental

---

91 Dickson RB and Lippman ME. Chapter 27: growth and regulation of normal and malignant breast tissue. In *The Breast: Comprehensive Management of Benign and Malignant Diseases*. Eds. Bland KI and Copeland EM. 2nd ed. Philadelphia : Saunders, 1998, p. 523; Editions of this book are as follows: Bland KI and Copeland EM. *The Breast: Comprehensive Management of Benign and Malignant Disorders*. Philadelphia: Saunders, 1991; Bland and Copeland. *The Breast: Comprehensive Management of Benign and Malignant Disorders*. 2nd ed. 2 vols. Philadelphia: W.B. Saunders, 1998; Bland and Copeland. *The Breast: Comprehensive Management of Benign and Malignant Disorders*. 3rd ed. 2 vols. St. Louis, MO: Saunders, 2004; Bland and Copeland. *The Breast: Comprehensive Management of Benign and Malignant Disorders*. 4th ed. 2 vols. Philadelphia: Saunders Elsevier, 2009.
92 Vogel V. "Chapter 16: epidemiology of breast cancer." In *The Breast: Comprehensive Management of Benign and Malignant Diseases*. Eds. Bland KI and Copeland EM. 2004. See n. 90, Table 16-1, pp. 343-4.

institutions that led to public health care information and policies that were damaging to public health. One especially egregious and well-documented case was the political pressure upon the NCI, which allowed a lung cancer epidemic to evolve into a major health care liability. For decades the epidemiological evidence of the cigarette-lung cancer link was suppressed.[93] The first study linking cigarettes to lung cancer was published in 1928. Even though thoracic surgeons were reporting huge increases in lung cancers after World War II, the NCI was largely silent and minimized smoking's risk in the development of lung cancer. This was shown to be due to pressure from southern senators. They complained that if it became widely known that cigarettes caused lung cancer, their states' economies, which were based on the production of tobacco and tobacco products, would collapse, causing financial ruin. In fact it was not the NCI that brought the cigarette-lung cancer link to public attention. Rather, it was the US Surgeon General, when in 1964 he made his first report to protect the public health, and required warnings on all cigarette packs.

Political pressure can also be brought to bear upon professional groups by governments to advance their political agendas. For example, during the presidency of Bill Clinton, a case was argued before the Supreme Court over whether the state of Nebraska was constitutionally entitled to ban partial birth abortion. The American College of Obstetrics and Gynecology (ACOG) had prepared a statement concerning partial-birth abortion, which was thought by legal counsel at the White House to be too problematic and a "disaster" for them, the term used by the future Supreme Court Justice, Elena Kagan, while working for Clinton. According to the initial ACOG statement, experts "could identify no circumstances under which the [partial-birth] procedure…would be the only option to save the life or preserve the health of the woman." This made it impossible for the White House to claim that there were medical reasons to support partial-birth abortions. ACOG's final statement added the phrase that Kagan wanted for purely political reasons, namely that the procedure may be "the best or most appropriate procedure in a particular circumstance to save the life or preserve the health of a woman." This information came to light several years later, when Kagan was interrogated in the confirmation hearings before being ratified as a Supreme Court Justice. She explained to the Senate judiciary committee that her meetings with ACOG were for the purpose of ensuring that ACOG had the opportunity to paint the whole picture.

---

93   Kessler DA. *A Question of Intent: A Great American Battle with a Deadly Industry.* New York, NY: Public Affairs, 2001.

This answer was characterized by Senator Hatch as a "real politicization of science."[94] Former Surgeon General C. Everett Koop wrote an open letter to all the senators urging that Kagan should be rejected for her disgraceful and unethical action in seeking the replacement of a medical statement with a political one.[95]

Political pressures are brought to bear by breast cancer advocacy groups with links to the abortion industry to deny the abortion breast cancer link. The Susan G. Komen Foundation is a breast cancer advocacy group in the United States, which has raised millions of dollars since its inception over twenty years ago. Its founder, Nancy Brinker, was also a board member of Planned Parenthood, a leading abortion provider. Planned Parenthood was also the recipient of grants from Komen. Komen denies the abortion-breast cancer link, as does the National Breast Cancer Coalition, an advocacy group that heavily lobbies the US Congress, influencing research funded by the Department of Defense.[96] The coalition maintains that there is no way to prevent breast cancer, despite the clear evidence that when fifteen million women stopped their hormone replacement therapy, breast cancer incidence began decreasing. Abortion is a large industry with trade organizations that lobby politicians to maintain a favorable environment in which to function.

Conclusion

There can be no doubt that a woman who is pregnant will increase her risk of breast cancer if she aborts that pregnancy. She will either remain childless, which in itself increases breast cancer risk, or she will delay her first full-term pregnancy, another known risk for breast cancer. She is also

---

94   AUL Action: The Legislative Action Arm of Americans United for Life. *Investigating the Confirmation Testimony of Elena Kagan Before the US Senate Judiciary Committee and the Negative Impact of Her Amendment of the 1997 Policy Statement of the American College of Obstetricians and Gynecologists (ACOG) on the Federal Administration of Justice and the US Supreme Court.* Washington, DC: AUL Action, July 15, 2010. http://www.aul.org/featured-images/Kagan-Ethics-Report.pdf.
95   Kiely KC. Everett Koop urges senators to block Kagan. USA Today, 19 July 2010. http://content.usatoday.com/communities/onpolitics/post/2010/07/everett-koop-urges-senators-to-block-kagan/1; Bravin J. Dr. Koop: keep Kagan off high court. Wall Street Journal, 19 July 2010. http://blogs.wsj.com/washwire/2010/07/19/dr-koop-keep-kagan-off-the-supreme-court/.
96   National Breast Cancer Coalition. Truth #30: I can influence what happens in Washington D.C. about breast cancer. 2011. http://www.breastcancerdeadline2020.org/know/31-myths-and-truths/truth-30-i-can-influence-capitol-hill.html.

deprived of breastfeeding her baby, which would further reduce her breast cancer risk.

By the end of a full-term pregnancy, a woman will cause 85 per cent of the Type 1 and 2 breast lobules she developed at puberty (where ductal and lobular cancers start respectively) to mature to Type 4 lobules, which are cancer-resistant. There are documented changes in the breast cells' genomes, which have been studied and provide the known molecular basis for the protective effect of a full-term pregnancy. In addition to the loss of the benefit of a full-term pregnancy, abortion increases her risk for breast cancer by increasing the number of breast cells where cancers can start. This fact is not only supported by the known biology of breast maturation, but through the world-wide epidemiological studies that have been done since 1957, which show that induced abortion increases breast cancer risk. After an abortion, a woman is more likely to have a premature delivery, which again increases her breast cancer risk. Scientific honesty makes it impossible to disregard over half a century of world medical literature confirming the abortion-breast cancer link. To dismiss those studies as flawed is scientifically untenable. On the other hand, the few studies recently acclaimed as disproving the abortion-breast cancer link have been guilty of major methodological flaws. They also fly in the face of the most recent studies from around the world, which continue to confirm the link between abortion and breast cancer. The fact that induced abortion significantly increases the risk of breast cancer deserves to become widely known to the public and to the medical profession. Women must be told of these risks so they can be fully informed before consenting to abortion.

Chapter 8

Prenatal testing and abortion for fetal anomaly

KEY POINTS

- The capacity to diagnose prenatally is now vastly disproportionate to the capacity to treat illnesses or disabilities.

- Prenatal diagnostic tests are most often used to prevent the birth of individuals with certain undesired characteristics through termination of pregnancy.

- Swift advances in diagnostic technologies are not matched by public and financial support for infants with disabilities and their families.

- Now that prenatal screening is standard medical practice, women who refuse testing may be seen as not "doing their motherly duty" to ensure the birth of a healthy child.

- In counselling, many have expressed disappointment that the information provided stresses only the negative aspects of having a child with a condition. Little emphasis is placed on the possible benefits of a disabled child to the family.

- One study found that 44 per cent of women had posttraumatic stress symptoms, and 28 per cent had symptoms of depression after terminating for fetal anomaly.[1] Many women are not fully informed of the risk of psychological distress after terminating a pregnancy.

---

1   Korenromp MJ, Page-Christiaens GC, van den Bout J, et al. A prospective study on parental coping 4 months after termination of pregnancy for fetal anomalies. Prenatal Diagnosis 2007; 27(8): 709-16.

SURVEILLANCE

Prenatal genetic diagnosis, while still a relatively new practice, is tracked through public health programs around the world. The flaws in surveillance and lack of transparency mean that the public has no idea of the effect of the national screening programs or the health policies that relate to prenatal programs. Public Health surveillance of diseases is a government initiative that collects data to track disease, does research, and recommends the policies and procedures necessary to prevent or eliminate the occurrence of a medical disorder, disease or condition. In the US the Centers for Disease Control performs this function, while in the European Union EUROCAT coordinates the information from twenty countries. In Canada Health Surveillance is part of the mandate of The Public Health Agency of Canada. The Canadian Congenital Anomaly Surveillance System (CCASS) is one of the twenty different surveillance programs within Public Health, and its mandate is to coordinate the information from a loose association of provincial programs that are charged with collecting data on congenital anomalies at the local or regional level.

The outcomes of pregnancies following prenatal diagnosis are not consistently reported. All surveillance programs report that they follow prenatally diagnosed children through birth, premature birth or elective termination after twenty weeks gestation. Yet there are problems with how this information is collected and disseminated. Brian Lowry of the Alberta Congenital Anomalies Surveillance System writes in the *Canadian Journal of Public Health* that "CCASS is a passive system with no verification capabilities."[2] He goes on to note that the data reported are inadequate since, due to privacy concerns, "no verification or follow-up of cases is possible and terminations of pregnancy are not included."[3] So, while reporting that the selective termination of affected fetuses is part of the data set in most instances, such information is not publicly available. A study by Liu and colleagues reported information on prenatal diagnosis and pregnancy termination. They concluded that fetal deaths due to termination for congenital anomaly increased in Canada between 1991 and 1998 by 578 per cent,[4] but no searchable reference was provided to account for the data. However, there has been a very recent report discussing the number of live births with congenital anomalies and the late termination

---
2   Lowry RB. Congenital anomalies surveillance in Canada. Canadian Journal of Public Health 2008; 99(6): 483-5.
3   Ibid.
4   Liu S, Joseph KS, Kramer MS, et al. Relationship of prenatal diagnosis and pregnancy termination to overall infant mortality in Canada. JAMA 2002; 287(12): 1561-7.

rates. It shows a clear correlation between the decreased number of children born with disabilities related to chromosomal or obvious physical defects (cleft palate and spina bifida being the most common) and the increase in late terminations.[5]

What some recent studies are measuring is the incidence of infants born with specific anomalies, before and after prenatal diagnosis programs were introduced. The results, as shown in the following table, show that the programs are decreasing the number of children born with certain conditions.

Table 8.1 **The impact of prenatal diagnosis programs on the incidence of children born with specific anomalies**

Study	Location	Condition	Outcome
Morris et al. [a] **2007**[i]	England/Wales	Neural Tube defect	Rate reduced from 3.6/1000 in 1964 to 2.31/1000 in 2004
Nordvig et al. 2005[ii]	Denmark	Down syndrome	98 per cent abortion rate after detection
Cochi et al. 2010[iii]	20 registries from 14 countries.	Down syndrome	Abortion rate for Down syndrome doubled 1993-2004.[b]
Khoshnood et al.[c] **2011**[iv]	16 European countries	Down syndrome	48.1 per cent abortion rate after detection

a: Estimated 52 per cent underreporting of terminations following prenatal screening with statistical decrease "due to screening and termination of affected pregnancies."
b: The rate of abortion with Down syndrome increased from 4.8/10,000 births in 1993 to 9.9/10,000 births in 2004.
c: Numbers vary from country to country. No selective abortions are done in Ireland, Malta and Poland.

i: Morris JK and Wald NJ. Prevalence of neural tube defect pregnancies in England and Wales from 1964 to 2004. Journal of Medical Screening 2007; 14: 55-9.
ii: Nordvig L, Secher NJ and Andersen S. Psykologiske aspekter, brugerholdninger og - forventninger I forbindelse med ultralydskanning I graviditeten. Medicinsk Teknologivurdering 2006; 6(13): p. 12.
iii: Cocchi G, Gualdi S, Bower C, et al. International trends of down syndrome 1993-2004: births in relation to maternal age and terminations of pregnancies. Birth Defects Research (Part A) 2010; 88: 474-9.
iv: Khoshnood B, Greenlees R, Loane M, and Dolk H and EUROCAT Working Group. Paper 2: EUROCAT public health indicators for congenital anomalies in Europe. Birth Defects Research Part A (Clinical and Molecular Teratology) 2011; 91(Suppl 1): S16-22.

5   Joseph KS, Kinniburgh B, Hutcheon JA, Mehrabadi A, Basso M, Davies C and Lee L. Determinants of increases in stillbirth rates from 2000 to 2010. CMAJ 2013; 185(8): E345-51.

What emerges from the surveillance information is a split understanding of the overall purpose of maintaining these statistics and the ultimate goal of surveillance itself. If the purpose of the prenatal screening and testing program is to eliminate genetic disorders in the population we see its results in the Danish study. That study analyzed the results of a nationwide screening initiative and reported the almost complete elimination of children diagnosed with Down syndrome. Yet, in the end, this costly program of prenatal screening resulted in the elimination of only 25 Down syndrome births.[6]

By contrast, in his introductory statement about surveillance of congenital anomalies in Canada, Brian Lowry wrote that surveillance was important in order to evaluate "preventative measures such as folic acid fortification."[7] Sadly, what the systematic collection of information on congenital conditions reveals is an increase in access to selective abortion services versus access to preventative measures. Increased support for pregnant mothers or for children with genetic disorders is not an outcome that is measured in any of the literature.

Prenatal Testing: Then and Now

Prenatal testing began in the late 1970s with the use of amniocentesis for the identification of fetuses with Down syndrome or spina bifida. Early research on the use of these procedures uncovered interesting results. British physicians in 1980 reported that the aim of such tests was the "detection of fetal abnormality, while the women wanted the reassurance of being told there were no abnormalities."[8] Seventy-five per cent of physicians reported that they required the women to agree to a termination of an affected pregnancy before proceeding with prenatal diagnosis and 80 per cent were prepared "to recommend" termination after twenty weeks gestation for both conditions. By 1993, a similar survey found that 34 per cent of physicians would require an undertaking to abort before referral for testing but that 95 per cent would be prepared "to recommend" termination after twenty weeks for either condition. What these results suggest is that while the understanding of women's autonomy of choice had become better recognized, the value of a disabled fetus dropped and the upper gestational limits for the abortion procedure increased to the edges of viability and beyond.

---

6   Nordvig, Secher and Andersen. See Table reference ii.
7   Lowry. See n. 2, p. 483.
8   Green JM. Obstetricians' views on prenatal diagnosis and termination of pregnancy: 1980 compared with 1993. BJOG 1995; 102(3): 228-32, p. 228.

Not only have the abortion limits been raised, but the ability to identify possible anomalies in the first trimester continues to expand with genetic research. As the impact of both the Human Genome Project and the advances in prenatal diagnosis reach from the laboratory to the doctor's office, the number of detectable conditions has gone up dramatically.[9] In addition to identifying chromosomal anomalies, prenatal screening can also detect conditions within the fetus that may be linked to non-heritable conditions. Some of these disorders are life-limiting, while others may result in delays in physical or cognitive developmental areas, or both. With this increase in possible identification has come a push to expand "a woman's right" to include prenatal testing. Offering early prenatal screening has become the norm for all pregnant women while the decision not to screen is now seen as unusual for Down Syndrome, Spina Bifida and Trisomy 13. Where previously pregnant women over the age of 35 were the cohort targeted for such screening, the Society of Obstetricians and Gynecologists of Canada (SOGC) has expanded the guidelines: "all pregnant women in Canada regardless of age should be offered through an informed consent process a prenatal screening test for the most common clinically significant fetal aneuploidies in addition to a second trimester ultrasound for dating, growth and anomalies."[10] This expansion of screening came at a time when genetic screening was already increasing in prevalence in Canada. In Ontario in 2000, over 40 per cent of women were screened prenatally; seven years later the rate of prenatal screening was over 60 per cent.[11]

Given these changes, a new set of clinical practice guidelines on prenatal screening has been laid down by the Society of Obstetricians and Gynaecologists of Canada and the Canadian College of Medical Geneticists. It is now recommended that "all pregnant women be offered prenatal screening, rather than just women aged 35 years or more."[12] While in the past legal precedents have placed an obligation on physicians to offer prenatal screening specifically to women over 35 years of age, legal scholars predict

---

9   Human Genome Management Information. About the human genome project. Information 2011. http://www.ornl.gov/sci/techresources/Human_Genome/project/about.shtml.
10 Summers AM, Langlois S, Wyatt P, and Wilson RD and Society of Obstetricians and Gynaecologists of Canada. Prenatal screening for fetal aneuploidy. Journal of Obstetrics and Gynaecology 2007; 29(2): 146-61.
11 Better Outcomes Registry and Network Ontario. *The Ontario perinatal surveillance system report 2008.* http://www.bornontario.ca/_documents/Publications/Annual%20Report%202008.pdf.
12 Pioro M, Roxanne M and Nisker J. Wrongful birth litigation and prenatal screening. CMAJ 2008; 179(10): p. 1027.

that successful legal actions against physicians will increase when they fail to offer prenatal tests, given their prevalence as standard practice.

Pioro and colleagues suggest that "the combination of this ability to choose and the legally sanctioned concept that the birth of a disabled child can constitute a harm may cause a woman to be viewed as harming a child simply by choosing to bring a disabled child to term."[13]

The capacity to diagnose prenatally is now vastly disproportionate to the capacity to ameliorate the various genetically related conditions. Rather than preventing or treating an illness or disability, the tests are most often used to prevent the birth of individuals with certain undesired characteristics. This prevention is carried out in North America and Europe through termination of pregnancy.

Although prenatal screening and subsequent termination are choices offered to pregnant women, Pediatric Neurologist Michael Shevell warns that "reasonable concerns exist that a publicly funded program of detection and counselling occurring at a time of funding limitations will be driven by a cost-containment emphasis that may weigh the scales of choice in one direction."[14]

At a time when families of children with disabilities and adults with disabilities are desperately seeking better services, how are scarce dollars best spent? Is the cost of universal prenatal screening justified by the monetary savings from not having to raise all those children who would have been born with Down syndrome and spina bifida? Merely to pose this question is to ask if the end justifies the means. Is the elimination of innocent unborn human life justified by the financial savings that will result? Morally, the answer can only be no.

Aside from the option of terminating the pregnancy, prenatal diagnosis may afford parents the opportunity to plan more effectively for the care for a disabled child. A mother who discovers that her child will have Down syndrome (Trisomy 21) for instance, may be able to seek community resources for infants and children with developmental disabilities.

In a minority of cases genetic amniocentesis is done because there is a pre-

---

13   Ibid., p. 1028.
14   Shevell M. Eugenics by another name? Canadian Journal of Neurological Sciences 2007; 34(4): p. 494.

existing history of a family member with a disease that has potential to limit the life expectancy of the child. This occurs with Trisomy 13 or Trisomy 18, for example. Knowledge of a life-limiting fetal abnormality can be very difficult for families to assimilate, since "instead of anticipating the arrival of a new baby, there is contemplation of the impending death of a loved one."[15] However, even in circumstances where neonatal death is common, families who receive prenatal diagnosis of such a condition can benefit from perinatal palliative care. Although not yet widely available, perinatal palliative care can provide appropriate care for child and supportive care for the family. Just as palliative care is given to the elderly at the end of life, so too the fetus is a patient worthy of treatment. Perinatal palliative care "focuses on enhancement of the quality of life for the child and support for the family,"[16] which in turn, can provide families with necessary psychological relief as they are given time to bond with their dying child and say goodbye in a nurturing environment.

---

15   Hoeldtke NJ and Calhoun BC. Perinatal hospice. AJOG 2001; 185: p. 526.
16   Leuthner S and Jones EL. Fetal concerns program: a model for perinatal palliative care. The American Journal of Maternal/Child Nursing 2007; 32(5): p. 273.

METHODS OF PRENATAL SCREENING AND DIAGNOSIS

Prenatal screening and diagnosis methods continue to evolve with the development of new technology.

Current Canadian guidelines recommend offering non-invasive screening for Down syndrome, Trisomy 18, and neural tube defects, in addition to a second trimester ultrasound, to all pregnant women. Women who are at high risk of genetic anomaly, or who will be 40 years old at the time of birth, are offered counselling and the option of diagnostic testing: amniocentesis or chorionic villi sampling (CVS)

The **non-invasive screening** can be done in the first and/or second trimester. A combination of tests from both the first and second trimester, known as integrated prenatal screening (IPS) is considered the most accurate result with the least number of false positives. The screening develops risk ratios based on biochemical markers from maternal blood tests, and also the measurement of nuchal translucency found in a first trimester ultrasound.

In addition to the above mentioned screening, a **second trimester ultrasound** is offered to all women between eighteen and 22 weeks. This ultrasound examines the complete anatomy of the fetus, and screens for gross congenital anomalies and "soft markers" which are associated with higher risk of some genetic anomalies.

If a woman is considered to be high risk due to age or family history, if the non-invasive screening reveals a high risk, or if the second trimester ultrasound shows evidence of anomalies, the woman is referred to a genetic counselling centre where she is offered counselling and invasive diagnostic genetic testing, often on the same day.

Amniocentesis and CVS are the two forms of diagnostic testing. In amniocentesis, amniotic fluid is removed from the uterus by inserting a needle through the maternal abdominal wall, guided by ultrasound. It can be done starting at fifteen to seventeen weeks gestation, and is considered highly accurate for detecting fetal aneuploidy and neural tube defects. Risks of amniocentesis include miscarriage (1/100 to 1/600), infection (1/3000 to 2/3000), amniotic fluid loss, bleeding and uterine irritability (one to five per cent).

During CVS, chorionic villi are removed by a needle through the abdomen or by a catheter through the cervix of the woman, guided by ultrasound. This procedure can be done starting as early as ten weeks gestation, until about 32 weeks. It is considered accurate for detecting fetal aneuploidy only, but the sample is sometimes contaminated with maternal cells, so sometimes a follow up amniocentesis is offered. Risks of CVS include a significant risk of miscarriage (one to six per cent), and a risk of harm to the fetus resulting in limb or facial anomalies (1/3000).

Research is ongoing in the field of prenatal genetic testing. A new chromosomal microarray analysis is being developed, which may soon be able to diagnose a genetic anomaly solely from a maternal blood sample, thus making genetic testing more widely available early in pregnancy, and less risky to the mother.

"Whether or not to have prenatal screening or prenatal diagnosis is each woman's choice."[17]

It is when the issue of induced abortion arises that one finds the most egregious violations of the concept of informed consent. In Chapter 20 on "Who are the experts? What 101 women told us" it is clear that women experiencing post-abortion emotional distress feel that they were not properly informed of the nature of the abortion procedure or the facts related to fetal development. Only two of the women we interviewed gave fetal abnormality as a reason for their abortions and yet 96 per cent of the cohort reported that they were not properly informed of the risks of the abortion procedure, or of prenatal development. Over two-thirds of the respondents identified pressure and coercion as a leading factor in their decision. From these findings it is obvious that there have been violations of the principle of informed consent (See also Chapter 5).

> "In a worst case scenario as was told to me, I would get a lot more information and not trust just two opinions. I didn't know anything about L'Arche. I was told there was only Children's Aid and institutions. I had experiences with Children's Aid and was afraid. I believed too much in what others thought I was capable of rather than what I thought I was capable of...now I know I was manipulated into what they thought was best for me and [they] manipulated me into thinking it was in my best interest too."
>
> "I was looking forward to this child until I got the news that the baby had Down syndrome. Then, the child became an 'it'...I was so defective that I couldn't produce a non-defective baby. I felt that if people knew, they would be horrified and I would be shunned."

It is considered gold-standard practice that doctors present the option of prenatal screening to all women but the choice to have it done remains with the pregnant woman. However, in the past few years many

---

17   Better Outcomes Registry and Network Ontario. *The Ontario perinatal surveillance system report 2008.* http://www.bornontario.ca/_documents/Publications/Annual%20Report%202008.pdf. Formerly known as the Fetal Alert Network.

women have come to feel increasingly obliged to have the test. Perhaps this misunderstanding comes from the language of the document where early screening for Down syndrome or Trisomy 18 is recommended "to determine whether invasive prenatal diagnosis tests are necessary."[18] What is meant by necessary? Analysis of this leads to the conclusion that earlier identification is done to make selective abortion more feasible.

While paying lip service to the choice being the woman's, the SOGC guidelines indicate that "screening programs should aim to provide a screen that at a minimum, offers women who present in first trimester a DR [detection rate] of Down syndrome of 75 per cent..."[19] The guidelines seek to have as many affected fetuses as possible identified but there is no mention of support for other outcomes. "Screening programs should show respect for the needs and quality of life of persons with disabilities. Counselling should be nondirective and should respect a woman's choice to accept or to refuse any or all of the testing or options offered at any point in the process."[20] And yet anecdotal evidence suggests that women who decline to terminate a disabled fetus are not provided with support or encouragement.

Doctors fear the potential legal ramifications if testing is not offered. In an article on the impact of the new Canadian guidelines on wrongful birth litigation, Pioro and colleagues conclude that "In Canada wrongful birth claims may increase if clinicians do not practice according to the new standard of care prescribed in the 2007 clinical practice guidelines on prenatal screening."[21] It is their legal opinion that there is liability if a physician does not offer prenatal screening and the child is born with a disabling condition "that could have been predetermined." The awareness of this liability may lead physicians to positively encourage screening rather than neutrally offering it as an option. At the same time there appear to be irreconcilable tensions between the physicians' obligation of respect for reproductive choice and the rights of disabled persons since "wrongful birth claims reinforce that view that the birth of a child with a disability is a harm for which one may be compensated."[22] If misinformation or the lack of complete, unbiased information leads to a decision to abort, there is little chance for a woman to take legal action if she later realizes that she would

---

18	Summers AM, Langlois S, Wyatt P and Wilson RD. See n. 10.
19	Ibid.
20	Ibid.
21	Pioro, Roxanne and Nisker. See n. 12, p. 1029.
22	Ibid., p. 1029.

have made a different decision with informed consent.

In a study of parents of disabled children and their response to technology in future pregnancy Kelly found that when it came to the use of

> ...reproductive technologies, the goal of which is to avoid the birth of an affected child, the majority of this sample of parents acted in ways that tended to remove them from the context of technologically imposed decision making and risk analysis.[23]

She went on to note that most of the parents refused testing in future pregnancies and her "...findings run counter to the rationale of risk reduction technologies of prenatal testing."[24]

There have, in fact, been *no* studies, which evaluate the outcome for mothers who decline screening, but there is nonetheless evidence of social pressure toward testing as an expected requirement of pregnancy. It is known that children are born annually with conditions that have either been a) prenatally detected but the family chose not to abort, or b) the family chose not to submit to the testing. Nordvig and colleagues noted noted that the women who declined screening accounted for only half of the children born with Down syndrome in Denmark after an expanded screening program was implemented.[25] The outcome measure for the Nordvig study considered only the reduction in number of births of children with Down syndrome. Success was defined as eliminating more disabled children from the Danish population. Nonetheless, children with Down syndrome were born both to women who were screened, and to women who declined screening.

Given that ultrasound is increasingly being used to evaluate the risk of fetal abnormalities, Nordvig and colleagues noted that

> the fact that a scan implies, intended or not, that fetal abnormalities might be detected, further implies that parents will have to consider whether to terminate the pregnancy. The ethical dilemma is intensified by the fact that ultrasound not always provides a hundred per cent accurate finding and that the findings sometimes might be difficult

---

23 Kelly SE. Choosing not to choose: reproductive responses of parents of children with genetic conditions or impairments. Sociology of Health and Illness 2009; 31(1): p. 84.
24 Ibid.
25 Nordvig, Secher and Andersen. See Table reference ii, p. 11.

to interpret. However, evidence has shown that ultrasound examinations in low-risk or unselected populations do not benefit mother or child; moreover, as a standard routine, ultrasound might have some drawbacks: increased worry, anxiety, insecurity etc. due to an increase of unclear findings or findings of uncertain clinical significance.[26]

Another study showed that, of the women whose fetuses were found to have an anomaly, 30 per cent expressed regret about their decision to screen[27] and would have preferred not to have screened. When parents who had one child with a disability already were asked whether they would choose to be screened during a subsequent pregnancy, many said no. In the words of one mother,

> If I had went as far as to consider having another child then I would have had it in my mind that no matter what it was, what happened, it would still be my child. Just like with her, I wouldn't have considered [prenatal testing] at all.[28]

Although it is unclear that prenatal screening was developed in response to women's desire for it, the comprehensive screening that is now routinely offered to all pregnant women influences society's perceptions of pregnancy and testing. Suter found that in California, where, as in Canada, they are legally required to *offer* the screening, more than one-third of women interviewed believed or suspected that the state *required* pregnant women to be screened.[29] Women risk being labeled as irresponsible or irrational by their physician and society if they refuse the test.[30] Nearly 30 years ago Katz Rothman wrote about the phenomenon of the "tentative pregnancy,"[31] and the view that a pregnancy must be validated through

---

26 Ibid., p. 11.
27 Green JM, Hewison J, Bekker HL, Bryant LD and Cuckle HS. Psychosocial aspects of genetic screening of pregnant women and newborns: a systematic review. Health Technology 2004; 8(33): iii, ix-x, 1-109.
28 Kelly. See n. 23, p. 89. Parents of children with disabilities need to be made more aware of agencies that are there to help them, such as Morning Light Ministry. See also Zambri B. *Hope in Turmoil*. 3rd ed., Mississauga, 2013 for more information.
29 Suter S. Genetics and the law: the ethical, legal and social implications of genetic technology and biomedical ethics: sex selection, non-directiveness and equality. University of Chicago Law school round table, 1996 473 N 34.
30 Seavilleklein V. Challenging the rhetoric of choice in prenatal screening. Ph.D dissertation. Halifax, NS: Dalhousie University, 2008.
31 Katz Rothman B. *The tentative pregnancy: prenatal diagnosis and the future of motherhood*. New York, NY: Viking, 1996.

prenatal testing before it is accepted. Because abortion is a norm, pregnancy becomes conditional until the child is proven "normal", and parental love moves from being unconditional to conditional.

Many have noted how difficult it is to "determine both what is material and what to disclose to each particular patient"[32] in order to obtain informed consent. While the standard among health care practitioners is to offer prenatal testing in the framework of a woman's autonomy and informed consent, many are questioning whether informed consent is being honoured. In 78 studies, the overwhelming conclusion was that the current procedures are inadequate for achieving informed consent.[33] Challenges in disclosure due to the lack of time that physicians have to explain the test coupled with social and legal pressures that might limit the voluntariness of the decision make informed consent very difficult to achieve. As the genetic counsellor Chris Trevors warns, "the difference is the volume of information you are getting... People look for health care providers to guide them on how to interpret this info, and if we can't, I don't think we should be offering it."[34]

> Much has been written on the complexity around the issues of diagnostic testing and the decision-making paradigm following a result that is positive for a disabling condition. True reproductive autonomy necessarily involves striving for a social context within which parents that choose not to undergo testing, or who choose to raise a child with a disability, would be supported.[35]

Lawson and Pierson note that, from the psychological perspective, the basis of decision making has been a rational-choice model, which has "informed protocols and the majority of investigations into the psychological processes involved in making decisions around prenatal testing and selective abortion."[36] The authors go on to argue that this approach may not be accurate, as the assumptions upon which it is based cannot encompass

---

[32] Polansky S. Overcoming the obstacles: a collaborative approach to informed consent in prenatal screening in Canada. Health Law Journal 2006; 14: 21-44.
[33] Seavilleklein. See n. 30.
[34] Collier R. Prenatal DNA test raises both hopes and worries. CMAJ 2008; 180(7): p. 180.
[35] Lawson KL and Pierson RA. Maternal decisions regarding prenatal diagnosis: rational choices or sensible decisions? JOGC 2007; 29(3): 240-6.
[36] Ibid.

the complexity of socio-medical and psychological implications of prenatal testing and the decision to abort. They suggest that the social context in which a woman lives as well as the societal attitudes towards the disability mean that the "individual pregnant woman is situated within interpersonal relationships (with her partner, her fetus and her physician) that are in turn imbedded within larger societal contexts (social legal and medical norms)."[37]

The influence of the woman's attending physician has been found to be correlated with whether or not prenatal testing is done. Many professionals as well as the literature they provide to women are biased in favour of screening. "There is often a bias toward the positive aspects of testing."[38] Polansky sees this social construction of choice as providing the "illusion of choice."[39]

The social context for decision-making has been expanded by the work of McCoyd, who suggests that "Burden Assessment" be considered as a foundational factor in the choices around selective abortion.[40] This model was adopted from a 1994 instrument used to evaluate the support needs of caregivers who must look after severely mentally ill family members.[41] It has been used by the WHO when considering the impacts of mental illness on families in India and has been translated into Swedish and Spanish. This scale is considered a valid and reliable measure of how individuals feel about the level of care and/or burden the family member places on them. It is based on experiential evidence and taps responsive feelings to those experiences. McCoyd has extrapolated the instrument into the realm of the "perceived burden" that led women to choose abortion following a diagnosis of fetal anomaly.

Some ethicists view the challenges to decision-making around genetic testing as being lodged in the cultural context of testing itself. One of them identified the way in which testing has moved from an option for women to a "need,"[42] as noted in the SOGC Guidelines, while another points out

---

37   Ibid.
38   Seavilleklein. See n. 30.
39   Polansky. See n. 32.
40   McCoyd JL. "I'm not a saint": burden assessment as an unrecognized factor in prenatal decision making. Qualitative Health Research 2008; 18(11): 1489-1500.
41   Reinhard SC. Burden assessment scale for families of the seriously mentally ill. Evaluation and Program Planning 1994; 17(2): 261-9.
42   Lippman A. Prenatal genetic testing and screening: constructing needs and reinforcing inequalities. American Journal of Law and Medicine 1991; 17(1-2): 15-50.

the way in which testing expectations have become "entrenched in cultural assumptions about the role and responsibilities of women and mothers,"[43] and may increase the difficulty women face in refusing screening.

Now that prenatal screening is standard medical practice, women who refuse testing may be seen as not "doing their motherly duty" to ensure the birth of a healthy child. One expert argues that even within the more restricted understanding of autonomy and informed consent, "reproductive autonomy is not being well protected in current prenatal screening practice..."[44] Another questions whether autonomy in decision making is even possible, given the complexity of information and the potential for individual differences in outcome.[45]

One study found that although the risk of conceiving a child with Down syndrome is not affected by socio-economic status, there is a statistically significant difference in birth rates. Women in lower socio-economic occupations were far less likely to seek testing, or to give birth.[46]

This reflects the clear evidence that, along with social and demographic factors, one of the main influences on a woman's decision to abort is the "attitude of the health care professional giving the post-diagnosis counselling."[47] Nordvig reiterates that these professionals "have significant influence upon women's decisions to accept risk assessment and to terminate an affected pregnancy."[48] Medical professionals may be predisposed to certain approaches to counselling. They may subtly promote prenatal testing and abortion out of a belief that patients desire the maximum information. Time constraints, fear of liability, little genetic training, and the habit of directiveness can also lead to a negative tone that medical professionals use when counselling after diagnosis.[49] These

---

43   Seavilleklein. See n. 30.
44   Ibid.
45   Polansky. See n. 32, p. 21.
46   Khoshnood B, De Vigan C, Vodovar V, Breart G, Goffinet F and Blondel B. Advances in medical technology and creation of disparities: the case of down syndrome. American Journal of Public Health 2006; 96(12): 2139-44.
47   Yilmaz Z. Ethical considerations regarding parental decisions for termination following prenatal diagnosis of sex chromosome abnormalities. Journal of Genetic Counselling 2008; 19(3); 345-52.
48   Nordvig, Secher and Andersen. See Table reference ii.
49   Dixon DP. Informed consent or institutionalized eugenics? how the medical profession encourages abortion of fetuses with down syndrome. Issues in Law & Medicine 2008; 24(1): 3-59.

pressures should be addressed in order to ensure proper counselling before and after prenatal testing. It has been determined that between 40 and 80 per cent of parents who are offered the option of perinatal palliative care—a supportive option for parents whose child has been diagnosed with a life-limiting anomaly—request this care and choose to continue their pregnancy.[50] The assurance of care for the duration of their child's life, no matter how long or short it might be, influences parents' confidence in parenting children with a genetic anomaly.

Prenatal Testing—Disability Rights

> Disability rights advocates are right to think of genetic counselling as a search and destroy mission because testing will likely ultimately lead to greater intolerance of disabilities and less money for research or treatment.[51]

There is a growing literature that addresses the ethical implications of prenatal testing from the perspective of disability rights.[52] Many researchers have attempted to construct a rationale that includes sensitivity to the rights of the disabled, but as the example of McCoyd shows, this is difficult to achieve when the clinician's orientation is fundamentally pro-choice: "I, like many, am troubled about the possibility that prenatal diagnosis and termination might act in a eugenic fashion and I advocate for the rights of people who are living with impairments and disabilities and yet...."[53] McCoyd goes on to note her support for women's decisions as well as her own orientation as "strongly pro-choice," while also stating her recognition of "prenatal bonding and mourning for lost pregnancies."[54] These inconsistencies she lodges in her respect for an individual woman's

---

50   Calhoun BC, Napolitano P, Terry M, Bussey C and Hoeldtke NJ. Perinatal hospice: comprehensive care for the family of the fetus with a lethal condition. Journal of Reproductive Medicine 2003; 58(11): 718-19; Breeze ACG, Lees CC, Kumar A, Missfelder-Lobos HH and Murdoch EM. Palliative care for prenatally diagnosed lethal fetal abnormality. Archives of Disease in Childhood; Fetal and Neonatal 2007; 92(1): F56-8.
51   Dixon. See n. 49, p. 21.
52   Shevell. See n. 14; Somerville M. Invited participant and written submission, "Consultation sur le dépistage prénatal du syndrome de down menée par le comissaire à la santé et au bien-être" (consultation on prenatal screening for down syndrome conducted by the commissionner for health and well-being), commissaire à la santé et au bien-être, Ministère de la Santé et des Services Sociaux du Québec, 12th May, 2008, Montréal.
53   McCoyd. See n. 40.
54   Ibid.

right to evaluate factors and choices in her life: "...and so I support fully, whatever informed, deliberative choice an individual makes."[55] As with so many other researchers in prenatal decision-making, she goes on to study women who have aborted, but not those who continued their pregnancy. Once a woman chooses not to be screened, she removes herself from the decision about what to do with a pregnancy that screens positive. From that point, few in the medical or genetic research establishment show interest in her or her child.[56]

North American society has adopted a dual attitude surrounding the question of disabilities. First, supports and services are provided when the following are at play:

- a person becomes disabled by accident

- a person is born with a prenatally undetectable condition such blindness, hearing impairment or cerebral palsy

But secondly, when a child is born with a genetic condition that could have been detected prenatally, the family are often faced with the question, "Didn't you know about prenatal testing?"[57] This exemplifies the concern raised by Dixon.[58] Choosing not to screen is seen as a reflection of ignorance, not nurturance; consequently, families of disabled children begin parenting a baby without emotional or social support for the child's birth. Why is it that so many of the guidelines for genetic counselling are couched in language that respects choice and pays lip service to respect for the disabled, when in reality the impetus is towards termination of an affected fetus and a concomitant lack of acceptance of the mother's decision to continue her pregnancy?

Those with disabilities, and those involved with them, make it clear that the concept is socially constructed, and not based directly upon the nature of the individual's differences. "The premise of the disability rights movement is that persons with disabilities are disadvantaged far more by negative social attitudes than by their disabilities."[59]

---

55   Ibid.
56   Dixon. See n. 49.
57   Friends of ours were asked this by a physician while in hospital after the birth of their child with Down syndrome.
58   Dixon. See n. 49.
59   Ibid.

The Roeher Institute at York University has raised questions about the unfettered use of prenatal testing in their document "Genetics Genie." Among the points they make is the concern that prenatal diagnosis is identified as inherently good and will somehow prevent human suffering. This judgment is dependent on a characterization of disability as something that universally causes suffering and distress, and that suffering is inherently bad.

> Advocates for persons who are differently abled stress that the wholesale elimination of those who are genetically different is in effect "biomedical elimination of diversity...based on market forces and the setting of norms and standards by non-disabled people.[60]

The Canadian Association for Community Living, Canada's largest federation supporting people with intellectual disabilities, comments as follows on the danger of the pressures around prenatal testing:

> The active devaluation of the lives of persons with disabilities is a disturbing trend. Misinformation about disability is a real concern for individuals and families who live with disability. The lack of public discussion about the impact of devaluation makes people with disabilities and their families extremely vulnerable… The increased demand for prenatal testing and the pressure prospective parents experience to terminate when an "anomaly" is detected risks leading us down a dangerous road reminiscent of our eugenic past.[61]

Germany, because of the nightmare of Nazism, is a nation that has suffered the effects of a eugenic mentality more severely than most. German ethics institutes warn of unrealistic notions of disability that are leading parents and physicians to favour termination after a genetic anomaly is detected.

> Should indications of a possible disability of the unborn children be found, the pregnancy will most of the time be broken off.... Mostly unrealistic ideas play a crucial role over the life with a

---

60   Crawford C. The genetics genie. Abilities Magazine. 2002-2003. Roeher Institute.
61   Canadian Association for Community Living. Family's heartbreaking plight sheds light on deeper issues. Press Release. April 9 2009.

disability child both with future parents and the physician.⁶²

Those who advocate for the disabled are concerned that the decisions after prenatal testing are often informed only by confusing medical results. They are often ill-informed about the holistic nature of the possible conditions and outcomes for the child that the tests indicate. Many have expressed disappointment that the information provided stresses only the negative aspects of having a child with such a condition. Little emphasis is placed on the possible benefits of a disabled child to the family.

Another little-noticed reality is that prenatal diagnosis is not always accurate. One of the authors knows of at least two women whose unborn children were diagnosed with Down syndrome. Ignoring the advice to terminate, they carried through with their pregnancies, and to their amazement delivered perfectly normal babies. One can only wonder at how many normal babies have been aborted because of a faulty diagnosis.

The experience of parents receiving prenatal diagnosis has received little research attention. One study of mothers who have a child with Down syndrome focused on the prenatal testing experiences. The mothers reported that they were scared and anxious after receiving the positive test results. Their physician had not adequately explained Down syndrome to them before or after the test. In fact, most mothers reported receiving misinformation or were directed toward a termination of pregnancy. The range of ability that their child might have was not discussed, and many reported insensitive language used by the counselling physician.⁶³ "Prospective parents tend to be told negative things ... like 'this child will ruin your life ... it will be hard on your life, hard on your kids, ruin your marriage'" reiterates Krista Flint of the Canadian Down Syndrome Society. "You don't hear about those who enrich the lives of others, who go to school, get married, get jobs."⁶⁴

Professionals within the disability community have spoken out

---

62   IMEW (institute mensch, ethik & wissenschaft). http://www.imew.de/index.php?id=513.. Retrieved July 23, 2009.
63   Skotko BG. Prenatally diagnosed down syndrome: mothers who continued their pregnancies evaluate their health care providers. AJOG 2005; 192(3): 670-7.
64   Abraham C. Simple test, complex questions. *Globe and Mail*. Toronto, February 7, 2009. http://www.theglobeandmail.com/news/national/simple-test-complex-questions/article1148236/?page=all.

about the lack of reality in viewing individuals with such conditions.[65] Yet Bromage identifies wide acceptance of selective abortion as a shift in attitudes to a postmodern "pursuit of aesthetic perfection."[66] This is a perspective shared equally by prospective parents and medical professionals. Thus maternity care organizations in North America now apparently favour phasing out maternal-age-based prenatal screening and replacing it with universal prenatal screening. Why? Because informed choice is of paramount importance to women and should be part of any change. Health care providers need to be engaged in and educated about any change to screening guidelines to offer women informed choices.[67]

Psychological Impact of Decisions Following Testing

Despite the shock and grief that many experience upon hearing the news of a fetal anomaly, the pregnant woman and her partner are usually urged to make the decision to terminate.[68] Very little time is allowed for couples to become informed about parenting children born with an anomaly and to consider carrying through with the pregnancy. This is in part due to the reluctance of most physicians to terminate a pregnancy after the age of viability—23.5 weeks.

One risk that may not be adequately disclosed to parents when they choose to undergo prenatal diagnosis is the potential for psychological distress following their decisions. As previously noted, 30 per cent of parents who received positive test results regretted their decision to screen.[69] In addition, while for many the termination of pregnancy is an attempt to eliminate suffering, it has been determined that 40 per cent of women who abort for fetal abnormality suffer long-term emotional distress. Nor does the distress diminish over time. A psychiatrist writes that

> women two to seven years after were expected to show a

---

65   Saxton M. Disability rights and selective abortion. In *Abortion wars: a half century of struggle: 1950 to 2000*. Ed., Rickie Solinger. Berkeley, CA: University of California Press, 1998.
66   Bromage DI. Prenatal diagnosis and selective abortion: a result of a cultural turn? Medical Humanities 2006; 32: 38-42.
67   Carroll JC. Maternal age-based prenatal screening for chromosomal disorders—attitudes of women and health care providers towards changes. Canadian Family Physician 2013; 59(1): e39-47.
68   Ring-Cassidy E and Gentles I. *Women's health after abortion: the medical and psychological evidence*. 2nd edition. deVeber Institute for Bioethics and Social Research. Toronto, 2003: p. 166.
69   Green. See n. 27.

significantly lower degree of traumatic experience and grief than women fourteen days after termination ...Contrary to hypothesis, however, the results showed no significant intergroup differences.[70]

Another study found that 44 per cent of women had post-traumatic stress symptoms, and 28 per cent had symptoms of depression after terminating for fetal anomaly.[71] Some women continue to grieve for years after terminating their pregnancy on account of fetal abnormalities. Their depression and grief can sometimes become too much to bear. After termination of pregnancy the rate of suicide increases for women, while suicides actually decrease for women who carry a child to term.[72] Others who, had they known in advance, might have decided to terminate, later changed their mind after the child arrived. One commented that if he and his wife had had prenatal testing, they would have terminated. "I know there would be no Sydney, and that tears me apart now. She's a wonderful, joyous child."[73]

The rationalization often given for termination after prenatal testing is "maternal necessity": that a fetal abnormality will "jeopardize her [a mother's] own health and future fertility."[74] However, while carrying a child with a disability might greatly influence a mother's psychological health, her physical health might not be affected. The very real risks to maternal psychological health have been discussed. Maternal physical health is sometimes cited,[75] but there is no supporting scientific evidence provided that usual fetal abnormalities for which abortions are requested,[76] such as Down syndrome and cleft palate have any deleterious physical health effects on the mother.

70 Kersting A. Trauma and grief 2-7 years after termination of pregnancy because of fetal abnormalities. Journal of Psychosomatic Obstetrics and Gynaecology 2005; 26(1): 9-14.
71 Korenromp, et al. See n. 1.
72 Gissler M, Berg C and Bouvier-Colle M. Injury deaths, suicides, and homicides associated with pregnancy, Finland 1987-2000. European Journal of Public Health 2004; 15(5): 459-63.
73 Shaw M. Airbrushing away diversity. Ottawa Citizen, March 2, 2008. http://www.canada.com/ottawacitizen/news/story.html?id=7ef9c418-70c1-49cc-bbbf-cb1ae997b326?.
74 Jackson-Lee S. Partial birth abortion ban act of 1997. Text from the Congressional Record. 1997. Page H8654. http://www.c-spanarchives.org/congress/?q=node/77531&id=6761323.
75 United Nations Population Division Department of Economic and Social Affairs. Abortion policies: a global review. http://www.un.org/esa/population/publications/abortion/doc/italy.doc.
76 Medical Practitioners Board of Victoria. Report on late-term terminations of pregnancy, April 1988. 1998. Acute Health Division, Department of Human Services. Victoria, Australia. http://www.dhs.vic.gov.au/ahs/archive/report/report7.htm.

A report on late-term abortions from the Medical Practitioner's Board of Victoria, Australia states, that, "there are a very small number of fetal conditions where the progression of the pregnancy may lead to significant maternal morbidity or mortality. These conditions are rare."[77] Only 56 cases of Mirror syndrome, a condition that might develop in a mother pregnant with a fetus who has certain genetic conditions, have been published since 1956.[78] Even these rare conditions have available treatments for the mother, with high success rates.

De Crespigny and Savulescu found that "the current practice often appears to depend primarily on the doctor's subjective assessment of the severity of the abnormality."[79] Given that physicians have significant influence when consulted by parents after the detection of fetal abnormality, it is a matter of professional responsibility for a physician not to make claims that have no supporting scientific evidence, such as recommending an abortion to preserve mother's physical health from the effects of a fetal abnormality when no relation between the two has been documented.

Conclusion: for the Betterment of Women

The rapid expansion of prenatal genetic testing has increased the amount of available medical information about a child before birth. However, this information is both complex and overwhelming. There is no ethical framework within which these results can be placed; consequently, families are dependent on the capacities of their attending physician or counsellor to interpret the myriad data and the implications surrounding the decisions that must be made. Prenatal diagnosis has brought to the physician's office increasing challenges in obtaining a fully informed consent, and in respecting a woman's autonomy while giving appropriate support and information. These new technologies have raised important questions about the value of disabled people in society, and the way that we care for the disabled. Diagnostic capabilities have far surpassed our ability to improve the lives of people with genetic conditions. The use of prenatal testing to diagnose and eliminate individuals with certain genetic

---

77   Ibid.
78   Braun T, Brauer M, Fuchs I, Czernik C, Dudenhausen JW, Henrich W and Sarioglu N. Mirror syndrome: a systematic review of fetal associated conditions, maternal presentation and perinatal outcome. Fetal Diagnosis and Therapy 2010; 27: 191-203.
79   De Crespigny L and Savulescu J. Is paternalism alive and well in obstetric ultrasound? Helping couples choose their children. Ultrasound in Obstetrics & Gynecology 2002; 20(3): 213-16.

conditions is eugenics.

Additionally, many women are not fully informed of the risk of psychological distress after terminating a pregnancy. Many could be saved the trauma of abortion if made more aware of their options. The "Prenatally and Postnatally Diagnosed Conditions Awareness Act" (S. 1810) that passed in the United States on October 8th, 2008 "is a positive step" toward ensuring that parents are provided with accurate information from appropriate sources about the conditions that may be detected through prenatal diagnosis.[80] More coordinated efforts to communicate the full range of knowledge about the genetic information to which we now have access, and increasing awareness about, and access to, options for improving the lives of the disabled and their families in society, may help to ensure that new prenatal genetic diagnosis technologies are used for the betterment of women, children and society.

---

80   The prenatally and postnatally diagnosed conditions awareness act. http://dredf.org/InfoSheetBrownbackKennedy.pdf.

Chapter 9

Physical complications: Infection and infertility

KEY POINTS

- Women who undergo an induced abortion later suffer a higher rate of Pelvic Inflammatory Disease (PID) than the general population.

- A risk factor for PID is pre-existing infection, one of the most common associated with PID and induced abortion being chlamydia trachomatis.

- In an attempt to prevent infection, antibiotics are commonly administered to women undergoing an induced abortion, but they are not always effective.

- The well-documented sequelae of PID include chronic pelvic pain, subfertility, infertility and ectopic pregnancy; other sequelae include intraamniotic infection, neonatal sepsis, and stillbirth.

- Although research on induced abortion and infertility is limited, there is evidence of a link between the two. A recent study from England documents a 620 per cent increase in subfecundity among women who terminated their pregnancies.

- There is a clear connection between PID and tubal disease, and between tubal disease and subfertility and infertility.

- PID is the most common cause of ectopic pregnancy, and there is accumulating evidence linking ectopic pregnancy to previous induced abortion—both surgical and medical.

- Sequelae of ectopic pregnancy include recurrent ectopic pregnancy, infertility and pregnancy-related death.

Pelvic Inflammatory Disease

Pelvic Inflammatory Disease (PID) is a general term used for an infection of the uterus lining (endometritis), of the uterine fallopian tubes (salpingitis), or of the ovaries. PID occurs when bacteria from the vagina or cervix moves up into the uterus, uterine tubes, or ovaries. "Pelvic inflammatory disease is an important consequence of both STIs [sexually-transmitted infections] and medical procedures that breach the cervical barrier,"[1] such as induced abortion.

It has been noted that women can contract infection "after surgical or medical abortion secondary to operative injury or retained products of conception (RPOC)," or that infection can come from "preexisting infections such as *Neisseria gonorrhea, chlamydia trachomatis,* and *Trichomonas vaginalis* or bacterial vaginosis (BV),"[2] which move from the lower to upper genital tract during an induced abortion. Mead noted that "infection after abortion is an ascending process, occurring more commonly in the presence of retained products of conception or operative trauma. Perforation of the uterus, with or without bowel injury, may be followed by severe infection."[3] There are also reports of Clostridia sordellii infections after medical abortions, which have resulted in fatalities of young and healthy women.[4]

Many different rates of infection following an abortion have been documented. A British study reported a range of five to ten per cent.[5] The Royal College of Obstetricians and Gynaecologists (RCOG) guidelines report a high risk of genital tract infection, including pelvic inflammatory disease, in up to ten per cent of cases of induced abortion.[6] It is difficult to arrive at a precise rate of infection following abortion because the definition of infection varies from one study to another, and from one country to another. American clinical guidelines report an infection rate of only 0.01 to 2.44 per cent.[7]

---

1 Dayan L. Pelvic inflammatory disease. Australian Family Physician 2006; 35(11): p. 861.
2 Rahangdale L. Infectious complications of pregnancy termination. Clinical Obstetrics and Gynecology 2009; 52(2): 198-204, p. 198.
3 Mead PB, Hager WD and Faro S, eds. *Protocols for infectious diseases in obstetrics and gynecology*, 2nd ed. Malden, MA: Blackwell Science, 2000: p. 124.
4 Lipworth, Katsouyani, Ekbom, et al. See Chapter 7, n. 34.
5 Penney GC, Thomson M, Norman J, et al. A randomised comparison of strategies for reducing infective complications of induced abortion. BJOG 1998; 105(6): 599-604.
6 Royal College of Obstetricians and Gynaecologists. *The care of women requesting induced abortion. Evidence-Based Clinical Guideline 7*, 2011: p. 42.
7 Achilles and Reeves. See Chapter 6, n. 57.

Risk factors: Pre-existing infection

"Many post-abortal infections occur in women without any identifiable risk factors apart from the abortion procedure."[8] However, cervical or vaginal infections—chlamydia trachomatis, Neisseria gonorrhea, Trichomonas vaginalis, and bacterial vaginosis (BV)—that are already present at the time of an induced abortion are known to be a significant risk factor.[9] Mycoplasma genitalium is another bacterium that has recently been shown to be associated with PID after induced abortion.[10]

The most common known pathogens that cause PID are chlamydia and Gonorrhea. One quarter of PID patients are identified as having chlamydia trachomatis.[11] A significant number of the women presenting for abortion have one of these infections.[12] Those women who have an STI and who undergo abortion are then at a greater risk of developing PID. One study found 22 out of 557 patients developed acute pelvic inflammatory disease after induced abortion. Of those 22 women, fourteen (63.6 per cent) had chlamydia trachomatis in their cervix before the procedure while eight (36.4 per cent) did not.[13] Another study examined women with chlamydia trachomatis or Neisseria gonorrhoea who had an induced abortion and found that "[c]linical signs of post-TOP [termination of pregnancy] pelvic inflammation developed in seven (28 per cent) women with chlamydial infection."[14]

---

8 Ibid., p. 299.
9 Lawton BA, Rose SB, Bromhead C, Gaitanos LA, MacDonald EJ and Lund KA. High prevalence of *mycoplasma genitalium* in women presenting for termination of pregnancy. Contraception 2008; 77(4): pp. 294-8.
10 Bjartling C, Osser S and Persson K. The association between *mycoplasma genitalium* and pelvic inflammatory disease after termination of pregnancy. BJOG: An International Journal of Obstetrics & Gynaecology 2010; 117(3): pp. 361-4.
11 Taylor BD and Hagger CL. Management of chlamydia trachomatis genital tract infection: screening and treatment challenges. Infection and Drug Resistance 2011; 4: 19-29.
12 Chen SM, van den Hoek A, Shao CG, et al. Prevalence of and risk factors for STIs among women seeking induced abortions in two urban family planning clinics in Shandong province, People's Republic of China. Sexually Transmitted Infections 2002; 78(3): e1-e3; Zhang RJ, Zhang XJ, Lu XJ, et al. Study on the correlation between induced abortion and reproductive tract infections. Zhonghua Liu Xing Bing Xue Za Zhi 2011; 32(1): 29-32.
13 Qvigstad E, Skaug K, Jerve F, Fylling P and Ulstrup JC. Pelvic inflammatory disease associated with chlamydia trachomatis infection after therapeutic abortion: a prospective study. British Journal of Venereal Diseases 1983; 59(3): pp. 189-92.
14 Smith CD, Carlin EM, Heason J, Liu TY, Jushuf IA and Hammond RH. Genital infection and termination of pregnancy: are patients still at risk? The Journal of Family Planning and Reproductive Health Care 2001; 27(2): p. 81.

Having an abortion dramatically increases the risk of developing PID for women who have chlamydia. Chen and colleagues derived probabilities from Blackwell's work,[15] and estimated that 30 per cent of women who have chlamydia will develop PID, of which 40 per cent will have been asymptomatic. Among women who have chlamydia and then have an induced abortion, the chance of developing PID doubles to 63 per cent.[16] An analysis of nine prospective studies showed overall that among women with a chlamydia trachomatis infection, those who underwent legal abortion had the highest rate of developing PID, ranging from 27 to 72 per cent.[17]

OTHER RISK FACTORS FOR ABORTION-RELATED PID

Heisterberg and colleagues provided evidence for an increased rate of complications in women who had never borne a child.[18] Nielsen has identified the risk factors for PID as: previous PID incident, no previously borne children, and a previous induced abortion.[19] Levallois and colleagues found that in a sample of Quebec women attending for abortion at Laval University Hospital those patients who were repeat abortion seekers and who had never been pregnant but had multiple sex partners developed pelvic infection nearly three times more frequently than others not having these characteristics.[20]

The evidence suggests that single, sexually active, never previously-pregnant young women are the most likely to suffer from PID following an induced abortion. An incident of PID in adolescence may mean that the woman will never achieve a successful pregnancy.

---

15   Blackwell AL, Thomas PD, Wareham K and Emery SJ. Health gains from screening for infection of the lower genital tract in women attending for termination of pregnancy. The Lancet 1993; 342(8865): pp. 206-10.
16   Chen S, Li J, and Van den Hoek A. Universal screening or prophylactic treatment for chlamydia trachomatis infection among women seeking induced abortions: which strategy is more cost-effective? Sexually Transmitted Diseases 2007; 34(4): 230-6.
17   Boeke AJ, van Bergen JE, Morre SA and van Everdingen JJ. The risk of pelvic inflammatory disease associated with urogenital infection with chlamydia trachomatis; literature review. Nederlands Tijdschrift voor Geneeskunde 2005; 149(15): 878-84.
18   Heisterberg L and Kringelbach M. Early complications after induced first-trimester abortion. Acta Obstetricia et Gynecologica Scandanavica 1987; 66(3): 201-4, p. 204.
19   Nielsen IK, Engdahl E, Larsen T. [Pelvic inflammation after induced abortion] Danish. Ugeskr Laeger 1992 September 28; 154(40): 2743-6.
20   Levallois P and Rioux JE. Prophylactic antibiotics for suction curettage abortion: results of a clinical controlled trial. AJOG 1988; 158(1): 100-5.

LACK OF FOLLOW-UP

As with other research on induced abortion, determining the rate of infection is confounded by lack of appropriate and timely follow up. Delay in the onset of symptoms is a critical factor when considering PID caused by chlamydia following abortion. Blackwell and colleagues found from their patient records that women continued to develop symptoms at eleven weeks, 24 weeks, and 36 weeks post-abortion.[21] Osser and Persson found the delay to be variable: If the woman was positive for chlamydia before the abortion, the time of onset for salpingitis (infection of the fallopian tubes) was 14.1 days and for endometritis (infection of the uterus) 8.2 days. As they report, "chlamydia-associated infections were diagnosed on the average three to ten days later than cases without chlamydia."[22] Such complications would not be identified by abortion clinics as immediate sequelae, or coded as being related to an abortion at all.

A recent study of women who screened positive for chlamydia at the time of an induced abortion in the UK showed that only 47.7 per cent of women attended follow-up.[23] Furthermore, Chen estimated that of women who have PID, the majority will be treated as outpatients, with merely fourteen per cent being hospitalized. Thus, their infections would not easily be traced back to the induced abortion.[24]

PREVENTION OF PELVIC INFLAMMATORY DISEASE AND CHLAMYDIA

There has been a growing literature discussing the efficacy of pre-abortion testing and treatment for chlamydia. Sawaya and colleagues report that, based on their meta-analysis, there is "a substantial protective effect of antibiotics in all subgroups of women undergoing therapeutic abortion, even women in low-risk groups."[25] At the same time, the European research suggests that a single antibiotic dose before abortion has little protective

---

21   Blackwell et al. See n. 15.
22   Osser S and Persson K. Postabortal pelvic infection associated with chlamydia trachomatis and the influence of humoral immunity. AJOG 1984; 150(6): p. 703.
23   Ayuk PT, Dudley S, McShane H, Rees M and Mackenzie IZ. Efficacy of follow up and contact tracing of women who test positive for genital tract chlamydia trachomatis prior to pregnancy termination. Journal of Obstetrics and Gynaecology 2004; 24(6): pp. 687-9.
24   Chen et al. See n. 16
25   Sawaya GF, Grady D, Kerlikowske K and Grimes DA. Antibiotics at the time of induced abortion: the case for universal prophylaxis based on a meta-analysis. Obstetrics & Gynecology 1996; 87(5 Part 2): p. 884.

effect and may not decrease post-abortion PID. Because the onset can occur any time up to nine months following the procedure, pretesting and aggressive antibiotic therapy for those infected is necessary to prevent its development.

Blackwell and colleagues utilize a ten-day regime of antibiotics, but recognize the limitation discussed by Brewer and problems with post-abortion compliance: "...although all were given a five-day course of prophylactic oxytetracycline (antibiotic), many left their tablets behind. Most women feel well after abortion. Others may not want to be reminded of it."[26]

Women with chlamydia have an increased risk of PID whether or not antibiotics are given. Some studies have shown that antibiotics do lower the risk, but often the difference is not statistically significant.[27] In fact, prophylactic antibiotics may not even protect against the majority of infections. Antibiotic prophylaxis became routine for surgical abortions in Planned Parenthood clinics in the United States in 2006, and for medical abortions in 2007. A study comparing three different regimens of antibiotic prophylaxis for women undergoing first-trimester surgical abortion revealed postoperative infection rates of 2.5 per cent, 7.1 per cent and 10.5 per cent.[28] Yet the risk of infection was reduced more by the change in procedure than by the addition of antibiotics.

The Society of Family Planning is now recommending that rather than being screened for STIs, all women undergoing surgical abortion should

---

26   Brewer C. Prevention of post-abortion infection. The Lancet 1993; 342(8874): p. 802.
27   Achilles and Reeves. See Chapter 6, n. 57. This review of 14 studies of antibiotic prophylaxis to prevent post-abortion infection reported that the difference was not statistically significant in 8 of the studies.
28   Caruso S, Di Mari L, Cacciatore A, et al. Antibiotic prophylaxis with prulifloxacin in women undergoing induced abortion: a randomized controlled trial. Minerva Ginecologica 2008; 60(1): 1-5. Among women with bacterial vaginosis at the time of their abortion, sixteen per cent who were not treated developed PID, while 8.5 per cent of those treated with metranidazole developed PID; Crowley T, Low N, Turner A, Harvey I, Bidgood K and Horner P. Antibiotic prophylaxis to prevent post-abortal upper genital tract infection in women with bacterial vaginosis: randomised controlled trial. International Journal of Obstetrics and Gynaecology 2001; 108(4): p. 402. After switching from vaginal to buccal administration of misoprostol for medical abortion, the rate of serious infection dropped from 0.93 to 0.25 per 1000 medical abortions. Antibiotic prophylaxis further reduced the rate of infection to 0.06/1000. Fjerstad M, Trussell J, Sivin I, Lichtenberg ES and Cullins V. Rates of serious infection after changes in regimens for medical abortion. NEJM 2009; 361(2): 145-51.

simply be treated with antibiotics.[29] Although this will undoubtedly provide some protective effect against PID, it carries a greater risk of the woman being re-infected by her partner if she has not been screened for STIs. In addition, there are known side effects to the antibiotics, as well as adverse reactions, and increased bacterial resistance to the antibiotics throughout the population.

SEQUELAE OF INFECTION

Levallois and colleagues report that "Pelvic infection is the most common complication of curettage abortion. Although the rate of post-abortal infections is low, it is of public concern for two reasons: First, abortion is a procedure commonly performed on young women; second, pelvic infection can lead to serious sequelae."[30] Sorensen and colleagues conclude that "[p]elvic inflammatory disease is the most frequent complication after induced abortion...." Contradicting Lavallois and colleagues, they refer to "...the high incidence of post-abortal PID, with potential long-term risks of chronic pelvic pain, dyspareunia, subfertililty and ectopic pregnancy."[31] The RCOG guidelines also point to the far-reaching consequences of infection: "Post-abortion infection may later result in tubal infertility or ectopic pregnancy as well as causing morbidity in the immediate post-abortion period."[32]

Chen estimated that eighteen per cent of women with PID will develop chronic pelvic pain, eight per cent will experience an ectopic pregnancy, and twelve per cent will be infertile.[33] Dayan reported similar risks for long term morbidity following PID: twenty per cent will develop tubal factor infertility, twenty per cent will develop chronic pelvic pain, and ten per cent will experience an ectopic pregnancy. This is a seven to ten times increase in the normal risk of ectopic pregnancy, and with each repeated episode of PID the risk of tubal damage and infertility increases by four to six times.[34] Women who did not have their PID treated immediately are

---

29   Achilles and Reeves. See Chapter 6, n. 57.
30   Levallois and Rioux. See n. 20, p. 100.
31   Sorensen JL, Thranov I, Hoff G, Dirach J and Damsgaard MT. A doubleblind randomized study of the effect of erythromycin in preventing pelvic inflammatory disease after first-trimester abortion. BJOG 1992; 99(5): p. 436.
32   Royal College of Obstetricians and Gynaecologists. See n. 6.
33   Chen, et al. See n. 16.
34   Dayan. See n. 1, pp. 858-62.

three times more likely to experience infertility or ectopic pregnancy,[35] so the consequences may be graver than previously thought.

INFERTILITY: LIMITATIONS TO ITS RESEARCH

Infertility is diagnosed variably between studies, as being unable to conceive after six months, a year or even two years of unprotected sex.[36] Research suggests that infertility affects seven per cent of couples, which translates into half a million people in Canada and 6.1 million in the United States.[37]

Research on abortion and subsequent infertility is limited by the inability to find an appropriate control group; thus studies have shown either that induced abortion increases the risk of infertility, or that is has no effect.[38] Case control and cohort studies compare women who experience infertility to women giving birth, or the time prior to a woman's subsequent pregnancy is measured, but these are inadequate. Results of studies have also been changed in an attempt to eliminate recall bias, but, as we shall see, this may in fact have introduced bias if the women had actually experienced abortions.

The sample of women experiencing infertility is often composed of women who visit infertility clinics. Only a quarter of those who experience infertility will be treated for it so the number of women experiencing negative sequelae of PID is underreported in the literature. Those who do not seek to become pregnant again after an induced abortion, or who do not seek medical treatment for infertility such as IVF (*in vitro* fertilization), may never know about their infertility or subfertility. The figures in the post-abortion literature, therefore, should be understood as representing the minimum of women who are infertile following abortion rather than the total percentage.

What is particularly interesting about the research from one study

---

35   95 per cent CI 1.27-6.11; Hillis SD, Joesoef R, Marchbanks PA, Wasserheit JN, Cates W Jr and Westrom L. Delayed care of pelvic inflammatory disease as a risk factor for impaired fertility. AJOG 1993; 168(5): 1503-9.
36   Norris S. Reproductive infertility: prevalence, causes, trends and treatments. Parliamentary Research Branch: In Brief, 2 January 2001: 1-4.
37   Ibid.
38   Thorp Jr. JM, Hartmann KE and Shadigan E. Long-term physical and psychological health consequences of induced abortion: review of the evidence. Obstetrical and Gynecological Survey 2002; 58(1): 67-79.

of infertility among women presenting for IVF treatment is the public admission that informing a woman of possible infertility before abortion is socially constructed and not part of medical information necessary for proper informed consent. In a most striking way the authors then go on to identify when and for whom it is appropriate to warn about possible future infertility: It is appropriate to tell a women when "the pregnancy timing is not quite right." However, it is inappropriate to tell "a young woman not able to contemplate forming a family with the child's father."[39]

PID AND TUBAL PATHOLOGY

The connection between PID and infertility is well known. Women with a history of pelvic inflammatory disease are at significantly increased risk of infertility.[40] In fact, ten to fifteen per cent of women who get PID may become infertile as a result.[41] One way that PID decreases a woman's fertility is through tubal disease, and a strong association was found between women with previous PID and current tubal disease in a meta-analysis of cohort studies and of case-control studies.[42] The link between tubal pathology and infertility or subfertility is also well documented. It is estimated that ten to 30 per cent of subfertility is due to tuboperitoneal factors.[43] The number of women experiencing a tubal problem is underestimated, as a woman could remain fertile with only one functioning uterine tube. Thus, women experiencing infertility and investigated for tubal pathology remain only a fraction of the number of women for whom one or both uterine tubes might have been compromised.

ABORTION AND INFERTILITY

One study found that tubal pathology is 60 per cent more likely after an induced abortion,[44] and a meta-analysis of three case-control studies

---

39   Hemminki E, Klemetti R, Sevon T and Gissler M. Induced abortions previous to IVF: an epidemiologic register-based study from Finland. Human Reproduction 2008; 23(6): p. 1322.
40   OR 15.76, 95 per cent CI 5.48-45.39; Torres-Sanchez L, Lopez-Carrillo L, Espinoza H and Langer A. Is induced abortion a contributing factor to tubal infertility in Mexico? Evidence from a case-control study. International Journal of Obstetrics and Gynaecology 2004; 111(11): 1254-60.
41   Centers for Disease Control and Prevention. Pelvic inflammatory disease (PID) - CDC fact sheet. 2011. 14 June 2012. http://www.cdc.gov/std/pid/stdfact-pid.htm.
42   OR 3.2, 95 per cent CI 1.6-6.6 and OR 5.5, 95 per cent CI 2.7-11.0, respectively; Luttjeboer FY, Verhoeve HR, van Dessel HJ, van der Veen F, Mol BWJ and Coppus SFPJ. The value of medical history taking as risk indicator for tuboperitoneal pathology: a systematic review. International Journal of Obstetrics and Gynaecology 2009; 116(5): 612-25.
43   Ibid.
44   OR 1.6, 95 per cent CI 1.3-1.9; Verhoeve HR, Steures P, Flierman PA, van der Veen F and Mol BW. History of induced abortion and the risk of tubal pathology. Reproductive BioMedicine Online 2008; 16(2): pp. 304-7.

showed a statistically significant 70 per cent increased risk of subsequent tubal pathology after induced abortion.[45] The authors of a recent study revealing a significant association between prior induced abortion and infertility[46] noted the increased risk of PID after induced abortion might be an explanation for the increase in infertility.[47] A study from Shanghai noted a significant association between infertility and prior induced abortion.[48] A Greek study showed induced abortion as an independent and significant risk factor for secondary infertility, with the risk increasing with the number of abortions.[49]

A study evaluating the risk of tubal infertility after abortion found a significant increased risk.[50] However, they reported no significant association after dropping four women from the analysis, merely because the women believed that induced abortion was associated with their infertility. This adjustment was said to have been made in order to eliminate recall bias, but that assumes that the women had not in fact had abortions. If the women actually had the abortions they said they had, then in reality it was the researchers who introduced bias into their study by dropping the women from it. It may be significant that a study on Greek women regarding induced abortion and breast cancer risk showed that Greek women did not have recall bias, supposedly because induced abortion was socially acceptable.[51]

An English study analyzed fecundity by "time to pregnancy". It compared fecundity *before* the pregnancy that was terminated with the "time to pregnancy" before the next birth. What emerged was a significant correlation between prior induced abortion and sub-fecundity.[52] The study of 2983 women revealed that those who aborted their pregnancies actually had *higher* than average fecundity before their abortions. But afterwards there was a "genuine reduction in the formerly high pregnancy of those who undergo termination of pregnancy." Buried in the findings is the

---

45 OR 1.7, 95 per cent CI 1.3-2.1; Luttjeboer, Verhoeve, van Dessel, et al. See n. 42.
46 OR 1.56, 95 per cent CI 1.03-2.38.
47 Che Y, Zhou W, Gao E and Olsen J. Induced abortion and prematurity in a subsequent pregnancy: a study from Shanghai. Journal of Obstetrics and Gynaecology 2001; 21(3): 270-3.
48 OR 1.56, 95 per cent CI 1.03-2.38; Che, Zhou, Gao and Olsen. See n. 47.
49 RR 2.1, 95 per cent CI 1.1-4.0 after one previous abortion, and RR 2.3, 95 per cent CI 1.0-5.3 after two previous abortions; Tzonou A, Hsieh CC, Trichopoulos D, et al. Induced abortions, miscarriages, and tobacco smoking as risk factors for secondary infertility. Journal of Epidemiology and Community Health 1993; 47(1): 36-9.
50 OR 4.29, 95 per cent CI 1.25-14.64; Torres-Sanchez et al. See n. 40.
51 Lipworth, Katsouyani, Ekbom, et al. See Chapter 7, n. 34.
52 Hassan MAM and Killick SR. Is previous aberrant reproductive outcome predictive of subsequently reduced fecundity? Human Reproduction 2005; 20(3): 657-64.

revelation that *the risk of sub-fecundity increased by no less than 620 per cent after induced abortion.*[53]

A record-linkage study showed a notable proportion, eleven to twelve per cent, of women who received infertility treatment had experienced one or more induced abortions in their history. Most had their abortions more than ten years previous to seeking fertility treatment.[54]

Ectopic Pregnancy

An ectopic pregnancy occurs when an embryo implants outside of the uterine cavity, generally in the fallopian tubes. Two per cent of pregnancies in the United States are ectopic, and six per cent of pregnancy-related deaths in the US are due to ectopic pregnancy. Ectopic pregnancy rates have been increasing in the last twenty years.[55]

Ectopic pregnancy poses a serious risk to women. Between 22 and 34 per cent of ectopic pregnancies rupture by the tenth week of gestation.[56] It is the leading cause of pregnancy-related death, accounting for ten per cent of all pregnancy related deaths.[57] It also reduces a woman's future fertility. Women with ectopic pregnancy have a twenty per cent chance of recurrent ectopic pregnancy, and a twenty to 40 per cent chance of infertility.[58]

PID and Ectopic Pregnancy

Why do induced abortions lead to ectopic pregnancies? Chung and colleagues "showed a highly significant association" between both retained products of conception and pelvic infection following induced abortion and the later occurrence of ectopic pregnancies. They conclude that these two medical complications of abortion lead to a five-fold increase in the rate of ectopic pregnancies.[59] The most common cause of an ectopic pregnancy

---

53   OR 7.2 (p 0.02): Ibid., p. 662.
54   Hemminki et al. See n. 39, pp. 1320-3.
55   Cunningham FG, Leveno KJ, Bloom SL, Hauth JC, Rouse DJ and Spong CY, eds. *Williams obstetrics*, 23rd Ed. New York: McGraw-Hill Companies, 2010.
56   Shannon C, Brothers LP, Philip NM and Winikoff B. Ectopic pregnancy and medical abortion. Obstetrics and Gynecology 2004; 104(1): 161-7.
57   Karaer A, Avsar FA and Batioglu S. Risk factors for ectopic pregnancy: a case-control study. Australian and New Zealand Journal of Obstetrics and Gynaecology 2006; 46(6): 521-7.
58   Tharaux-Deneux C, Bouyer J, Job-Spira N, Coste J and Spira A. Risk of ectopic pregnancy and previous induced abortion. American Journal of Public Health 1998; 88(3): 401-5.
59   Chung CS, Smith RG, Steinhoff PG and Mi MP. Induced abortion and ectopic pregnancy in subsequent pregnancies. American Journal of Epidemiology 1982; 115(6): 879-87.

is pelvic infection.[60] Induced abortions increase the incidence of pelvic infections, which cause scarring within the fallopian tubes. The scar tissue interferes with normal tubal motility or flexibility. As a consequence, the fertilized ovum is entrapped and then implants in the tube. The presence of post-abortion pelvic inflammatory disease is predictive of a greater likelihood of an ectopic pregnancy.

Chen estimates that eight per cent of women who have a PID infection will experience an ectopic pregnancy.[61] As noted above, Dayan reports that ten per cent of women will experience an ectopic pregnancy following PID, a seven- to tenfold increase in the normal risk.[62] Although medical abortion is not considered as great a risk as surgical abortion for developing PID, Bouyer and colleagues hypothesized that the increase in ectopic pregnancy subsequent to medical abortion could be attributed to the fact that most women undergoing surgical abortion were routinely treated with antibiotic prophylaxis to prevent PID, whereas such prophylaxis was not routine among women undergoing medical abortion.[63]

ECTOPIC PREGNANCY AND ABORTION

Evidence linking ectopic pregnancy to previous induced abortion is overwhelming. One study showed 50.5 per cent of women with ectopic pregnancy had previous induced abortions, while only 6.3 per cent of controls had a previous abortion.[64] Another study found an odds ratio of 2.0 for ectopic pregnancy following induced abortion—in other words double the risk of ectopic pregnancy after an induced abortion.[65] The largest recent study, a case-control study from France, included 803 cases and 1683 controls. It showed a significant association between medically-induced abortion and subsequent ectopic pregnancy.[66] This risk was tripled if a woman had undergone both surgical and medical abortion, as

---

60   Tenore J. Ectopic pregnancy. American Family Physician 2000; 61(4): 1080-8.
61   Chen et al. See n. 16, pp. 230-6.
62   Dayan. See n. 1, pp. 858-62.
63   Bouyer J, Coste J, Shojael T, Pouly JL, Fernandez J, Gerbaud L and Job-Spira N. Risk factors for ectopic pregnancy: a comprehensive analysis based on a large case-control, population-based study in France. American Journal of Epidemiology 2003; 157(3): 185-94.
64   Smith C, Bush J and Sutija VG. Adverse obstetric history and ectopic pregnancy. Journal of Reproductive Medicine 2007; 52(9): 801-4.
65   Fernandez H and Gervaise A. Ectopic pregnancies after infertility treatment: modern diagnosis and therapeutic strategy. Human Reproduction Update 2004; 10(6): 503-13.
66   OR 2.8, 95 per cent CI 1.1-7.2. Bouyer et al. See n. 63.

occurs when a medical abortion fails[67] (See also Chapter 13). In addition, a study from India found that women with prior abortions had a more than six times greater rate of ectopic pregnancy than women with no history of induced abortion. The authors concluded that their study "clearly demonstrates the adverse effects of induced abortions on subsequent pregnancy, with increased incidence of [spontaneous] abortion, placenta previa, intrauterine growth retardation, preterm deliveries and low birth weight babies."[68] Previous induced abortion has also been noted as a risk factor for the rare occurrence of a cervical pregnancy, an ectopic pregnancy that occurs in the cervix.[69]

Table 9.1 **Induced Abortion as a risk factor for ectopic pregnancy**

Number of prior induced abortions	Crude OR	95 per cent CI	P value
None	1		<0.001
1	1.3	1.0-1.6	
≥2	3.0	1.7-5.3	

Type of prior induced abortions

None	1		<0.001
Surgical only	1.4	1.1-1.8	
Medical only	2.6	1.2-5.9	
Both	8.9	1.0-79.0	

Source: Bouyer J, Coste J, Shojael T, Pouly JL, Fernandez J, Gerbaud L, Job-Spira N. Risk factors for ectopic pregnancy: A comprehensive analysis based on a large case-control, population-based study in France. American Journal of Epidemiology 2003; 157(3): pp. 185-94.

---

67   Ibid.
68   Dhaliwal LK, Gupta KR and Gopalan S. Induced abortion and subsequent pregnancy outcome. Journal of Family Welfare 2003; 49(1): 50-5.
69   Hanstede MF, van Hof DB, van Groningen K and de Graaf IM. Severe complication after termination of a second trimester cervical pregnancy. Fertility and Sterility 2008; 90(5): e5-e7.

Neonatal Sepsis

A case-control study of neonatal sepsis with the Washington State Birth Registry showed a significant increase in the risk of neonatal sepsis following an induced abortion, even after controlling for the effect of parity.[70] The authors hypothesized that a subclinical infection could be introduced at the time of an induced abortion and remain present until being transmitted to the newborn in a subsequent pregnancy.[71]

Intraamniotic Infection

Intraamniotic infection (IAI) occurs in two to five per cent of births (sudden onset in labour), and more often in preterm births. Infants born when there is IAI are at a twofold risk of death, and more than twofold risk of sepsis. Women who labour with IAI are at three times the risk of cesarean delivery, and higher risk of postpartum endometritis. Previous induced abortion has been associated with a 300 per cent increased risk of intraamniotic infection.[72]

Stillbirth

Another study found that the rate of stillbirth increased 379 per cent after an induced abortion that was followed by an infection.[73]

Conclusion

The rate of infection for women undergoing an induced abortion is reported to be as high as ten per cent. Pelvic inflammatory disease (PID) is a consequence both of sexually transmitted infections (STIs) and medical procedures like surgical abortion that introduce bacteria from the vagina or cervix into the uterus, uterine tubes or ovaries. Women with an STI who procure an induced abortion are therefore up to 72 per cent more likely to contract PID; this association is most commonly seen among women with chlamydia.

---

70   OR 1.45, (95 per cent CI 1.03-2.04).
71   Germain M, Krohn MA and Daling JR. Reproductive history and the risk of neonatal sepsis. Pediatric and Perinatal Epidemiology 1995; 9(1): 48-58.
72   OR 4.0 (95 per cent CI 2.7-5.8); Krohn MA, Germain M, Mühlemann K and Hickok D. Prior pregnancy outcome and the risk of intraamniotic infection in the following pregnancy. AJOG 1998; 178(2): 381-5.
73   OR 4.79 (95 per cent CI 1.46-15.68); Zhou W and Olsen J. Are complications after an induced abortion associated with reproductive failures in a subsequent pregnancy? Acta Obstetricia et Gynecologica Scandinavica 2003; 82(2): 177-81.

Even with the administration of antibiotics prior to an induced abortion, women still risk the sequelae of infection. The consequences most discussed in the literature are subfertility, infertility and ectopic pregnancy. Studies also show that PID can cause tubal pathology that renders a woman infertile. Ectopic pregnancy is one of the leading causes of pregnancy-related deaths, and because of the scarring caused by PID, the risk of ectopic pregnancy rises seven- to tenfold in infected women. Most strikingly of all, there is now a strong correlation between abortion and subsequent ectopic pregnancy. Evidence linking ectopic pregnancy to previous induced abortion is overwhelming. Abortion has also been associated with neonatal infection, intraamniotic infection and stillbirth. Women who are considering an abortion ought to be, and have the right to be, informed of these recent findings.

Chapter 10

Physical complications: Injury, miscarriage, placenta previa

KEY POINTS

- The rate of perforation of the uterus during induced abortion is higher than often recognized.

- Perforation of the uterus can result in scarring and lead to infertility from Asherman's syndrome (intrauterine adhesions).

- Dilation of the cervix during a surgical abortion can render the cervix incompetent, resulting in miscarriage or preterm births in subsequent pregnancies.

- The risk of placenta previa also rises after one or more induced abortions.

UTERINE PERFORATION

The rate of uterine perforation during induced abortion was reported by the Royal College of Obstetricians and Gynaecologists as moderate—from one to four per 1000 (0.1-0.4 per cent).[1] Elsewhere Leibner notes "Although uterine perforation with intra-abdominal injury is a well-described complication of vacuum aspiration termination of pregnancy, most postabortion perforations go undetected."[2] Women may remain asymptomatic or may develop abdominal discomfort many weeks after the abortion, which may signal damage to surrounding organs such as the small bowel.

Kaali and colleagues discovered this to be true during a study of 6408 first-trimester abortions.[3] They found that the resulting true uterine perforation rate was actually about seven times higher than practitioners typically suspected. They suspected a rate of 2.8 per 1000 procedures if "the instrument was passed beyond the expected distance." However, Kaali also checked the number of perforations found in patients whose abortions were performed along with laparoscopic sterilization. They detected a perforation rate of 15.6 per 1000 procedures, which was "sevenfold higher than the perforation rate recognized with traditional methods" (i.e., surgeon's suspicion and patients' symptoms). They also noted that "...most traumatic uterine perforations during first-trimester abortions are unreported or even unsuspected."[4] The presence of such injuries is only detected later when scarring prevents implantation of a subsequent pregnancy or when women have difficulty conceiving or carrying a pregnancy to term.

This raises the question, what happens to women who have an abortion without sterilization by laparoscopy? It may be assumed that their rate of undetected perforation is also seven times higher than conventionally expected. But, insofar as they were not also sterilized, they would not likely know about it; nor would they know that this complication could impair their fertility. Untreated uterine perforations may produce scar tissue that can affect the implantation of an embryo in a future pregnancy.

---
1   Niinimaki, Pouta, Bloigu, et al. See Chapter 6, n. 15. This rate included studies by Zhou (rate: 2.3/1000), and an Australian study (rate 0.86/1000): Pridmore BR and Chambers DG. Uterine perforation during surgical abortion: a review of diagnosis, management and prevention. Aust N Z J Obstet Gynaecol 1999 August; 39(3): 349-53.
2   Leibner EC. Delayed presentation of uterine perforation. Annals of Emergency Medicine 1995 November; 26(5): 643-6, p. 643.
3   Kaali SG, SzigetvariIA and Bartfai GS. The frequency and management of uterine perforations during first-trimester abortions. AJOG 1989 August; 61(2): pp. 406-8.
4   Ibid., p. 407.

Asherman's Syndrome:

Asherman's syndrome (intrauterine adhesions or IUA, also known as *synechia uteri*), results from scar tissue that develops following curettage of the pregnant or recently pregnant uterus. "Gestational changes bring about the softening of the uterus; consequently, the traumatizing effect of eventual curettage is more intense". Therefore, it is possible that the depth of curettage may cause "denudation of the basal layer, the regenerative reservoir of the endometrium."[5] The incidence of Asherman's syndrome is increasing worldwide.[6] Asherman's often presents as abnormal menses, infertility or recurrent miscarriage, but is also most likely underreported on account of possibly varying degrees of severity of the disorder. Women experiencing reduced menstrual flow may not recognize it as a sign of Asherman's syndrome.

Those who generate data on Asherman's syndrome often do not examine induced abortion as an independent factor, but combine it with D&Cs for miscarriages or postpartum retained placentas. A recent study that did separate induced abortion reported that the risk of developing Asherman's syndrome after an elective abortion is 13 per cent, but that risk increases to 39 per cent after repeated abortions.[7] This risk is most often cited for D&C abortions, but Asherman's has also been found to occur after vacuum aspiration abortion.[8]

Among women being investigated for infertility, intrauterine adhesions were the most common abnormal uterine finding.[9] One study of women with Asherman's syndrome seeking treatment for infertility (70.4 per cent) or repeated pregnancy loss (29.6 per cent) collected data on the assumed causes of their Asherman's syndrome. The largest cohort, 42 per cent,

---

5   Schenker JG. Etiology of and therapeutic approach to synechia uteri. European Journal of Obstetrics and Gynecology and Reproductive Biology 1996 March; 65(1): 109-13, p. 109.
6   Yu D, Wong Y, Cheong Y, Xia E and Li T. Asherman syndrome—one century later. Fertility and Sterility 2008; 89(4): 759-79.
7   March CM. Asherman's syndrome. Seminars in Reproductive Medicine 2011 March; 29(2): 83-94.
8   Dalton VK, Saunders NA, Harris LH, Williams JA and Lebovic DI. Intrauterine adhesions after manual vacuum aspiration for early pregnancy failure. Fertility and Sterility 2006; 85(6): 1823.e1-e3.
9   Lasmar RB, Barrozo PR, Parente RC, et al. Hysteroscopic evaluation in patients with infertility. Rev Bras Ginecol Obstet 2010 August; 32(8): 393-7.

developed Asherman's syndrome after a prior D&C induced abortion.[10] Another study found that 42.4 per cent of patients with Asherman's syndrome presenting for infertility treatment had a history of induced abortion.[11]

Asherman's is treated by hysteroscopicadhesiolysis, with a post-treatment pregnancy rate as high as 89.6 per cent and a live birth rate of 77 per cent.[12] However, Asherman's has a recurrence rate of between 3.1 per cent and 23.5 per cent, rising to between 20 per cent and 62.5 per cent for severe adhesions.[13] It hardly needs saying that the best way to prevent Asherman's is to avoid curettage as much as possible.

UTERINE RUPTURE

Evidence of uterine rupture during or following an abortion comes only from case reports.[14]

HYSTERECTOMY

Immediate complications of induced abortion may on rare occasions necessitate a hysterectomy.[15] Castadot notes that pelvic infection with at least three days fever at 38°C, bleeding requiring transfusion, and a second surgery due to problems from the first represent 88 per cent of all major complications. He writes, "Sometimes a hysterectomy is the only alternative."[16] Without this surgery the patient will die from hemorrhage

---

10 Fernandez H, Fadheela A, Chauveaud-Lambling A, Frydman R and Gervaise A. Fertility after treatment of Asherman's syndrome stage 3 and 4. Journal of Minimally Invasive Gynecology 2006; 13: 398-402.
11 Yu D, Li TC, Xia E, Huang X, Liu Y and Peng X. Factors affecting reproductive outcome of hysteroscopicadhesiolysis for Asherman's syndrome. Fertility and Sterility 2008; 89(3): pp. 715-22.
12 Yu et al. See n. 6, pp. 759-79.
13 Ibid.
14 Royal College of Obstetricians and Gynaecologists. *The care of women requesting induced abortion. Evidence-based clinical guideline number 7*, 2004.
15 Trott E, Ziegler W and Levey J. Major complications associated with termination of a second trimester pregnancy: a case report. Delaware Medical Journal 1995 May; 67(5): pp. 294-6; Mittal S, Misra SL. Uterine perforation following medical termination of pregnancy by vacuum aspiration. International Journal of Gynaecology and Obstetrics 1985 February; 23(1): pp. 45-50.
16 Castadot RG. Pregnancy termination: techniques, risks, and complications and their management. Fertility and Sterility 1986 January; 45(1): pp. 5-17.

or peritonitis. With this surgery the patient is rendered sterile. It is not clear how often outcomes that produce sterility occur. Numerous occurrences are reported from patient records identified in a 1996 survey of official medical and legal files.[17] But Ferris and colleagues eliminated hysterectomy from their study because there was only one case.[18] If the removal of such cases is common research practice it is difficult to pinpoint the actual numbers of women who experience this complication.

Likewise, the coding system of hospitals may make it difficult to determine any link between a hysterectomy and a recent induced abortion. In one case an ectopic pregnancy, "discovered after an unsuccessful uterine aspiration…resulted in a hysterectomy, performed in part for voluntary sterilization."[19] Hysterectomy may be an immediate consequence of an abortion when lacerations or abrasions to the uterus occur, or when bleeding from a severed uterine artery can be stopped only by removing the entire uterus. Such incidents have also been documented when damage occurs to the bowel or small intestine.

How often does this happen? A major unknown factor in assessing the number of emergency hysterectomies that are required is whether a patient who experienced severe bleeding after discharge from a day patient abortion clinic would return to the clinic. It is the policy of most private day clinics to instruct the patient to go to a hospital if complications arise. In such cases, the problems she experiences may not enter the abortion statistics.

> "I have seen post-TA [therapeutic abortion] bleeds in ER [Emergency Room] and they are not readily identified."[20]

---

17   Crutcher M. *Lime 5: Exploited by Choice*. Denton, Texas: Life Dynamics, 1996.
18   Ferris LE, McMain-Klein M, Colodny N, Fellows GF and Lamont J. Factors associated with immediate abortion complications. CMAJ 1996 June 1; 154(11): pp. 1677-85.
19   Jacot FR, Poulin C, Bilodeau AP, et al. A five-year experience with second-trimester induced abortions : no increase in complication rate as compared to the first trimester. AJOG 1993 February; 168 (2): pp. 633-7.
20   The deVeber Institute of Bioethics. Survey of Canadian physicians on women's health after induced abortion. Unpublished. Toronto: The deVeber Institute, 1997.

CERVICAL TRAUMA

The Royal College of Obstetricians and Gynaecologists reports that the risk of cervical trauma after surgical abortion may be as high as one in 100.[21] Cervical trauma is more frequent during Dilation and Evacuation (D&E) abortions in the second trimester (0.1 per cent to 2.1 per cent).[22] Aside from increasing gestational age and mechanical dilation of the cervix, the absence of a previous pregnancy (nulliparity) and provider inexperience are also risk factors for cervical lacerations.[23]

During the course of a normal pregnancy, the cervix needs to resist the tendency to dilate under the downward pressure of the infant in the uterus. A decrease in cervical resistance leads to the premature dilation of the cervix with a subsequent late second trimester spontaneous abortion as the cervix becomes incompetent. Cervical incompetence has been defined as: "a cervix that shows a painless dilation and shortening during the second trimester of pregnancy with resultant recurrent pregnancy loss or delivery."[24] Women with short cervixes are more likely to have a miscarriage or preterm birth. Molin examines the problem of decreased cervical resistance following induced first-trimester abortions. His study suggests that cervical resistance is correlated with the ability to continue subsequent pregnancies to term, and that a "fall in resistance to dilatation corresponds to a tear in the cervical tissue of more than two millimeters."[25] He has found that if the cervix is dilated to nine millimetres during an induced abortion prior to the evacuation of the fetus, there will be a fall in cervical resistance in 12.5 per cent of patients. Dilating the cervix to eleven millimetres leads to decreased cervical resistance in two-thirds (66.7 per cent) of the women. This finding did not change according to whether or not the woman had borne a child.

Injury to the cervix can cause later spontaneous abortions. Zlatnik and colleagues determined that such cervical incompetence was associated with

---

21 Royal College of Obstetricians and Gynaecologists 2004. See n. 14.
22 Diedrich and Steinauer. See Chapter 6, n. 22.
23 Ibid., pp. 205-12.
24 Anum EA, Brown HL and Strauss III JF. Health disparities in risk for cervical insufficiency. Human Reproduction 2010 November; 25(11): pp. 2894-900.
25 Molin A. Risk of damage to the cervix by dilatation for first-trimester induced abortion by suction aspiration. Gynecologic and Obstetric Investigation 1993; 35(3): pp. 152-4.

a wide cervical canal.[26] Slater and colleagues reported lower birth weights in subsequent pregnancies when in a previous abortion the dilatation of the cervix was greater than twelve millimetres. It was also found that the subsequent pregnancies were shorter in duration, although the difference was not statistically significant.[27]

A recent study of women pregnant again after abortion (primiparous) showed a sharp increase in cervical insufficiency with each prior induced abortion over the baseline rate of cervical insufficiency: a 149 per cent increase after one previous pregnancy termination,[28] a 366 per cent increase after two terminations,[29] a 707 per cent increase after three terminations,[30] and an 1136 per cent increase after four or more terminations.[31] This trend was also evident among women pregnant more than one time (multiparous). The authors pointed to cervical trauma from the prior abortions as the presumed cause of the women's current cervical insufficiency. Other medical scientists have hypothesized that "cervical lacerations during the abortion procedure may cause cervical incompetence leading to higher mid-trimester abortions and preterm deliveries in future pregnancy."[32]

MISCARRIAGE

"Minor trauma caused to the uterus by induced abortion, as well as uterine infection, might delay the implantation of the embryo, and then result in miscarriage."[33] This trauma could include uterine perforation, and could have led to Asherman's syndrome.

Research findings on miscarriage after induced abortion are mixed. Some studies show no correlation between induced abortion and

---

26   Zlatnik FJ, Burmeister LF, Feddersen DA and Brown RC. Radiological appearance of the upper cervical canal in women with a history of premature delivery II. Relationship to clinical presentation and to tests of cervical compliance. Journal of Reproductive Medicine 1989 August; 34(8): 525-30.
27   Slater PE, Davies AM and Harlap S. The effect of abortion method on the outcome of subsequent pregnancy. Journal of Reproductive Medicine 1981 March; 26(3): pp. 123-8.
28   OR 2.49 (95 per cent CI 2.23-2.77).
29   OR 4.66 (95% CI 4.07-5.33).
30   OR 8.07 (94% CI 6.77-9.61).
31   OR 12.36 (95% CI 10.19-15.00): Anum et al. See n. 24, pp. 2894-900.
32   Dhaliwal, Gupta and Gopalan. See Chapter 9, n. 68.
33   Sun Y, Che Y, Gao E, Olsen J and Zhou W. Induced abortion and risk for subsequent miscarriage. International journal of epidemiology 2003; 32: pp. 449-54.

subsequent miscarriage.[34] However, other studies have found statistically significant increases in miscarriage after two abortions in France;[35] after vacuum aspiration abortion in China;[36] and after one previous induced abortion in the UK.[37] Sun and colleagues estimated that fifteen per cent of first-trimester miscarriages in Shanghai were attributable to prior induced abortions.[38] One study showed a significant correlation between previous first-trimester induced abortion and subsequent miscarriage if the time between the induced abortion and the following pregnancy was less than three months.[39]

PLACENTA PREVIA

Placenta previa occurs when the placenta implants in the lower uterine segment, near or covering the cervix. Between 0.3 and 0.8 per cent of pregnancies are affected by placenta previa, which is also the leading cause of uterine bleeding during the third trimester of pregnancy. It increases the likelihood of preterm birth, low birth weight and perinatal death.[40]

Why does induced abortion increase the risk of placenta previa if a woman conceives again? For the simple reason that "vacuum aspiration or dilation and curettage may cause scarring and adhesions in the uterus that impede proper placentation in subsequent pregnancies."[41]

Research in this field has been of limited value because spontaneous and induced abortions are often not separated in the literature.[42] Nevertheless,

---

34 Parazzini F, Chatenoud L, Tozzi L, Di Cintio E, Benzi G and Fedele L. Induced abortion in the first trimester of pregnancy and risk of miscarriage. BJOG 1998; 105: pp. 418-21; Thorp Jr., Hartmann and Shadigan. See Chapter 9, n. 38.
35 (OR 4.43, 95 % CI 1.46-13.36): Infante-Rivard C and Gauthier R. Induced abortion as a risk factor for subsequent fetal loss. Epidemiology. 1996 September; 7(5): pp. 540-2.
36 (OR 1.55, 95 per cent CI 1.08-2.23): Sun Y, Che Y, Gao E, Olsen J and Zhou W. Induced abortion and risk for subsequent miscarriage. International journal of epidemiology 2003; 32: pp. 449-54.
37 (OR 1.72, 95 per cent CI 1.27-2.31): Maconochie N, Doyle P, Prior S and Simmons R. Risk factors for first trimester miscarriage—results from a UK population-based case-control study. BJOG 2007 February; 114(2): pp. 170-86.
38 Sun et al. See n. 33, pp. 449-54.
39 (OR 4.06, 95 per cent CI 1.98-8.31): Zhou W, Olsen J, Nielsen GL and Sabroe W. Risk of spontaneous abortion following induced abortion is only increased with short interpregnancy interval. Journal of Obstetrics and Gynaecology 2000; 20(1): pp. 49-54.
40 Thorp Jr., Hartmann and Shadigan. See Chapter 9, n. 38.
41 Hung, Hsieh, Hsu, et al. See Abstract II: The Medical Impact, p. 92, n. 1.
42 Crane JMG, Van den Hof MC, Dodds, and Armson. Maternal complications with placenta previa. American Journal of Perinatology 2000; 17(2): 101-5.

evidence of an association between placenta previa and prior induced abortion is accumulating. One study showed that induced abortion increased the risk of placenta previa by 30 per cent,[43] while a meta-analysis revealed an increased risk of 70 per cent.[44] Other studies have confirmed these findings,[45] and pointed out that the risk of developing placenta previa is even greater after a second-trimester abortion.[46] A review of eight American studies showed a 50 per cent increased risk of placenta previa after induced abortion.[47]

Furthermore, within the past decade two studies[48] have shown that the risk of placenta previa increases with each induced abortion that a woman undergoes.

Table 10.1 **Risk of placenta previa after D & C abortion**

Number of previous D&C abortions	Risk of placenta previa (Cochran-Armitage trend test, exact p=0.01)
1	1.4 (95 per cent CI 0.8-2.6)
2	2.0 (95 per cent CI 1.0-4.0)
≥3	2.8 (95 per cent CI 1.0-8.1)

Source: Johnson LG, Mueller BA and Daling JR. The relationship of placenta previa and history of induced abortion. International Journal of Gynecology and Obstetrics 2003 May; 81(2): 191-8.

---

43   (OR 1.3.95 % CI 1.01-1.66): Taylor VM, Kramer MD, Vaughan TL and Peacock S. Placenta previa in relation to induced and spontaneous abortion: a population-based study. Obstetrics and Gynecology 1993 July; 82(1): 88-91, p. 91.
44   (RR 1.7, 95 per cent CI 1.0-2.9): Ananth CV, Smulian JC and Vintzileos AM. The association of placenta previa with history of cesarean delivery and abortion: a meta-analysis. AJOG 1997 November; 177(5): 1071-8.
45   Sheiner E, Shoham-Vardi I, Hallak M, Hershkowitz R, Katz M and Mazor M. Placenta previa: obstetric risk factors and pregnancy outcome. Journal of Maternal-Fetal Medicine 2001; 10: pp. 414-19.
46   Dhaliwal, Gupta and Gopalan. See Chapter 9, n. 68.
47   OR 1.5 (95 per cent CI 1.3-1.9): Faiz AS and Ananth CV. Etiology and risk factors for placenta previa: an overview and meta-analysis of observational studies. Journal of Maternal-Fetal and Neonatal Medicine 2003; 13: pp. 175-90.
48   Johnson LG, Mueller BA and Daling JR. The relationship of placenta previa and history of induced abortion. International Journal of Gynecology and Obstetrics 2003; 81(2): pp. 191-8.

Table 10.2 **Risk of placenta previa after induced abortion**

Number of previous induced abortions	Adjusted OR	95 per cent CI
0	1.0	Referent
1-2	1.3	1.1-1.6
3-4	2.0	1.4-2.9
≥ 5	3.0	1.3-7.1

Source: Hung TH, Hsieh CC, Hsu JJ, Chiu TH, Lo LM and Hsieh TT. Risk Factors for Placenta Previa in an Asian Population. International Journal of Gynecology and Obstetrics 2007 April; 97(1): 26-30.

The authors state that if both spontaneous and induced abortions could be reduced, the incidence of placenta previa could also be reduced proportionately.[49]

PLACENTA PROBLEMS IN THE THIRD STAGE OF LABOUR IN SUBSEQUENT BIRTHS

Women with one or more previous first-trimester induced abortion(s) have been found to be at a 159 per cent higher risk of prolonged third-stage labour in subsequent pregnancies. This risk is even higher for women who had their abortion towards the end of the first trimester.[50] The rate at which the placenta had to be removed manually, the uterine cavity manually revised, and the womb scraped (curettage) after the third stage increased by 23 per cent after one or more previous induced abortions.[51]

---

49 Ananth, Smulian and Vintzileos. See n. 44.
50 OR 2.59 (95 per cent CI 1.06-6.37): Zhou W, Gao E, Che Y and Olsen J. Induced abortion and duration of third stage of labour in a subsequent pregnancy. Journal of Obstetrics and Gynaecology 1999; 19(4): 349-54.
51 OR 1.23 (95 per cent CI 1.10-1.38): Haldre K, Rahu K, Karro H and Rahu M. Previous history of surgically induced abortion and complications of the third stage of labour in subsequent normal vaginal deliveries. Journal of Maternal-Fetal and Neonatal Medicine 2008 December; 21(12): 884—8.

CONCLUSION

In the past fifteen to twenty years the medical literature has increasingly documented the immediate hazards of surgical abortion: perforation of the uterus, causing scarring, which in turn can result in Asherman's syndrome and infertility. The risk of placenta previa in a subsequent pregnancy is also increased. The necessity to force open the cervix (dilation) during a surgical abortion can weaken the cervix and render it incapable of performing its primary function during pregnancy: holding in the baby. A weakened or "incompetent" cervix will mean a higher rate of miscarriage and premature births. Women ought to, and deserve to be, informed of these very real hazards stemming from surgical abortion.

Chapter 11

Physical complications: Autoimmune diseases

KEY NOTES

- Induced abortion is associated with a greater frequency of fetal microchimerism; in other words, a greater number of fetal cells are detected in women who have undergone induced abortion than in other women who have brought their pregnancy to term.

- Some researchers suggest that fetal microchimerism may cause, or contribute to, autoimmune diseases in women.

- Therefore, the consistently rising incidence of autoimmune diseases in women over the past four decades may well be attributable to the increased incidence of induced abortion.

INTRODUCTION

Autoimmune diseases occur when the body's immune system mistakenly attacks and destroys healthy tissue. Over 80 disorders have been identified, and between five and eight per cent of Americans are affected by them.[1] Autoimmune diseases are the third most common category of disease after heart disease and cancer, and their prevalence is increasing.[2] Thyroid disorders and rheumatoid arthritis represent over 50 per cent of the cases.[3]

MICROCHIMERISM

Research into the causes of autoimmune diseases is ongoing. One mechanism that has been proposed is fetal microchimerism. Fetal microchimerism is regarded as a kind of "trans-placental stem cell transplant," which is becoming a plausible explanation of the large diversity of tissue pathology and the yearly increase in autoimmune diseases in women.[4] Fetal microchimerism begins at four to five weeks gestation (28 to 35 days) when fetal immune cells transfer across the placenta into the mother's bloodstream and, with a great capacity for dividing and maturing, circulate and reside in her tissues.[5] This fetal-maternal transfer of cells is a normal part of pregnancy, since for the fetus to survive the mother's immune system must not attack it.[6] It is common for fetal cells to linger in postpartum women before being lost, but fetal microchimerism has remained in some women for over 27 years after delivery.[7]

There are several hypotheses about the role of microchimeric cells in autoimmune diseases: "Most reports present evidence that microchimerism is present in a higher proportion of subjects with autoimmune disease

---

1 Progress in Autoimmune Diseases Research, Report to Congress, National Institutes of Health, The Autoimmune Diseases Coordinating Committee, March 2005. http://www.niaid.nih.gov/topics/autoimmune/documents/adccfinal.pdf.
2 Fairweather D. Autoimmune Disease: Mechanisms. *Encyclopedia of Life Sciences*. Chicester, UK: John Wiley & Sons, Ltd., 2007, pp. 1-7. Online edition: www.els.net.
3 Rose NR and Mackay IR, eds. *The autoimmune diseases*, 3rd ed. San Diego: Academic Press, 1998, as cited in "Prevalence and Incidence of Autoimmune diseases" (Health Grades Inc., 2011), http://www.rightdiagnosis.com/a/ai/prevalence.htm.
4 Miech RP. The role of fetal microchimerism in autoimmune disease. International Journal of Clinical and Experimental Medicine 2010; 3(2): 162-8.
5 Ando T and Davies TF. Postpartum autoimmune thyroid disease: the potential role of fetal microchimerism. Journal of Clinical Endocrinology & Metabolism 2003; 88(7): 2965-71.
6 Ibid.
7 Ibid.

and/or that a higher number of microchimeric cells are detected in these subjects compared to controls."[8] However, as Johnson indicates, "varied and sometimes conflicting data led to two other hypotheses regarding fetal cell microchimerism. One is that the observed fetal cells are merely innocent bystanders and have no impact on maternal health. The other, the "good microchimerism" hypothesis, suggests that persistent fetal cells, instead of inducing a maternal immune response, provide a rejuvenating source of fetal progenitor cells that may have the capacity to participate in maternal tissue repair processes."[9]

While some researchers suggest that fetal-maternal cell transfusion can contribute to tissue repair,[10] others suspect that microchimerism may increase the risk of developing autoimmune diseases, especially if the fetal cells implanted in maternal tissue spark a graft vs. host response, as when a donated organ is rejected by the recipient's autoimmune system. The foreign fetal cells could cause the woman's immune system to attack and destroy healthy tissue:

> Chronic graft-versus-host disease (cGvHD) that results from stem cell transplantation has clinical similarities with some autoimmune diseases. These observations, together with the bi-directional trafficking of cells during pregnancy, have suggested the possible role of fetal-maternal or maternal-fetal microchimerism in the pathogenesis of auto-immune diseases. Examples are systemic sclerosis (SSc), juvenile idiopathic inflammatory myopathies (JIIM), Graves' disease, Hashimoto's thyroiditis, Sjogren's syndrome (SS), primary biliary cirrhosis (PBC) and systematic lupus erythematosus (SLE).[11]

Another recent study notes that "fetal microchimerism has been adversely implicated in scleroderma, an autoimmune disease with clinical similarity to graft-versus-host disease after

---

8 Sarkar K and Miller FW. Possible roles and determinants of microchimerism in autoimmune and other disorders. Autoimmunity Reviews 2004; 3(6): 453-63, p. 455.
9 Johnson KL and Bianchi DW. Fetal cells in maternal tissue following pregnancy: what are the consequences? Human Reproduction Update 2004; 10(6): 497-502, p. 498.
10 Adams KM and Nelson JL. An investigative frontier in autoimmunity and transplantation. JAMA 2004 March; 291(9): 1127-31.
11 Sarkar and Miller. See n. 8, p. 455.

hematopoietic cell transplantation."[12]

In addition, "women have a predilection to autoimmune disease, and human leukocyte antigen (HLA) class II genes are known to be important both in autoimmune disease and in GvHD [graft vs. host disease]. Considered together, these observations led to the hypothesis that microchimerism and HLA genes of host and non-host cells are involved in autoimmune disease."[13] Similarly, "women with RA [rheumatoid arthritis] had microchimerism with RA-associated HLA alleles, but not with non-RA-associated HLA alleles, more often and at higher levels compared with healthy women. These observations are the first to indicate that microchimerism can contribute to the risk of an autoimmune disease by providing HLA susceptibility alleles."[14]

Microchimerism and Non-Autoimmune Diseases

"Microchimerism has also been associated with non-autoimmune human diseases. Examples are polymorphic eruptions of pregnancy (PEP), pre-eclampsia, infectious hepatitis, non-autoimmune thyroid disorders, blood cancers and cervical cancer."[15]

Abortion and Microchimerism

Not only is fetal loss in elective abortions "accompanied with the loss of suppression of the maternal immune system by Early Pregnancy Factor, which may be another factor in the setting the stage for the future development of autoimmune disease."[16] There is further evidence from Bianchi and colleagues' testing of 23 women undergoing induced abortion for fetal cell microchimerism. Samples within one hour after termination of pregnancy revealed a "significant fetal-maternal transfusion of cells" from the 21 male fetuses to the mother, while no transfusion was detected from the two female fetuses.

---

12   Yan Z, Lambert NC, Guthrie KA, et al. Male microchimerism in women without sons: quantitative assessment and correlation with pregnancy history. American Journal of Medicine 2005; 118(8): p. 900.
13   Stevens A and Nelson JL. Maternal and fetal microchimerism: implications for human diseases. Neo Reviews 2002; 3(1): e11-e19, p.e11.
14   Rak JM, Maestroni L, Balandraud N, et al. Transfer of the shared epitope through microchimerism in women with rheumatoid arthritis. Arthritis & Rheumatism 2009; 60(1): 73-80, p. 73.
15   Sarkar and Miller. See n. 8, p. 457.
16   Miech. See n. 4, p. 166.

> If one assumes a blood volume of 4.5 litres in a pregnant woman at thirteen weeks of gestation, an equivalent of 436,500 nucleated fetal cells is present in the woman after termination. Some of these cells will be relatively undifferentiated and may have the ability to proliferate. Therefore a consideration of the biologic consequences of pregnancy and the potential for the development of fetal cell microchimerism must now extend to women who have undergone elective termination of pregnancy in the first or second trimester.[17]

The study also notes that transfusion occurs in much greater volume after elective abortion than after a normal pregnancy.

Male microchimerism is measured in women who have had an induced abortion but have not had any live-born male children. Yan and colleagues estimate that women with previous induced abortion are eight times more likely to have microchimerism than other healthy women.[18]

Although microchimerism occurs more frequently after surgical abortion, it is also found after medical (meaning drug-or chemically-induced) abortion: "The phenomenon of increased fetal cell trafficking following a medical abortion was also confirmed in a murine model [an experiment with mice]. ... The amount of fetal DNA found in maternal circulation following a first-trimester abortion was found to be higher in women who underwent a surgical abortion than in women who had a chemical abortion."[19] In addition, induced abortion results in greater frequency of fetal microchimerism than spontaneous abortion (miscarriage).[20]

Miech proposes that the reason for high levels of fetal microchimerism in women following an induced abortion might be that "there is an increased fetal-to-maternal transfer of fetal undifferentiated progenitor

---

17 Bianchi DW, Farina A, Weber W, et al. Significant fetal-maternal hemorrhage after termination of pregnancy: implications for development of fetal cell microchimerism. AJOG 2001; 184(4): 703-6, p. 705.
18 Yan et al. See n. 12, pp. 899-906.
19 Miech. See n. 4, p. 166.
20 Boyon C, Collinet P, Boulanger L, et al. Fetal microchimerism: benevolence or malevolence for the mother? European Journal of Obstetrics & Gynecology and Reproductive Biology 2011; 158(2): pp. 148-52.

cells during an abortion procedure as the placenta is being destroyed."[21] He states that "fetal microchimerism is increased in women who had a termination of pregnancy and may be associated with the development of autoimmune disease later on in life. Furthermore, the consistently rising incidence of autoimmune diseases in women over the past four decades may be attributed to the increase in the utilization of abortion."[22]

Conclusion

More research is needed to determine the exact nature of the relationship between microchimerism and autoimmune diseases. Studies to date indicate that if the fetal-maternal transfusion of cells increases a woman's chances of contracting an autoimmune disease, a history of induced abortion will also increase her chances of contracting an autoimmune disease. This is because microchimerism occurs after induced abortion with much greater frequency than after a normal, completed pregnancy.

---

21   Miech. See n. 4, p. 166.
22   Ibid., p. 162.

Chapter 12

Physical complications: Maternal mortality from abortion

KEY POINTS

- Large-scale, data-linkage studies from Scandinavia, Britain and the USA have documented a significantly higher maternal mortality from induced abortion than from childbirth.

- A recent US study claiming that abortion is safer than childbirth is based on faulty methodology and incomplete data.

- Thanks to the politicization of the abortion issue in North America many abortion-related deaths are attributed to other causes.

- Only jurisdictions that keep systematic records of births, abortions and deaths can provide accurate statistics for maternal abortion-related mortality. Neither the US nor Canada keeps such records.

INTRODUCTION

How likely is a woman to die after an induced abortion? Is she less likely to die than if carries her pregnancy to term and delivers her child? A recent US study argues that induced abortion is more than fourteen times safer than giving birth, and that abortion is therefore good for women's health. To arrive at this conclusion Raymond and Grimes used a deceptively simple approach. They first estimated the mortality among women who gave birth, based on statistics gathered by the Centers for Disease Control and Prevention (CDC). They then divided that figure into the number of live births as reported on birth certificates. This yielded a figure of 8.8 maternal deaths per 100,000 live births.[1] To estimate abortion-related mortality, the authors divided the number of legal abortion-related deaths in the US reported by the CDC, by the number of legal abortions *estimated* by the Guttmacher Institute. This yielded a maternal death rate of only 0.6 per 100,000 abortions.

These findings are open to serious question, and are in fact contradicted by four large-scale studies from the US and other countries. As Raymond and Grimes themselves acknowledge, both abortion and childbirth can cause mortality and morbidity long after the end of pregnancy, yet they confine their attention to the period immediately following the abortion or birth.

By contrast, a study of 408,000 British women over a five-year period found that women who had induced abortions were 225 per cent more likely to attempt suicide than women admitted for normal delivery.[2] This study also found that the rate of attempted suicide *prior to pregnancy* was similar for both groups. In other words, women prone to attempt suicide were not more likely to have abortions and attempt suicide again.

Two Scandinavian studies have uncovered a much higher mortality after abortion than after childbirth. Unlike either the US or Canada, Finland and Denmark keep accurate centralized registries for abortion, as well as for all births and deaths. A study of all Finnish women who died over an eight-year period found the following variations in maternal mortality after pregnancy[3]:

---

1 Raymond EG and Grimes DA. The comparative safety of legal induced abortion and childbirth in the United States. Obstetrics & Gynecology 2012 February; 119(2): 215-19.
2 Morgan CL, Evans M and Peters JR. Suicides after pregnancy: mental health may deteriorate as a direct effect of induced abortion. BMJ 1997 March; 314(7084): pp. 902-3.
3 Gissler M, et al. Pregnancy associated deaths in Finland 1987-1994: definition problems and benefits of record linkage. Acta Obstet Gynecol Scand 1997; 76: 651–7.

Table 12.1 **Maternal deaths within twelve months of end of pregnancy, per 100,000 women in Finland**

After giving birth	26.7
After miscarriage or ectopic pregnancy	47.8
After induced abortion	100.5

In other words, the maternal death rate after abortion was nearly four times greater than the maternal death rate after childbirth. They further noted that 73 per cent of all pregnancy-associated deaths could not have been identified from death certificates alone.[4] The researchers also found that within one year of the end of pregnancy, the suicide rate associated with childbirth was six times lower than the suicide rate associated with abortion.[5]

A recently published investigation of the impact of abortion in Denmark has come up with similar findings.[6] This large-scale, 25-year study employed a rigorous methodology based on data linkage to complete pregnancy and abortion records. Surveying the entire female population born between 1962 and 1993, the authors compared mortality rates linked to induced abortion, miscarriage ("natural losses"), and live births. Covering the period from 1980 to 2004, the study included over a million women. Those who had experienced induced abortion or miscarriages suffered more than three times the risk of death of women who had only experienced birth. The researchers also uncovered "rather alarmingly high rates of death … among women who had not experienced any pregnancies", much higher than among women who gave birth.[7] Those in the oldest age group experienced increased risk from one, two or three induced abortions of

---

4   Gissler M, Berg C, Bouvier-Colle MH and Buekens P. Methods for identifying pregnancy-associated deaths: population-based data from Finland 1987-2000. Paediatric and Perinatal Epidemiology 2004; 18(6): 448-55.
5   Gissler M, Hemminki E and Lonnqvist J. Suicides after pregnancy in Finland, 1987-94: register linkage study. BMJ 1996 December; 313(7070): 1431-4.
6   Coleman PK, Reardon DC and Calhoun BC. Reproductive history patterns and long-term mortality rates: a Danish, population-based record linkage study. European Journal of Public Health 2013; 23(4): 569-74; Reardon DC and Coleman PK. Short and long term mortality rates associated with first pregnancy outcome: population register based study for Denmark 1980-2004. Medical Science Monitor 2012; 18(9): PH71-76.
7   Colemen et al. European Journal of Public Health 2013: 569-74. See n. 6.

49 per cent, 96 per cent and 152 per cent respectively. Giving birth had a protective effect, with the women who gave birth twice, experiencing the greatest reduction in mortality—108 per cent reduced risk.[8]

The fourth large-scale study comes from California. It too is methodologically rigorous, based exclusively on data linkage.[9] Medical records were linked to death certificates for 173,279 low-income women who underwent a state-funded delivery or induced abortion in 1989. Four years later the annual suicide rate among the women who terminated their pregnancies was found to be 160 per cent higher (7.8 compared to 3.0 per 100,000) than among the women who gave birth. When deaths after delivery and abortion were compared over an eight-year period it was found that the women who aborted had a 30 per cent higher mortality than the women who delivered their children (738 vs. 586 per 100,000). This higher mortality was not the effect of previous psychiatric history. When the effects of previous psychiatric history were removed, the relative risk for woman who had abortions actually increased, compared with that of delivering women.

Given the agreement among these large-scale studies from several countries, why do some North-American researchers continue to assert that abortion is safer than childbirth? One reason is that they confine their attention to the six weeks (42 days) after the termination or birth event. But there are several more reasons why abortion-related maternal mortality is generally underreported. Codes in hospitals report only the *presenting* cause of death, not the *underlying* reason. In the case of abortion-related death the presenting cause might be a hemorrhage, infection, embolism, or ectopic pregnancy. In fact, the reporting systems in the United States, Canada, and the World Health Organization are so imprecise that deaths related to a previous abortion are hard to track: death certificates are inaccurately completed and, either to protect the privacy of the woman and her family, or to avoid a possible lawsuit, hospital staff or doctors may deliberately avoid coding an abortion-related death.

Another reason for underreporting bias is that many of the statistics provided by the Centers for Disease Control (CDC) come from unreliable

---

8   Ibid.
9   Reardon DC, Ney PG, Scheurer FJ, Congle JR, Coleman PK. Suicide deaths associated with pregnancy outcome: A record linkage study of 172,279 low income American women. Archives of Women's Mental Health 2001; 3(4 Supplement 2): p. 104.

hospital and clinic records. Statistics from abortion providers in Canada tend to underreport negative findings, perhaps in order to promote the impression that abortion is a safe procedure. Worse still, in the US there is *no* reporting requirement for negative outcomes relative to abortion clinics or coroners. In countries where the study of abortion is not politically charged, there is little attempt to create such an impression. Researchers in Eastern Europe, for example, candidly admit that the high frequency of abortion there has contributed to the "deleterious" population decline and that maternal mortality remains "unacceptably high". "It is particularly worrying," write Mogilevkina and colleagues, "that in Russia, Ukraine, Belarus, Estonia, Latvia and Lithuania "induced abortions make up twenty per cent to 35 per cent of all maternal mortality".[10]

UNDERREPORTING OF MATERNAL DEATHS IN THE US AND CANADA

In the United States and Canada, as well as in the World Health Organization (WHO) there has been a general and systematic underreporting of maternal deaths—deaths of women during pregnancy or delivery, or in the six weeks following the termination of a pregnancy. According to one analysis of mortality statistics, "more than half of such deaths...are probably still unreported", and the Centers for Disease Control's Pregnancy-Related Mortality Surveillance System "does not identify all pregnancy-related deaths".[11] In other words, women have died as a result of pregnancy, but their pregnancy was never connected to official death records.

The system used in linkage studies to identify maternal deaths works back from a recorded birth. Because of this, it "cannot identify pregnancy-related deaths that do not generate a record of pregnancy outcome (e.g. ectopic pregnancies ...induced or spontaneous abortions)".[12] In any event, Centers for Disease Control (CDC) reports combine maternal deaths by miscarriages and induced abortions into a single category and these combined numbers are accepted as accounting for all maternal deaths

---

10   Mogilevkina I, Markote S, Avakyan Y, Mrochek L, Liljestrand J, Hellberg D. Induced abortions and childbirths: trends in Estonia, Latvia, Lithuania, Russia, Belarussia and the Ukraine during 1970 to 1994. Acta Obstetricia et Gynecologica Scandanavica 1996 November; 75(10): 908-11, p. 910.
11   Berg CJ, Atrash HK, Koonin LM, Tucker M. Pregnancy-related mortality in the United States, 1987-1990. Obstetrics & Gynecology 1996 August; 88(2):161-7, pp. 161, 166.
12   Jacob S, Bloebaum L, Shah G, Varner MW. Maternal mortality in Utah. Obstetrics & Gynecology 1998 February; 91(2):187-91, p. 190.

from abortion, even though demographic researchers recognize that there is systematic underreporting.

More than a decade ago, a Canadian health researcher found that the problem of underreporting of maternal and abortion-related deaths was not limited to the United States and Canada, but was also the result of flawed reporting guidelines from the World Health Organization (WHO). WHO's claim that legal abortion (an abortion procedure performed by a licensed practitioner) is safe depends on a voluntary system of death certification that has been shown to be inherently unreliable. WHO's statistics come from physicians who are not told that they must specify the type of abortion that led to maternal death—spontaneous, induced, legal or illegal.[13] Physicians are not even told that they must specify that the terminal illness (e.g. sepsis) followed an abortion. WHO itself has admitted the barriers to accurately estimating abortion deaths in a number of countries. "Maternal deaths are hard to identify precisely because this requires information about deaths among women of reproductive age, pregnancy status at or near the time of death, and the medical cause of death. All three components can be difficult to measure accurately, particularly in settings where deaths are not comprehensively reported through the vital registration system and where there is no medical certification of cause of death."[14] The problem is particularly acute in the US, where Horon noted that physicians fail to report recent or current pregnancies on a minimum of 50 per cent of death certificates.[15]

How the Reporting System Works

In the US the success of the CDC system depends entirely on whether a report is made in the first place. Unless induced abortion is identified as an immediate cause of death, it will not be investigated or recorded by the CDC. Inaccuracies may creep into the reporting process in a number of ways. For example, the great majority of abortions in the US are performed in free-standing abortion clinics. A woman whose post-abortion condition is life-threatening will be admitted to a general hospital through an

---

13   Bégin I. Mortality and Morbidity Coding in Canada and the World—Pitfalls and Shortcomings. 1999. Ottawa (unpublished paper).
14   World Health Organization. *Maternal mortality in 2000-estimates by UNICEF, WHO, & UNFPA*. Geneva: Department of Reproductive Health & Research. 2004.
15   Horon I. Under-reporting of maternal deaths on death certificates and the magnitude of the problem of maternal mortality. American Journal of Public Health 2005; 95: p. 479.

emergency department. The attending emergency room doctor will not be the physician who performed the abortion and may not record a subsequent death as resulting from an abortion.

Furthermore, if a woman dies from her abortion, it is not usually the abortion provider but a casualty officer or the family doctor who must complete the death certificate, and it is this information upon which the death may or may not be reported to the CDC.[16] In Canada it has been noted that "if complications ensue after a patient has been discharged from hospital, the condition is treated as a separate case and does not appear in the original abortion record".[17]

In addition, inadequate information may be provided on the physician's or coroner's report. For example, the death may be noted as related to a previous abortion, but insufficient detail may make it impossible to determine whether the abortion was induced or spontaneous. In general, Canadian Medical Certificates of Death have been found to contain major errors 32.9 per cent of the time.[18] Given the politicization of the issue in North America, it is not surprising that the records of abortion-related deaths are incomplete.

Among other factors, hospital coding may not reflect the international numbering system. A woman who dies from a hemorrhage may have the event recorded simply as "hemorrhage" but with no code that would connect the bleeding to an earlier induced abortion. Codes such as embolism or cardiomyopathy can stand alone, with no reference to an induced abortion as the cause. Hospital staff may avoid using the full coding in order to protect the privacy of the deceased patient, and/or the family, or to avoid legal or political entanglement. Incomplete, indirect, or subtle coding, if it occurs, may also assist the abortion practitioner who otherwise might run a greater risk of civil liability. Malpractice is a significant issue for all physicians, but in recent years concerted civil litigation by women injured

---

16   Henshaw SK and Van Vort J. Abortion services in the United States, 1991 and 1992. Family Planning Perspectives 1994 May-June; 26(3): 100-6, 112.
17   Wadhera S and Millar WJ. Second trimester abortions: trends and medical complications. Health Reports 1994; 6(4): 441-54.
18   Myers KA, Farquhar DR. Improving the accuracy of death certification. CMAJ 1998 May 19; 158(10): pp. 1317-23.

by abortion has made abortion providers particularly vulnerable.[19] For example, in Cincinnati, Ohio Planned Parenthood recently settled out of court in a suit brought against them for alleged physical harm, as well as emotional and psychological distress suffered by a fourteen-year-old girl upon whom they had performed an abortion. Although she was a minor at the time, the abortion agency did not inform her parents of the abortion, or the legal authorities that she was in an illegal and criminal sexual relationship with an adult, her 21-year-old soccer coach. The plaintiffs also alleged that immediately after the abortion the girl was given a Depo-Provera (birth-control) shot and a supply of condoms. Neither the abortionist nor any other agent of Planned Parenthood obtained the informed and voluntary consent of the girl before providing these medical "services". In a highly significant ruling, the Common Pleas Court judge found that the Planned Parenthood doctor breached a legal duty by not holding an "informed consent" meeting with the girl before the abortion.[20] The case dragged on for seven years, 2005 to 2012, when it was finally resolved to the satisfaction of the plaintiffs.[21]

A review of death statistics and the medical coding methods used to attribute death to maternal causes found that the health records of eighteen American states, and four of seven Canadian provinces surveyed do not permit deaths to be classified as maternal if they occur more than 42 days after the termination of a pregnancy. Thus, if a woman has died from abortion-related complications such as ectopic pregnancy more than six weeks after her abortion, abortion will not be noted; the only cause of death referred to would be "ectopic pregnancy". If death is immediate, it is not required to specify on the death certificate what kind of an abortion was performed, and if maternal death happens 43 days after an abortion, the death will not be linked to it. As this situation makes clear, accurate reporting on maternal abortion-related deaths is not, at present, a reality in North America.

---

19   Collett TS. Abortion malpractice: Exploring the safety of legal abortion. *Life and Learning; vol. V.* Koterski JW, ed. Fifth University Faculty for Life Conference; 1995 June; Marquette University: pp. 243-72.
20   Perry K. Abortion provider loses ruling. *Cincinnati Enquirer*, Dec. 9, 2010, p. C1.
21   Jamie and Brenda Wallace, parents of Jane Roe, a minor vs. Planned Parenthood Southwest Ohio region, et al. Court of Common Pleas, Civil Division, Hamilton County, Ohio. Case No. A0502691 (2007). We are grateful to Brian Hurley, one of the prosecuting attorneys, for providing details and court documents related to the case.

Doubtful Data

To recapitulate, death certificates may not connect the direct cause of death with the preceding abortion event. A death from cardiac arrest may be listed as such, and not as a cardiac arrest due to a reaction to the anaesthetic given during an abortion. Jacob found that in the statistics of maternal mortality, the greatest errors in classification occurred for women who had recently undergone an induced abortion.[22]

Conclusion

Large-scale studies based on data linkage from the US, Britain, Denmark and Finland, have shown that women who undergo induced abortion have a sharply increased death rate compared to women who give birth. Having an induced abortion also greatly increases a woman's chance of later attempting or committing suicide, while carrying a baby to term greatly reduces that likelihood. As two recent researchers write, "pregnant women considering their options deserve accurate information about comparative risks."[23] Yet their own study purporting to show that induced abortion is safer than childhood is based on faulty methodology and incomplete data, and is in any case limited to the period immediately after childbirth or termination of pregnancy. It completely ignores four data-linkage studies, which are based on a far more objective and neutral methodology, as well as complete and reliable data. Those and other studies effectively explode the myth that abortion is safer for a woman than childbirth.

---

22 Jacob S et al. Maternal mortality in Utah. Obstetrics & Gynecology 1998 February; 91(2): pp. 187-91
23 Raymond and Grimes. See n. 1, pp. 215-19.

Chapter 13

Medical or drug-induced abortion: How safe?

KEY POINTS

- 'Medical', meaning chemically-induced, abortion has become more widely practised in recent years as an alternative to surgical abortion.

- The failure rate of medical abortion ranges between four and sixteen per cent, making it much less reliable than surgical abortion.

- One of the drugs used in medical abortion—misoprostol—has been linked to fetal malformation in later pregnancies.

Introduction

Medical or chemically-induced abortion has become more widespread over the last decade as some women seek an alternative to surgical abortion. One attraction is that it can be done privately, without anyone finding out. On the other hand it can be a difficult experience for women since the treatment takes longer, involves artificial labour, and (when successful) ends in the delivery of a bruised, dead fetus.[1] There are a number of drugs available for use in chemically-induced ("medical") abortion. Currently, the three widely used regimens are: mifepristone (RU486) combined with misoprostol, methotrexate combined with misoprostol, and misoprostol alone.

Since the discovery and development of the antiprogesteron drug mifepristone (RU486) in 1988, chemically-induced ("medical") abortion has increased steadily.[2] The drug is currently approved in 30 countries, mostly in the developed world.[3] Mifepristone is widely used for first-trimester medical abortion (up to the ninth week of pregnancy) in many countries. Its low cost and easy availability make it an attractive alternative to surgical abortion in some developing countries.[4] It is estimated that medical abortion accounts for 21 per cent of all first-trimester abortions in the US but only three per cent of all abortions in Canada in 2004.[5] Medical abortion accounts for 48 per cent of all abortions in England and Wales, a percentage over three times higher than a decade ago.[6] Medical abortion is thought to constitute one-third of all abortions in China.[7]

---

1 Grossman D, Blachard K, Blumenthal P. Complications after Second Trimester Surgical and Medical Abortion. Reproductive Health Matters 2008; 16(31): p. 179.
2 Jones R and Henshaw K. Mifepristone for early medical abortion: Experiences in France, Great Britain, and Sweden. Perspectives on Sexual and Reproductive Health 2002; 34(3): pp. 154-160.
3 Bartz D, Golberg A. Medication Abortion. Clinical Obstetrics and Gynecology 2009; 52(2): pp. 140-50.
4 Nguyen N, Winikoff B, Clark S et al. Safety, Efficacy and Acceptability of Mifepristone-Misoprostol Medical Abortion in Vietnam. IFPP 1999; 25(1): pp. 10-14; Vietnamese Ministry of Health. *A strategic assessment of policy, programme and research issues relating to abortion in Vietnam: a draft report.* Hanoi, Vietnam: Author, 1997.
5 Jones RK, Kost K, Singh S, Henshaw SK and Finer LB. Trends in Abortion in the United States. Clinical Obstetrics and Gynecology 2009; 52(2): pp. 119-29; Health Care Statistics Section, Health Statistics Division. *Therapeutic Abortion Survey.* Ottawa: Statistics Canada, June 2007: 2004-A.
6 National Statistics: Department of Health. *Abortion statistics, England and Wales: 2012.* London: HMSO, 2013, p. 14.
7 Sedgh G, Henshaw SK, Singh S, Bankole A, Drescher J. Legal Abortion Worldwide: Incidence and Recent Trends. IFFP 2007; 33(3): 106-16.

Regimens and Outcomes

Mifepristone + Misoprostol

Mifepristone is an antiprogesterone, which means that it can block progesterone from binding to its receptor. Progesterone, a steroid hormone, plays an active role in maintaining pregnancy by preparing the uterus for implantation of the fetus. Because pregnancy cannot be initiated or continued without progesterone, the antiprogesterone effect of mifepristone causes an abortion. The abortive effects of mifepristone include cervical dilation, decidual necrosis (death of cells in the mucus membrane lining the uterus), shedding of the uterine lining, and an increase in sensitivity towards prostaglandin, a steroid hormone that causes uterine contraction in pregnancy.[8] Although mifepristone can interrupt pregnancy, it alone is insufficient to expel the fetus from the body.[9] Taking advantage of the heightened sensitivity towards prostaglandin, mifepristone is commonly used with a synthetic prostaglandin analog such as misoprostol to induce uterine contraction, leading to the expulsion of the fetus.[10] Without mifepristone, the incidence of complications and side effects from repeated doses of misoprostol would dramatically increase.[11] Mifepristone is also an antiglucocorticoid. Glucocorticoids are hormones that help to diminish the immune response such as inflammation. Thus, as an antiglucocorticoid, mifepristone has the potential to diminish inappropriately the immune response causing the individual to be susceptible to infections. Mifepristone is usually administered in a clinic and patients are usually asked to return 24 to 72 hours later, when misoprostol is administered.

A successful medical abortion is defined as a complete expulsion of the fetus without surgical intervention. Failure can result from: 1) an incomplete abortion, after which the fetus is dead but has not been completely expelled; 2) severe bleeding often requiring a blood transfusion, or other life-threatening conditions requiring surgical intervention; 3) ongoing pregnancy; 4) the patient's request for surgical intervention, usually because of bleeding. The success rate varies from 86 per cent to 96

---

8   Bygdeman M, Swahn ML. Progesterone Receptor Blockage: Effect on uterine contractility and early pregnancy. Contraception 1985; 32(1): pp. 45-51; Hammond C. Recent advances in second-trimester abortion: an evidence-based review. AJOG 2009; 200(4): pp. 347-56.
9   Bartz and Golberg. See n. 3.
10   Ibid.
11   Ibid.

per cent depending on the regimen and the gestational age (the duration of the pregnancy).[12]

The lowest success rate (86 per cent) was reported in a prospective, non-randomized study. It compared the outcome of medical abortion using mifepristone + misoprostol regimen with that of surgical abortion. Within the medical abortion group of 178, fourteen resorted to suction curettage because of bleeding, nine needed it for ongoing pregnancy, while five resorted to it to remedy an incomplete abortion. The failure rate increased with increasing gestational age.[13]

Other studies reported a much higher success rate than Jensen, using a different protocol. Cochrane's meta-analysis of randomized control studies, for example, reported an overall success rate of 96 per cent for first-trimester abortion (up to 63 days of gestation). Moreover, in many studies—unlike Jensen's—patients were given multiple doses of misoprostol to ensure that the abortion was complete.[14] In a retrospective study of 932 abortions cases in Britain, Child and colleagues found a 9.8 per cent failure rate for medical abortion in which mifepristone and misoprostol were used, compared to 5.5 per cent for surgical abortion. Furthermore, women who previously delivered three or more births were more at risk of failed medical abortion than surgical.[15]

Researchers found higher failure rates in developing countries.[16] They also noted that the failure rate of medical abortion increased with increasing gestational age. In Cuba the failure rate rose from seven per cent at six weeks to 22 per cent at eight weeks.[17]

---

12 Jensen, Astley, Morgan and Nichols. See Chapter 6, n. 17; Ashok P, Templeton A, Wagaarachchi P, Fleet G. Factors affecting the outcome of early medical abortion: a review of 4132 consecutive cases. BJOG 2002; 109: pp. 1281-9; Tang O, Xu J, Cheng L, Lee S, Ho P. Pilot study on the use of sublingual misoprostol with mifepristone in termination of first trimester pregnancy to 9 weeks gestation. Human Reproduction 2002; 17(7): pp. 1738-40; Bartz and Golberg. See n. 3, pp. 140-50; Child TJ, Thomas J, Rees M, MacKenzie IZ. A comparative study of surgical and medical procedures: 932 pregnancy terminations up to 63 days gestation. Human Reproduction 2001; 16(1): pp. 67-71.
13 Jensen, Astley, Morgan and Nichols. See Chapter 6, n. 17.
14 Kulier R, Gulmezoglu AM, Hofmeyr GJ, Cheng LN, Campana A. Medical methods for first trimester abortion. Cochrane Database of Systematic Reviews 2004,Issue 1. Art. No. CD002855.
15 Child et al. See n. 12, pp. 67-71.
16 Winikoff B, Sivin I, Coyaji K, et al. Safety, efficacy and acceptability of medical abortion in China, Cuba, and India: A comparative trial of mifepristone-misoprostol versus surgical abortion. AJOG 1996; 176(2): pp. 431-7.
17 Ibid.

Table 13.1 **Overall Failure Rate - Medical vs. Surgical Abortion**

	China (%)	India (%)	Cuba (%)	Britain (%)
Medical	8.4	5.2	16.0	9.8
Surgical	0.4	4.0	0.0	5.5

Sources: Winikoff B, Sivin I, Coyaji K, et al. Safety, efficacy and acceptability of medical abortion in China, Cuba, and India: A comparative trial of mifepristone-misoprostol versus surgical abortion. American Journal of Obstetrics and Gynecology 1996; 176(2): pp. 431-7; Child TJ, Thomas J, Rees M, MacKenzie IZ. A comparative study of surgical and medical procedures: 932 pregnancy terminations up to 63 days gestation. Human Reproduction 2001; 16(1): pp. 67-71.

Although medical abortion is generally not recommended beyond nine weeks' gestation of pregnancy, second-trimester (beyond 69 days or nine to ten weeks' gestation) abortions do occur on a large scale. Second-trimester medical abortion constitutes ten to fifteen per cent of all induced abortion worldwide.[18] One study found that "the risk of death [for the mother] increased exponentially by 38 per cent for each additional week of gestation."[19]

Misoprostol Alone

Misoprostol has been studied and used extensively for cervical dilation, postpartum hemorrhage, and induction of labour and abortion.[20] Misoprostol-alone regimen is considered an attractive alternative to the widely-used mifepristone-misoprostol regimen because it is cheap and can be stored without refrigeration.[21] Other abortifacients such as mifepristone and gemeprost are more expensive and require refrigeration. Since misoprostol alone is not approved for use in abortion in many countries including the United States, it is considered off-labelled.[22] There are only a few randomized controlled studies that compare the misoprostol alone regimen with other combined regimens.

---

18 Gemzell-Danielsson K, Lalitkumar S. Second trimester medical abortion with mifepristone—misoprostol and misoprostol alone: a review of methods and management. Reproductive Health Matters 2008; 6(31): pp. 162-72.
19 Barlett LA, Berg CJ, Shulman HB et al. Risk factors for legal induced abortion-related mortality in the United States. Obstetrics and Gynecology 2004; 103(4): pp. 729-37.
20 Bartz and Golberg. See n. 3, pp. 140-50.
21 Ibid.
22 Ibid.

The 2004 Cochrane systematic review concluded that misoprostol alone is less effective than other combined regimens (e.g., methotrexate + misoprostol, mifepristone + misoprostol, tamoxifin + misoprostol).[23] Use of the misoprostol alone regimen in the second trimester is less common and failure rates are sharply higher than in the first trimester. One study found that misoprostol alone in the second trimester failed nineteen per cent of the time.[24]

In summary, the available randomized studies suggest that misoprostol alone regimen is less effective than other combined regimens. It may take repeated doses of misoprostol to achieve pregnancy termination, and the repeated doses may increase the incidence of side effects such as vomiting, diarrhea, abdominal pain, severe bleeding, and nausea.

Methotrexate + Misoprostol

Methotrexate is a folic acid antagonist that inhibits DNA synthesis and is normally used as a cancer treatment because of its ability to inhibit the growth of rapidly dividing cells.[25] In an abortion methotrexate inhibits the growth of the rapidly developing embryo, leading to the embryo's death. Methotrexate is used in Canada instead of mifepristone owing to a death that occurred during mifepristone's clinical trial.[26] Side effects from methotrexate include nausea, vomiting, headaches, and mouth sores.[27] A major drawback is that it may take up to four weeks to complete an abortion for women using this drug, compared to up to 48 hours for mifepristone.[28] If a complete abortion does not occur in four weeks using methotrexate, surgical intervention is often required.[29] In Cochrane's meta-analysis, methotrexate combined with misoprostol showed an overall success rate of over 90 per cent.[30]

---

23   Kulier et al. See n. 14.
24   Autry AM, Hayes EC, Jacobson GF, and colleagues. A comparison of medical induction and dilation and evacuation for second-trimester abortion. AJOG 2002; 187(2): pp. 393-7.
25   Kulier et al. See n. 14.
26   Laliberte J. Still no mifepristone for Canada: is it safe? National Review of Medicine 2005; 2(16): p. 1.
27   Moreno-Ruiz NL, Borgatta L, Yanow S, et al. Alternatives to mifepristone for early medical abortion. International Journal of Gynaecology and Obstetrics 2005; 96(3): pp. 212-18.
28   Bartz and Golberg. See n. 3, pp. 140-50.
29   Ibid.
30   Kulier et al. See n. 14.

DEATHS

Medical abortion is widely assumed to be a 'safe and effective procedure.' Yet in 2005, four American deaths were linked to medical abortion[31] after the women succumbed to toxic shock associated with clostridium sordellii (bacteria) infection. In Canada, one woman died during a mifepristone-misoprostol trial from the same bacterial infection.[32] By the end of 2006, in the United States, eight reported deaths were associated with the use of mifepristone.[33]

Although the connection between medical abortion and septic shock syndrome remains unclear, medical researchers have found that intrauterine delivery of misoprostol in rats "significantly worsened mortality from C. Sordellii uterine infection." Misoprostol inhibited the production of an important inflammatory cytokine, TNF α.[34] This cytokine, found in both humans and animals, is crucial in controlling bacterial infections. In addition, misoprostol inhibited the ability of macrophages (important cells in the immune system) to eliminate C. Sordelli and suppressed the ability of local endothelial cells to defend the body from invading microbes. Investigators concluded that "high local concentrations of misoprostol suppress innate immune defenses against C. Sordellii within the mice's reproductive tract."[35] If misoprostol does indeed disrupt the innate immune system, women undergoing medical abortion will be vulnerable to potentially life-threatening infections.

SIDE EFFECTS

Its side effects are one of the most disturbing features of medical abortion. In a recent literature review of medical abortion in the second trimester, Grossman and colleagues found that women who underwent medical abortion experienced a 29 per cent rate of adverse effects, while those undergoing surgical abortions experienced a four per cent rate. The adverse effects included nausea, vomiting, severe stomach pain and bleeding,

---

31 Fischer M, Bhatnagar J et al. Fatal toxic shock syndrome associated with clostridium sordellii after medical abortion. NEJM 2005; 353:2352-60, p. 2352.
32 Laliberte J. See n. 26, p. 1.
33 Gary M, Harrison D. Analysis of severe adverse events related to the use of mifepristone as an abortifacient. Annals of Pharmacotherapy 2006; 40: pp. 191-7.
34 Aronoff D, Hao Y, Chung J, et al. Misoprostol impairs reproductive tract's innate response to c. sordellii. Journal of Immunology 2008; 180: pp. 8222-30.
35 Gary and Harrison. See n. 33, pp. 191-7.

infection, uterine perforation and uterine rupture.[36] Several other studies of first and second trimester medical abortions have come up with similar findings.[37] The severity of side effects varies according to the regimen and gestational age; the greater the gestational age, the greater the risk of complications.[38]

Other serious complications such as ectopic pregnancy can also occur. During the first year of clinical use of mifepristone and misoprostol in the US, five ectopic pregnancies linked to medical abortion were reported, with one resulting in death.[39] One major study[40] found that nine per cent of women who undergo medical abortion suffer emergency complications. Another systematic analysis of morbidity and mortality of mifepristone found that infection and hemorrhaging were the leading complications. The authors also discovered that the reporting to the Food and Drug Administration of adverse events due to mifepristone is "grossly deficient" and inadequate.[41]

Misoprostol is used in many third-world countries because it is cheaper and more available than other abortion methods. Yet when a medical abortion fails, the children who survive are at great risk of developing Möbius syndrome, a congenital neurological disorder associated with facial paralysis.[42] One study has determined that 49 per cent of mothers with

---

36   Grossman D, Blachard K, Blumenthal P. Complications after second trimester surgical and medical abortion. Reproductive Health Matters 2008; 16 (31): 173-182.
37   Winikoff B, Sivin I, Coyaji KJ, Cabezas E, Xiao B, Gu S, Du MK, Krishna UR, Eschen A, Ellertson C. Safety, efficacy, and acceptability of medical abortion in China, Cuba, and India: a comparative trial of mifepristone-misoprostol versus surgical abortion. AJ OG 1997 Feb; 176(2):431-7; Tang OS, Xu J, Cheng L, Lee SW, Ho PC. Pilot study on the use of sublingual misoprostol with mifepristone in termination of first trimester pregnancy up to 9 weeks gestation. Human Reproduction 2002 July; 17(7):1738-40; Gemzell-Danielsson K, Lalitkumar S. Second trimester medical abortion with mifepristone-misoprostol and misoprostol alone: a review of methods and management. Reproductive Health Matters 2008 May; 16 (31 Suppl):162-72. doi: 10.1016/S0968-8080(08)31371-8.
38   Henshaw RC, Naji SA, Russell IT, Templeton AA. A comparison of medical abortion (using mifepristone and gemeprost) with surgical vacuum aspiration: efficacy and early medical sequelae. Human Reproduction 1994; 9(11): 2167—72.
39   Hausknecht R. Mifepristone and misoprostol for early medical abortion: 18 months experience in the United States. Contraception, 2003; 67: pp. 463-5.
40   Child et al. See n. 12.
41   Gary and Harrison. See n. 33.
42   Gonzalez C, Marques-Dias MJ, Kim CA, et al. Congenital abnormalities in Brazilian children associated with misoprostol misuse in first trimester of pregnancy. The Lancet 1998; 351: pp. 1624-7; Marques-Dias MJ, Gonzalez CH, Rosemberg S. Möbius sequence in children exposed *in utero* to misoprostol: neuropathological study of three cases. Birth Defects Research (Part A) 2003; 67(12): pp. 1002-7.

Möbius infants used misoprostol in the first trimester.[43] In other words, about half of the babies who suffered from Möbius in these cases were survivors of medical abortion. Consider the significance of this finding for Brazil, where it is estimated that three-quarters of all abortions are induced by misoprostol, but up to 80 per cent fail. It is known that approximately twenty per cent of those infants who survive medical abortion develop Möbius syndrome.[44] A recent systematic review has confirmed the strong association between fetal exposure to misoprostol and later development of Möbius syndrome.[45]

Risk to the fetus from misoprostol is of concern because many women decide to carry their pregnancy to term after a failed medical abortion. Yet the relative lack of research and the absence of discussion on this topic in many reviews of medical abortion reviews, suggest a lack of concern. Much effort is now dedicated to improving the efficacy of medical abortion but little attention is paid to its many infant survivors.

Finally, there are few studies on the effect that misoprostol or mifepristone has on the women and their babies after failed medical abortion. In most studies, surgical abortion is provided for participants if medical abortion fails. However, affordable surgical abortion is not always possible, a reality in developing nations, nor is it always desirable. What happens to the woman and her baby then? What are the consequences if a woman changes her mind and decides to go on with her pregnancy? These are questions that require further investigation, as they are vital in helping patients make informed decisions.

Conclusion

As the ratio of medical abortions to all induced abortions continues to rise, it is important that we know more about its safety and effectiveness. Mifepristone-misoprostol and methotrexate-misoprostol regimens have been shown to be relatively effective in terminating pregnancy while the misoprostol-alone regimen has been reported to be less effective. The

---

43   Pastuszak AL, Schüler L, Speck-Martins CE, et al. Use of misoprostol during pregnancy and Möbius syndrome in infants. NEJM 1998; 338: pp. 1881-5.
44   Miller G. Neurological Disorders: The Mystery of the Missing Smile. Science 2007; 316(5826): pp. 826-7.
45   Pizzo T, Knop F Mengue S. Prenatal exposure to misoprostol and congenital anomalies: Systematic review and meta-analysis. Reproductive Toxicology 2006; 22(4): pp. 666-71.

overall failure rate of chemical abortion is not less than four per cent, while some studies suggest that in poor countries it may be as high as 80 per cent. Minor side effects are common, while serious and lethal complications such as fatal toxic shock syndrome, hemorrhages, and ectopic pregnancies are also familiar phenomena. Much current effort is dedicated to making the drugs more available globally. However, the lack of research on the teratogenicity (ability to cause birth defects) of the three commonly-used drugs is troubling. What happens if medical abortion fails and surgical abortion is not available, or not desired? Given the increasing resort to medical abortion in developing countries, these realities generate a serious health crisis, especially where there is limited public health care.

Chapter 14

Multi-fetal pregnancy reduction (MFPR)

KEY POINTS

- For couples who cannot conceive, there is a very strong motivation to do whatever is medically recommended in order to have a child.

- *In vitro* fertilization (IVF) is often used in cases of long-term infertility, sometimes requiring as many as nine cycles of treatment before conception takes place. The result is often three or more implanted fetuses.

- Multi-fetal pregnancy reduction (MFPR) is a form of abortion (a needle stab to the heart) to reduce the number of fetuses produced by IVF. MFPR does not guarantee that the remaining fetuses will remain healthy, but it usually results in at least one live birth.

- Parents' reactions to the loss of some of the fetuses conceived are similar to those experienced after abortion for genetic reasons: sadness, guilt, and depression.

- Too often medical professionals do not obtain genuine informed consent from parents, or give them a choice about the number of fetuses to be kept alive.

- More unbiased research needs to be done into the effects of MFPR on couples and on their future family life with the surviving babies.

INTRODUCTION

Multi-fetal pregnancy reduction (MFPR) is the unexpected and ironical result of the desperate desire of many infertile couples to have a child. Here is how one woman has expressed her distress at not being able to conceive:

> You can't have a baby—a numbness beyond desperation. Baby lust—do you know how it feels to want a baby so much that every other activity in life, everything you've worked for and planned for—jobs, friends, family, marriage, seem hollow as a tin can? To be in emotional pain so extreme that when you see a pregnant woman's stomach or a newborn baby the pain becomes physical?[1]

Reproductive technologies, specifically *in vitro* fertilization (IVF), have answered the emotional pain of many such women. Ironically, IVF often brings couples face-to-face with abortion: Assisted reproduction typically entails the implantation of multiple embryos, with the expectation by medical staff that the number of fetuses will later be reduced in a process by which selected fetuses are terminated by puncturing their heart.

The justification for aborting these fetuses is that it will increase the chances of carrying at least one embryo to term, but the research on which this is based is usually carried out by the practitioners and advocates of the procedure. Furthermore, analysis of the results has not shown that MFPR actually improves the chances for a healthy birth. Many critics are calling for a limit on the number of embryos that are implanted at each fertilization.

There is also the question of whether MFPR involves "informed consent" on the part of the parents because the medical profession has tended to assume that parents would not want several babies and doctors may not offer parents a choice about how many babies they can keep. The aftermath of MFPR for some parents, now apparent as they seek therapy, is feelings of pain, frustration, sadness, and guilt, and a sense that they have been coerced by the medical staff into aborting some of their babies. Up to this point there are few studies looking into the impact of multi-fetal abortions on family life with the surviving babies. It is clear that further research needs to be done on the wider impact of MFPR.

---

1   Blomain K. "You Can't Have a Baby—A Numbness Beyond Desperation." [Customer Review of An Empty Lap: One Couple's Journey to Parenthood, by Jill Smolowe]. October 31, 1997. http://www.amazon.com/exec/obidos/tg/stores/detail//books/0671004379/customer- reviews/107-9690183-1333303.

IN VITRO FERTILIZATION AND PREVALENCE OF PREGNANCY REDUCTION

Just as reproductive technologies have changed obstetrical practice, so too have they led to a type of abortion that affects a different population of pregnant women from those who do not want to be pregnant. These women want very much to have a child, and it is ironic that they and their partners who are suffering the problems of infertility must often come face-to-face with abortion.

With the challenge of infertility in North America has come the medical response that has grown into a major fertility industry. But IVF is not only medically invasive; it is far from being a "sure thing". Parents desperate to have a baby often undergo several cycles of treatment in an effort to achieve a successful pregnancy. Each treatment may increase the odds of having a baby, but each attempt entails psychological, physical and financial costs.

The financial cost in Canada is outlined in the table below:

Table 14.1 **Success rate and financial costs of *in vitro* fertilization in Canada**

Number of cycles	Percentage of live births	Financial cost in $
First	6-43	8800
After 3	52	26,400
After 6	72	52,800
After 12	85	105,600

Sources: Gnoth C, Maxrath B, Skonieczny T, Friol K, Godehardt E, Tigges J. Final ART success rates: a 10 years survey. Human Reproduction 2011; 26(8):2239-46; IVF.CA accessed at http://www.ivf.ca/faq.htm

The above data show that between fifteen and 57 per cent of those who begin Artificial Reproductive Therapy (ART) never achieve a pregnancy that leads to the birth of a living infant.

In 2003 the Centers for Disease Control reported that the number of embryos implanted was influenced by the age of the mother.[2] The older the mother the larger was the number of embryos transferred:

Table 14.2 **Average number of embryos transferred to each mother in the US**

Age of Women	Number of embryos transferred	Percentage of the Time
under 35 years	3 or more	46
	2 or more	95
35-37 years	3 or more	70
	2 or more	93
38-40 years	3 or more	69
	2 or more	90
41-42 years	3 or more	70
	2 or more	88
over 42 years	3 or more	63
	2 or more	83

Source: Wright VC, Chang J, Jeng G, Macaluso, M. Assisted reproductive technology surveillance - United States, 2003.Division of Reproductive Health National Center for Chronic Disease Prevention and Health Promotion. May 26, 2006; 55(SS04);1-22. http://www.cdc.gov/mmwr/preview/mmwrhtml/ss5504a1.htm

---

2   Wright VC, Chang J, Jeng G, Macaluso, M. Assisted reproductive technology surveillance - United States, 2003.Division of Reproductive Health National Center for Chronic Disease Prevention and Health Promotion. May 26, 2006; 55(SS04); 1-22. http://www.cdc.gov/mmwr/preview/mmwrhtml/ss5504a1.htm

As a result of multiple embryos being implanted the number of twin deliveries has increased by 65 per cent and higher order births by 400 per cent in the last two decades.[3] In 2003, 51 per cent of infants born after ART treatment were in multiple birth deliveries.[4] Then Stone, Berkowitz and colleagues published trends in MFPR at their clinic, indicating that while four per cent of their cases from 1986 to 1999 started as twins, that number had jumped to fifteen per cent of cases between 1999 and 2006. This is happening in spite of the fact that French authors continue to report that "there is generally no medical indication for MFPR in twins."[5] No matter what the starting number of fetuses in a pregnancy, the most recent research indicates that over 40 per cent of MFPRs at Berkowitz's clinic now end as singleton pregnancies, and this percentage continues to rise.[6]

In an attempt to reduce the risk of fetal loss or infant morbidity the practice of MFPR has been refined to reduce the number of fetuses implanted, which explains the recent increasing trend.

JUSTIFICATION FOR MFPR

The medical justification for performing multi-fetal pregnancy reduction is philosophically similar to the "lifeboat" theory: it is morally acceptable to sacrifice some "innocent" fetal lives in order to increase the chances of survival, or decrease the risk of serious morbidity, for the ones who remain.[7] Multiple pregnancies are often associated with increased complications because of the high rate of preterm birth, as well as other complications such as malformations, twin-to-twin transfusion syndrome, preeclampsia, gestational diabetes, postpartum hemorrhage, and fetal or maternal death. MFPR reduces these risks. This is why Lee and colleagues state that "these results suggest that MFPR of higher-order pregnancies to twins is a *medically*

---

3   Antsaklis A, Anastasakis E. Selective reduction in twins and multiple pregnancies. Journal of Perinatal Medicine 2011; 39:15-21.
4   Wright VC, Chang J, Jeng G, Macaluso M. Assisted reproductive technology surveillance—United States, 2003.MMWR Surveillance Summary 2006; 55(4):1-22.
5   Sentilhes L, Audibert F, Dommerques M, Descamps P, Frydman R, Mahieu-Caputo D. Multifetal pregnancy reduction : indications, technical aspects and psychological impact. Presse Medicale 2008; 37(2 Pt 2): 295-306.
6   Stone J, Belogolovkin V, Matho A, Berkowitz RL, Moshier E, Eddleman K. Evolving trends in 2000 cases of multifetal pregnancy reduction: a single-center experience. AJOG 2007; 197: 394.e1-394.e4.
7   Berkowitz RL, Lynch L, Stone J, Alvarez M. The current status of multi-fetal pregnancy reduction. AJOG 1996 April; 174(4): 1265-72; p. 1270.

justifiable procedure"[8] (emphasis added).

Using the information from chorionic villi sampling or amniocentesis, many doctors recommend that higher order pregnancies be reduced to twin or singleton pregnancies by the strategic feticide of one or more of the developing fetuses. This practice has become so widespread in the ART industry that vulnerable couples desperate to have a live child feel compelled to agree to this procedure. Doctors often frame the choice in terms of infant health. Parents are presented with an option of having several unhealthy babies or one or two healthy ones. The way this procedure is presented and the fact that this is recommended to all women with multiple Artificial Reproductive Therapy (ART) pregnancies reflects the industry belief that "… MFPR of higher-order pregnancies to twins is a medically justifiable procedure."[9]

From this widely accepted practice comes a push to have reductions done well past the age of viability. Hern presented case studies of selective termination at 32 or more weeks gestation for fetal anomaly,[10] while Shalev and colleagues propose doing MFPR at 28 to 30 weeks,[11] as well as calling for reduction of even naturally occurring twin pregnancies to a singleton pregnancy. The rationale for this is since abortion is legal and available in the US it is a woman's right to have one of her twins terminated and the other continue to term.

While many researchers end their studies with a call for curbs on the number of embryos that are implanted (which would reduce the likelihood of higher order multiple births to near-natural levels),[12] many other continuing studies are committed to the improvement of the techniques for MFPR. What is interesting about the studies in this area is the high degree of overlap between researchers. The twelve most prolific writers in this

---

8   Lee JR, Ku SY, Jee BC, Suh CS, Kim KC, Kim SH. Pregnancy outcomes of different methods for multifetal pregnancy reduction: A comparative study. J Korean Med Sci. 2008; 23(1): 111-18.
9   Ibid.
10   Hern WM. Selective termination for fetal anomaly/genetic disorder in twin pregnancy at 32+ menstrual weeks. Fetal Diagnostic Therapy 2004; 19: 292-5.
11   Shalev J, Meizner I, Rabinerson D, Mashiach R, Hod M, Bar-Chava I, Peleg D, Ben-Rafael Z. Improving pregnancy outcome in twin gestations with one malformed fetus by postponing selective feticide in the third trimester. Fertility and Sterility 1999; 72(2): 257-60.
12   Cohen J. How to avoid multiple pregnancies in assisted reproduction. Human Reproduction 1998 June; 13(Supplement 3):197-214; discussion 215-18; p. 197.

field all cite each other and often collaborate on research.[13] This self-referral or "incestuous citation"[14] is similar to that found in the general abortion literature. As in the other abortion areas the majority of these researchers are themselves practitioners of the MFPR procedure and some are also advocates for it, and are cited as experts on the probity of the procedure.

The procedure for aborting some of the fetuses in multiple pregnancies has been improved and expanded to the point that all major teaching hospitals in North America and Western Europe now routinely offer couples MFPR as an option for management of multiple pregnancies. One problem, however, is that the couple who never imagined themselves actually having a single child, and who have succeeded thanks to advanced IVF techniques, may feel themselves to be faced with what auto dealers call a "mandatory option" in dealing with their unexpected bounty. For many couples their new situation is very uncomfortable, not least because the gestational age at which these abortions are occurring has steadily increased to the point where Evans and colleagues are supporting the use of the technique into the third trimester (after 26 weeks of pregnancy).[15]

COMPARED TO GENETIC ABORTIONS

In an attempt to make the use of MFPR a more readily-accepted part of obstetrical practice, the literature links the procedure to the already well-tolerated practice of abortion for genetic or fetal abnormality. The proponents of this technique believe the linkage addresses two important concerns: First, they conclude that most patients will not tolerate multiple births, so the use of MFPR will avoid the "trauma"[16] of the abortion of a wanted pregnancy on the grounds that the patient will choose to abort one or more of the embryos rather than give birth to several children. Second, MFPR will lead to the ultimate goal of having one's own child. This ethical justification has also been articulated by Chevernak and colleagues who

---

13 Cassidy E. Multifetal Pregnancy Reduction (MFPR): The psychology of desperation and the ethics of justification. In Life and Learning IX: Proceedings of Ninth Annual Meeting, University Faculty for Life in Trinity International University 1999, ed. Koterski, JW; 1999 331-46. Washington, D.C.: University Faculty for Life, 2000.
14 Crutcher M. *Lime 5: Exploited by Choice*. Denton, Texas: Life Dynamics, 1996.
15 Evans MI, Goldberg JD, Horenstein J, Wapner RJ, Ayoub MA, Stone J, et al. Selective termination for structural, chromosomal, and Mendelian anomalies: international experience. AJOG 1999 October;181(4): 893-7.
16 Evans MI, Quintero RA, Fletcher JC. Ethical issues surrounding multifetal pregnancy reduction and selective termination. Clinical Perinatology 1996 September; 23(3): 437-51.

express it in terms of three goals:

1. achieving a pregnancy that results in a live birth of one or more infants with minimal neonatal morbidity and mortality;
2. achieving a pregnancy that results in the birth of one or more infants without antenatally detected anomalies;
3. achieving a pregnancy that results in a singleton live birth.[17]

The research literature assumes that parents faced with the potential birth of three to seven children are "free" to choose to abort most of them to achieve a family size of their choice. However, individuals acting out of desperation are not "free", and without freedom there is no true choice. The psychological impact of coercive choice is well documented in the decision-making literature. Miller delineated several models that apply to the decision to abort[18] and Cassidy expanded upon these in relation to decision-making in abortions for fetal abnormality.[19] The consensus among psychologists is that major life decisions based on perceived or overt coercion result in significant psychological distress.

In North America the prevailing model for making medical decisions is based on the concept of "personal autonomy" and informed consent, which have become cornerstones for the ethical acceptability for all medical procedures.[20] Often however, the decisions taken by couples to reduce the number of fetuses can be seen as lacking true personal autonomy because of parental desperation, medical coercion, and a lack of informed consent.

LACK OF INFORMED CONSENT

A couple's capacity to give full assent is badly compromised owing to the pre-existing psychological trauma brought on by long-term infertility and the IVF process itself. As the number of these multi-fetal abortions

---

17   Chervenak FA, McCullough LB, Wapner R. Three ethically justified indications for selective termination in multifetal pregnancy: A practical and comprehensive management strategy. Journal of Assisted Reproduction and Genetics 1995 September; 12(8): 531-6; p. 531.
18   Miller WB. An empirical study of the psychological antecedents and consequences of induced abortion. Journal of Social Issues 1992 Fall; 48(3): 67-93.
19   Cassidy E. Psychological decision-making models: an extension of Miller's abortion decision models to miscarriage and genetic abortion in light of the human genome project [Unpublished Conference Paper]. University Faculty for Life, 1997 June.
20   Beckwith FJ. Absolute autonomy and physician-assisted suicide: Putting a bad idea out of its misery. Joseph Koterski SJ, ed. Life and Learning VII. Seventh University Faculty for Life Conference; 1997; Loyola College, Baltimore. Washington, D.C.: University Faculty for Life, 1998.

grows, the families involved are now coming forward to discuss pursuant issues that are only just beginning to be dealt with in the clinical therapy and post-abortion healing literature. Kluger-Bell describes a family of triplets whose IVF resulted in a quad pregnancy. As her client notes "...I really didn't feel like I had a whole lot of choice about reducing it. And I was pretty much told by the doctors, 'Oh, well, you're not going to *carry* that many babies.' And most likely it would have to be reduced to two. And not knowing anything about it, we thought that was just the way it was." It was only when this family firmly expressed their desire to have all four babies that the doctors agreed to leave three. The MFPR was successful, "but emotionally there's still an ache that will probably always be there. We had been trying for so many years to create life, it was very contradictory and painful...no one ever said we could *consider* keeping all four...why wasn't that an option?"[21]

Ninety-nine per cent of the women who go through fetal reduction had achieved pregnancy through infertility treatment. Therefore, they represent a group which Tabsh describes as "...highly motivated to have a successful pregnancy outcome. They tend to be compliant with the medical plan for their care..."[22] and will therefore, as Macones and Wapner imply, assent to whatever approach will most likely assure them of a healthy child. In general, women seeking such an outcome will do anything the medical experts deem necessary.[23]

The attitude of infertility patients towards multiple births was not investigated until the mid-nineties. It was then that Gleicher and colleagues found that the medical profession's implementation of MFPR was being made without input from patient populations:

> [Infertile patients] express a considerable desire for multiple births...The medical profession so far has assumed that the decision to minimize multiple births...was reflective of patient desires. This study suggests otherwise.[24]

---

21 Kluger-Bell K. *Unspeakable Losses: Understanding the Experience of Pregnancy Loss, Miscarriage, and Abortion*. New York: W.W. Norton, 1998, pp. 92-4.
22 Tabsh KM. A report of 131 cases of multifetal pregnancy reduction. Obstetrics & Gynecology 1993 July; 82(1): 57-60.
23 Macones GA, Schemmer G, Pritts E, Weinblatt V, Wapner RJ. Multifetal reduction of triplets to twins improves perinatal outcome. AJOG 1993 October; 169(4): 982-6.
24 Gleicher N, Campbell DP, Chan CL, Karande V, Rao R, Balin M, et al. The desire for multiple births in couples with infertility problems contradicts present practice patterns. Human Reproduction 1995 May; 10(5): 1079-84.

Britt and Evans note that doctors often pose the choice to parents as having, for example, four "unhealthy babies", or two "healthy" ones, in which case the decision is "simple." Rather than offering a clear choice, some medical professionals give parents the sense of *"having to reduce."*[25]

The ethical justification for MFPR is the desperate desire of parents to have a healthy baby. But what is the psychological price?

To desperate people, the avenue that promises the greatest hope may appear to be the morally best option, especially if pregnancy reduction is presented as the medically appropriate decision—the decision that will guarantee them one live baby. To refuse such an option requires freedom from coercion and access to other management approaches that provide alternatives. It is clear that these couples do not meet the criterion for free choice and, indeed, the actual level of coercion in this procedure is striking in the recent literature on surrogacy.

MEDICAL OUTCOMES OF MULTIFETAL PREGNANCY REDUCTIONS

The main rationale for MFPR is the birth of at least one healthy child. Does MFPR actually guarantee this? This is a matter of debate. Berkowitz has written of the politics and ethics of reducing twins to singletons, stating that "no data suggest that this procedure significantly improves perinatal outcome,"[26] however since abortion was available on demand in the United States, it was a woman's right to have one twin terminated and the other continue to term. By 2005, Berkowitz's colleagues Evans and Britt reported an increase in the use of MFPR to terminate one twin, and stated that in order to improve outcomes, "reduction of twins to a singleton is now a reasonable consideration."[27]

Nonetheless, Groutz and colleagues found that "contrary to previous studies we found a higher incidence of pregnancy complications after MFPR compared with spontaneous twins...."[28] Souter and Goodwin did a meta-

---

25   Britt DW, Evans MI. Sometimes doing the right thing sucks: Frame combinations and multi-fetal pregnancy reduction difficulty. Social Science & Medicine 2007; 65: 2342-56.
26   Berkowitz RL. From twin to singleton. BMJ 1996; 313: 373.
27   Evans MI, Britt DW. Fetal reduction. SeminPerinatology 2005; 29:321-329.
28   Groutz A, Yovel I, Amit A, Yaron Y, Azem F, Lessing JB. Pregnancy outcome after multifetal pregnancy reduction to twins compared with spontaneously conceived twins. Human Reproduction 1996 June; 11(6): 1334-6; p. 1334.

analysis of all 83 articles published on the procedure since 1989 and found that "there is a general consensus that reducing triplets to twins results in significant secondary benefits: lower cost and fewer days in hospital and a decrease in a variety of moderate morbidities associated with prolonged hospitalizations and preterm delivery for mother and baby. However, *it is not clear that couples are more likely to take home a healthy baby, if they undergo multi-fetal pregnancy reduction.*"[29] (emphasis added).

Why should this be so? It is because, after MFPR, there is still a significant risk of fetal loss. A Swedish study identified the presence of post-procedure full miscarriage in 21 per cent of the cases undertaken in that country, a further eighteen per cent died in the womb or shortly after birth, or were born with defects.[30] Likewise, Elliott has suggested that studies of properly managed triplet pregnancies "show an equal or better outcome with non-reduced triplets compared with selective reduction."[31] In addition, Stone and colleagues found that fetal loss occurred among eleven per cent of women who started with five or more fetuses, 5.5 per cent for those who started with four, 5.1 per cent for those who started with three, and 2.1 per cent for those who started with two fetuses. It was also found that multiple pregnancies increased the risk of prematurity as well as a number of maternal, fetal and neonatal health risks, including a very high risk of preterm birth (50 per cent among those who undergo MFPR and give birth to twins, and thirteen per cent among those who give birth to a singleton after MFPR).[32]

PSYCHOLOGICAL OUTCOMES OF MFPR

Given the difficulties inherent in the MFPR procedure, it is not surprising that even following the achievement of the goal of parenting a child, couples who have participated in MFPR decisions experience grief and emotional distress similar to that which accompanies the loss of a child. Follow-up studies of these families point to the fact that the parents do not experience significant psychiatric disturbance, and that "the birth of healthy children

---

29 Souter I, Goodwin TM. Decision making in multifetal pregnancy reduction for triplets. American Journal of Perinatology 1998 January; 15(1): 63-71; p. 63.
30 Radestad A, Bui TH, Nygren KG, Koskimies A, Petersen K. The utilization rate and pregnancy outcome of multifetal pregnancy reduction in the Nordic countries. Acta Obstetricia et Gynecologica Scandanavica 1996 August; 75(7): 651-3.
31 Elliott JP. Multifetal reduction of triplets to twins improves perinatal outcome. AJOG 1994 July; 171(1): 278.
32 Stone J, Ferrara L, Kamrath J, Getrajdman J, Berkowitz R, Moshier E, Eddleman K. Contemporary outcomes with the latest 1000 cases of MFPR. AJOG 2008; 199(4): 406 e1-4.

helps reduce the traumatic impact of fetal reduction".[33] What is not stressed in the literature, however, is the following:

- There are significant attrition and refusal rates in study samples.
- Couples who miscarried the whole pregnancy following the procedure are unwilling to participate in follow up.
- There is as yet no study of the full psychological impact on the children who are described by practitioners as "the surviving fetuses."

Given these limitations, the studies that do address the psychological outcomes find that a significant proportion of their sample experience psychological distress following the procedure. The affective reactions are immediate, and intense grief reactions are characterized by repetitive and intrusive thoughts and images of the terminated fetus(es).

Schreiner-Engel and colleagues report that twenty per cent of those willing to participate in follow up experienced long-term *dysphoria*. "Their continued feelings of guilt appeared due to a wishful belief that some better solution should have been found." The characteristics of the most disturbed group were those who were young, religious, came from larger families, wanted more than two children, and viewed the ultrasound of the pregnancy more frequently. The authors conclude that "seeing multiple viable fetuses on repetitive sonograms may interfere with the ability of women to maintain an intellectualized or emotionally detached stance toward the multi-fetal pregnancy."[34] Curiously, the researchers assume that women who have undergone the stress and emotional impact of infertility and subsequent treatment can—and somehow should—be detached from the one thing that has been a driving force in their lives, pregnancy. This expectation goes against all that is known about maternal-infant attachment and psychosocial understanding of the nature of pregnancy.[35] Garel and colleagues had a 44 per cent interview refusal rate among reduction patients. Of those who agreed to be seen at one and two years post-procedure, one-

---

33   McKinney M, Downey J, Timor-Tritsch I. The psychological effects of multi-fetal pregnancy reduction. Fertility and Sterility 1995 July; 64(1): 51-61, p. 59.
34   Schreiner-Engel P, Walther VN, Mindes J, Lynch L, Berkowitz RL. First-trimester multi-fetal pregnancy reduction: acute and persistent psychologic reactions. AJOG 1995 February; 172(2Pt 1): 541-7; pp. 545-6.
35   Campion B. An argument for continuing a pregnancy where the fetus is discovered to be anencephalic. In *Life and Learning IX: Proceedings of Ninth Annual Meeting, University Faculty for Life in Trinity International University 1999*, ed. Koterski, JW. Washington, D.C.: University Faculty for Life, 2000.

third reported "persistent depressive symptoms related to the reduction, mainly sadness and guilt. The others made medical and rational comments expressing no emotion."[36]

In these reactions, the link becomes apparent between the lack of affect as an outcome of elective abortion and a similar lack of emotion among women who undergo abortion in the form of MFPR. Another issue of concern is the psychological impact this will have on parenting interactions with surviving children. About such parents, McKinney and colleagues noted: "Conscious and unconscious responses to the procedure included ambivalence, guilt, and a sense of narcissistic injury, increasing the complexity of their attachment to the remaining babies."[37] No research has yet been done on the long-term implications of parental distress on the psychological development of these children nor have any studies addressed the dynamics of Post-Abortion Survivor Syndrome.

Laffont and Edelmann concluded that long-term infertility that is treated by *in vitro* fertilization (IVF) superimposes cycles of hope and disappointment on the already depressed and vulnerable psyche of couples who are having difficulty conceiving.[38] The process can take up to nine cycles of treatment because few couples conceive on the first attempt. Indeed, the overall success rate of IVF is a matter of continuing controversy. Oddens and colleagues found that for women involved in this treatment psychological well-being may deteriorate after unsuccessful treatment cycles.[39] Both partners experience psychological swings during treatment, and Boivin and colleagues observed that "spouses appeared equally...to respond...with ambivalent feelings involving emotional distress and positive feelings of hope and intimacy."[40] Other researchers find that women report greater negative reactions to IVF failures than men. The coping mechanisms utilized by some women to face the cycles of failure,

---

36 Garel M, Stark C, Blondel B, Lefebvre G, Vauthier-Brouzes D, Zorn JR. Psychological reactions after multifetal pregnancy reduction: A 2-year follow-up study. Human Reproduction 1997 March; 12(3): 617-22; p. 617.
37 McKinney MK, Tuber SB, Downey JI.Multifetal pregnancy reduction: psychodynamic implications. Psychiatry 1996 Winter; 59(4): 393-407, p.393.
38 Laffont I, Edelmann RJ. Psychological aspects of in vitro fertilization: A gender comparison. Journal of Psychosomatic Obstetrics & Gynecology 1994 June; 15(2): 85-92.
39 Oddens BJ, den Tonkelaar I, Nieuwenhuyse H. Psychosocial experiences in women facing fertility problems—a comparative survey. Human Reproduction 1999 January; 14(1): 255-61.
40 Boivin J, Andersson L, Skoog-Svanberg A, Hjelmstedt A, Collins A, Bergh T. Psychological reactions during in-vitro fertilization: Similar response pattern in husbands and wives. Human Reproduction. 1998 November; 13(11): 3262-7, p. 3262.

identified by Lukse and Vacc,[41] are the same denial and desensitization often seen in post-abortion psychopathology.

Following this cyclical emotional roller coaster, the fortunate couple may find themselves pregnant. In increasing numbers, however, these pregnancies are "higher order" with three or more implanted fetuses. "The international rates of triplet or higher order pregnancies after assisted reproduction are 7.3 per cent at conception."[42] In order to deal with such pregnancies, women must put themselves in the care of high-risk obstetrical experts who know the latest research on the new technologies used in the management of multiple pregnancies.

Conclusion

There is still a great deal to be found out on the effects of multifetal pregnancy reduction on parents and on the surviving children of the pregnancy. What research has been done suggests similar reactions to induced abortion; namely, feelings of grief and loss, minimized somewhat by the carrying to term of at least some of the fetuses. Certainly, to enable parents to make decisions about such births, more research needs to be undertaken, and findings need to be shared with them in order for their consent to be truly informed in compliance with current criteria for medical procedures.

---

41   Lukse MP, Vacc NA. Grief, depression, and coping in women undergoing infertility treatment. Obstetrics & Gynecology 1999 February; 93(2): 245-51.

42   Cohen 1998. See n. 12.

Chapter 15

Premature or preterm births after abortion

KEY POINTS

- Women who have had one or more induced abortions have a significantly higher rate of prematurity or preterm birth, and low birth weight in subsequent pregnancies.

- Children who are born prematurely, or with low, or very low birth weights suffer from significantly higher rates of:

  - Infant mortality
  - Cerebral palsy
  - Intellectual impairment
  - Autism
  - Epilepsy
  - Blindness

- The practice of induced abortion is thus responsible for significantly higher social and health costs by causing a higher percentage of children to be born preterm, or with low birth weight.

IS INDUCED ABORTION RESPONSIBLE FOR A HIGHER RATE OF PREMATURE DELIVERY OF SUBSEQUENT PREGNANCIES?

The great majority of women who have had an induced abortion wish to get pregnant again.[1] That is why it is of the utmost importance that women contemplating an abortion should be aware of the possible consequences of that abortion for a subsequent pregnancy.

Thanks to two recently-published systematic reviews it is now settled science that women who have had one or more induced abortions significantly increase their chances of later giving birth to a preterm or low-birth-weight child. Shah and colleagues analyzed 37 sound studies, and determined that the adjusted estimate of increased risk of low birth weight births was 24 per cent after one abortion, and 47 per cent after more than one abortion. The adjusted risk of preterm birth—meaning under 37 weeks' gestation—increased by 27 per cent after one abortion, and 62 per cent after two or more abortions.[2] Swingle and colleagues reviewed 21 sound studies and concluded that one induced abortion increased the adjusted risk of a subsequent preterm birth by 25 per cent, while two or more abortions increased the risk by 51 per cent (Adjusted risk, means after other variables such as income, age and marital status have been taken account of). More important, they found that women with prior induced abortions have 64 per cent higher risk of a very preterm delivery (under 32 weeks' gestation) compared to women with no prior induced abortions.[3] Both these studies confirm the "dose-response" effect; in other words, the more abortions a woman has, the greater her risk of later having a preterm and/or low birth weight child. Why should this be so? The explanation is that in a surgical abortion the cervix is forced open, thereby weakening it. The more abortions a woman has, the weaker her cervix is likely to become.

The real-life impact of the link between abortion and prematurity is suggested by the experience of black American women. For some time it has been known that they have an almost four times greater risk of delivering an extremely preterm baby (under 28 weeks' gestation) than

---

1   Shah PS, Zao J. Induced termination of pregnancy and low birth weight and preterm birth: a systematic review and meta-analyses. BJOG: An International Journal of Obstetrics & Gynaecology May 2009; 116(11): 1425-42, p. 1439.
2   Ibid, pp. 1436-9.
3   Swingle HM, Colaizy TT, Zimmerman MB, Morriss FH. Abortion and the risk of subsequent preterm birth. Journal of Reproductive Medicine 2009 February; 54(2): pp. 95-108.

non-black American women.[4] Strikingly, it has recently come to light that they also have a more than four times greater rate of induced abortion than non-black American women.[5] These findings are reinforced by a massive Scottish study of more than a million pregnancies over a 26-year period, recently presented to the European Society of Human Reproduction and Embryology conference in Stockholm. Scottish women who have had only one abortion are 37 per cent more likely to have a premature birth than those pregnant for the first time.[6] Finally, earlier this year a Canadian study of over 6000 women revealed that those who had already experienced a miscarriage, abortion or ectopic pregnancy were 40 per cent more likely to have a preterm birth from their next pregnancy.[7] Another Canadian study, published a few weeks later, found that women who reported one prior induced abortion had an increased risk, ranging from 45 to 117 per cent, of subsequently bearing a preterm child. The risks were even higher for women with two or more previous abortions.[8]

Table 15.1 **Increased risks of preterm birth after one induced abortion**

Weeks gestation	adjusted odds ratio (OR)
32	1.45
28	1.71
26	2.17

Source: Hardy G, Benjamin A, Abenhaim HA. Effect of induced abortions on early preterm births and adverse perinatal outcomes. J Obstetrics and Gynaecology of Canada 2013 February; 35(2): p. 141.

---

4   Behrman RS, Butler AS, Alexander GR. *Preterm birth: causes, consequences, and prevention.* Washington, DC: National Academy Press, 2007, p. 76.
5   Rooney B, Calhoun BC, Roche LE. Does induced abortion account for racial disparity in preterm births, and violate the Nuremberg Code? Journal of American Physicians and Surgeons 2008; 13(4): pp. 102-4.
6   Bhattacharya S, Lowit A et al. Reproductive outcomes following induced abortion: a national register-based cohort study in Scotland. BMJ Open 2012; 2:e000911.doi:10.1136/bmjopen-2012-000911, p. 1.
7   Heaman M, Kingston D, Chalmers B, Sauve R, Lee L, Young D. Risk factors for preterm birth and small-for-gestational age births among Canadian women. Paediatric and Perinatal Epidemiology 2013; 27(1): 54-61, p. 58 (Table 2). The adjusted OR was 1.4; the unadjusted OR was 1.5, meaning a 50% greater risk of having a preterm birth. (p. 57, Table 1).
8   Hardy G, Benjamin A, Abenhaim HA. Effect of induced abortions on early preterm births and adverse perinatal outcomes. JOGC 2013 February; 35(2): 138-43, Table 2, p. 141.

What Are the Health Risks That Accompany Premature Births?

Infants who do not reach a gestational age of 37 weeks or more have a much lower chance of reaching adulthood than those who do, as Table 15.2 illustrates.

Table 15.2 **Percentage of infants who survive to adulthood by gestational age**[9]

Gestational age in weeks	Percentage who survive to adulthood
22-27	17.8
28-30	57.3
31-33	85.7
34-36	94.6
37 and higher	96.5

Source: Moster D, Lie RT, Markestad T. Long-term medical and social consequences of preterm birth. NEJM July 2008; 359(3): 262-73, p. 262.

In addition, after studying more than 900,000 children born in Norway over a sixteen-year period, Moster and colleagues found that prematurity entailed the risk of serious medical disabilities such as cerebral palsy, intellectual impairment, and disorders of psychological development, behaviour and emotion, as well as other major disabilities such as blindness or low vision, hearing loss, and epilepsy. In fact it has been known for some time that preterm birth is *the* most important risk factor for cerebral palsy. An important Swedish study demonstrated that if the mother of a premature baby has had *any* prior induced abortions, her premature baby, on average, has a 60 per cent higher risk of cerebral palsy than a premature baby whose mother has had *no* previous induced abortions.[10] The lower the gestational age at birth, the higher the risk of disabilities in every category. Moster also

---

9   Moster D, Lie RT, Markestad T. Long-term medical and social consequences of preterm birth. NEJM July 2008; 359(3): 262-73, p. 262.
10   Jacobsson B, Hagberg G, Hagberg B, Ladfors L, Niklasson A, Hagberg H. Cerebral palsy in preterm infants : a population-based case-control study of antenatal and intrapartal risk factors. ActaPaediatrica 2002; 91: 946-51, p. 948 (table 2).

observed a significant association between autism and very low gestational age, but the findings were based on a small number of cases. A more recent study, however, by Limperopoulos and colleagues, in the highly respected journal *Pediatrics*, has confirmed the Dr. Dag Moster study by finding that extremely preterm newborns have a high autism risk.[11] Indeed, more than a decade ago, a paper in the *Journal of Perinatal Medicine* reported that a woman who terminates one or more pregnancies has at least a 179 per cent increased risk of delivering a baby later diagnosed with autism.[12] Furthermore, a much higher proportion of young adults born prematurely were receiving disability pensions than those who were born at term. Children born prematurely had a lower chance of attaining a high level of education or landing a well-paying job. They were less likely to find a life partner or have children.[13] These findings are summarized in the following table.

Table 15.3 **Percentage increase in medical disabilities according to gestational age at birth**

Gestational age	Percentage increased risk by disability		
	Cerebral palsy	Intellectual impairment	Other major disabilities
23-27 weeks	7790	930	1860
28-30 weeks	4480	320	830
31-33 weeks	1310	110	130
34-36 weeks	170	60	50
37+ weeks	0	0	0

---

11   *Sources:* Moster D, Lie RT, Markestad T. Long-term medical and social consequences of preterm birth. NEJM July 2008; 359(3): 262-73, p. 262; Limperopoulos C, Bassan H, Sullivan NR, Soul JS, Robertson RL, Moore M, Ringer SA, Volpe JJ, du Plessis AJ. Positive screening for autism in ex-preterm infants: prevalence and risk factors. Pediatrics 2008 April; 121(4): 758-65, p. 758.
12   Two models are used in this study. In the first, Burd and colleagues found a 236% increased risk of autism. However, when birthweight was eliminated as a variable in the second model, there was a 179% increased risk of autism. Burd used two models because the first model, while highly significant, was a poor fit with the data in the study's sample. "Eliminating birthweight decreased the model chi-square but produced a substantial improvement in goodness of fit". Burd L, Severud R, Kerbeshian J, Klug MG. Prenatal and perinatal risk factors for Autism. Journal of Perinatal Medicine 1999; 27(6): 441-50, p. 447.
13   Moster et al. See n. 9, pp. 265-6.

In a meta-analytic review of the relationship of cerebral palsy to gestational age, Himpens and colleagues came up with similar findings.[14] Finally, it is sobering to realize that as long as forty years ago the direct link between induced abortion and subsequent prematurity was already well known to Hungarian physicians. Hungary fully legalized abortion in 1956, and by the early 1970s had the highest abortion rate in the world. In December 1973 Professor Jenö Sárkány revealed that studies over the previous fifteen years had shown that women who had abortions had a much higher likelihood of bearing children with a variety of health problems, including prematurity.[15]

PRETERM BIRTHS AND AUTISM

The prevalence of typical autism across the world has risen rapidly in the past half-century, and is now said to be about two to four per 1000 children. Virtually all parts of the world have experienced an increased prevalence of autism, but in the US, the rise has been particularly dramatic.[16] There, the Centers for Disease Control and Prevention (CDC) reports that the prevalence of Autism Spectrum Disorder (ASD) has reached two per cent, or one child in fifty.[17] Part of the increase over the past half-century may be due to changing diagnostic methods and greater public awareness of autism, but this is unlikely to explain the phenomenal rise in its recorded incidence since the 1990s. One risk factor for autism is maternal age: the older the mother the higher the chance that her child will be born with autism. Sex is also a risk factor: boys are four to five times more likely to be born with autism than girls. Being born preterm or with a low birth weight is also associated with an increased risk of later development of autism. Limperopoulos and colleagues reported that 25 per cent of children born prematurely had positive screening results for autism.[18] This is more than twelve times higher than the general rate of autism in North America. The researchers cautiously concluded that both early gestational

---

14 Himpens E, Broeck CV, Oostra A, Calders P, Vanhaesebrouck P. Prevalence, type, distribution and severity of cerebral palsy in relation to gestational age : a meta-analytic review. Developmental Medicine and Child Neurology 2008 March; 50(5): pp. 334-40.
15 Népesedéspolitikánknéhánykérdése: A KülönbUtódokért Magyar Hirek 1973; 26(10). We are grateful to Dr. Elizabeth Demeter for translating this article.
16 Duchan, Patel, DR. Epidemiology of Autism Spectrum Disorders. Pediatric Clinics of North America 2012 February; 59(1): p. 27.
17 Blumberg SJ et al. Changes in prevalence of parent reported Autism Spectrum Disorder in school-aged U.S. children. National Health Statistics Reports, number 5, 2013 March 20: 1-11; p. 1. http://www.rescuepost.com/files/blumberg-et-al-2013-i-in-50-nchs-1.pdf
18 All the information in this paragraph is drawn from Limperopoulos et al. See n. 11.

age (prematurity) and birth weight, as well as maternal age were "possible predictor variables" for autism.[19]

As we have seen, induced abortion results in a significantly higher rate of low birth weight or preterm births in subsequent pregnancies. Therefore, it is logical to infer that abortion is a factor in the documented increasing risk of autism. To date there are only a few studies that directly address the question of an abortion-autism link. Burd and colleagues found that the children of mothers who had experienced one or more induced abortions had a 236 per cent increased risk of being born with autism.[20] A large study by Lyall and colleagues found that 21.2 per cent of mothers of children with ASD (autism spectrum disorder) reported previous abortions, while only 15.6 per cent of mothers with no ASD children reported previous abortions.[21] When adjusted for mother's age, the abortion-related risk was 47 per cent higher than it was for mothers who had no history of induced abortion. The "fully-adjusted" risk (OR) for induced abortion was 1.26, meaning a 26 per cent higher risk. A smaller, "prospective" study was carried out on a subgroup of women who were tracked since 1993. For these women, no statistically significant relationship was found between induced abortion and autism. This may be because of the small sample size, and also because the researchers controlled for "recall bias".[22] In our chapter on breast cancer above, we have shown that recall bias was not a factor that changed the results of studies showing increased risk of breast cancer after abortion.

Finally, a study by Eaton and colleagues found that the unadjusted risk for autism among mothers who had experienced a previous abortion was 1.35 and the adjusted risk was 1.10.[23] The unadjusted risk for mental retardation was 1.86, while the adjusted risk was 1.72. In one part of their report they acknowledged that "a history of provoked abortion increases risk for mental retardation and learning disorders." Yet later in the same report they drew back, stating, "it would be an improper extrapolation from the data, for example, to conclude that provoked [i.e. induced] abortions

---

19   Ibid., pp. 758-65.
20   Burd et al. See n. 12, pp. 441-50. The Adjusted Odds Ratio (OR) was found to be 2.79.
21   Lyall K, Pauls DL, Spiegelman D, Ascherio A, Santangelo SL. "Pregnancy complications and obstetric suboptimality in association with Autism Spectrum Disorders in children of the Nurses' Health Study II." Autism Research 2012 February;5(1): pp. 21-30.
22   Ibid.
23   Eaton WW, Mortensen PB, Thomsen PH, Frydenberg M. Obstetric complications and risk for severe pychopathology in childhood. Journal of Autism and Developmental Disorders 2001; 31(3): 279-85, p. 285.

were causing mental retardation or learning disorders in later pregnancies." They hypothesized that previous abortions may have been induced in order to eliminate a defective fetus. They also raised the possibility that a history of induced abortion may reflect an existing "lifestyle of the mother that places all her babies at greater risk."[24] We have already seen that a significant percentage of abortions were undertaken by women whose lifestyle was not different on average from that of women who did not undertake to terminate their pregnancies.[25]

Although research into the link between induced abortion and the later birth of a child with autism is in its early stages, the results that have been published so far give reason to believe that there may be a correlation between the two. No one disputes that a history of abortion increases the likelihood that a woman will later give birth prematurely. No one disputes that children born extremely prematurely experience a much higher rate of autism than children who are born after the normal 37 weeks' gestation. More than that, three studies have now documented a higher risk that women with a history of abortion will give birth to a child with autism. To these should be added a fourth study which has noted in passing that prior abortions were "significantly more common" among women who bore autistic children than among women who did not.[26] While all these findings might be considered preliminary, they deserve to be made widely known, and to become the subject of public discussion. Instead, researchers seem to be bending over backwards to minimize a finding that points to the deleterious consequences of abortion.

A very preterm birth can also have bad consequences for the mother. According to a study in the *British Journal of Cancer* it doubles her lifetime risk of having breast cancer.[27]

---

24 Ibid., p. 285.
25 See above, pp.202, 204. See also pp. 280-1.
26 Wilkerson DS, Volpe AG, Dean RS, Titus JB. Perinatal complications as predictors of infantile autism. International Journal of Neuroscience 2002; 112: 1085-98, p. 1091. The authors unfortunately did not quantify this finding, though they did report that the value of p was <0.05.
27 Melbye M, Wohlfahrt J, Andersen A-MN, Westergaard T, Andersen PK. Preterm delivery and risk of breast cancer. British Journal of Cancer 1999; 80(3/4): 609-13.

Conclusion

It is settled science that induced abortion greatly elevates the subsequent risk of bearing a premature baby. Two systematic reviews published in the *British Journal of Obstetrics and Gynaecology* and the *Journal of Reproductive Medicine*, as well as two recently completed, massive studies from Scandinavia and Britain have established that preterm and low-birth-weight children have a much greater chance of dying in childhood than children who spend 37 or more weeks in the womb, or weigh over 2500 grams at birth. These preterm or low-birth-weight children also have a much higher incidence of medical disabilities, most notably cerebral palsy and intellectual impairment. They fare worse in the educational system, on the job market, and in finding a life partner. Furthermore, four studies have documented a link between autism and prior abortions. Abortion may well be a major factor in the alarming increase over the past half century in the percentage of children born with autism.

The association between having one or more induced abortion(s) and later giving birth to a premature child has also been clearly established, most recently by two major Canadian studies this year.[28] The more abortions a woman has, the greater her chances of later delivering a preterm or low-birth-weight child. The reason is that induced abortion can result in a weakened cervix, which later can lead to premature deliveries. The most important prematurity risk imparted by prior induced abortions is infection, most significantly womb infections. Surgical abortions also elevate the risk of uterine scar tissue (also known as adhesions) and cervical insufficiency (also called incompetent cervix), both of which raise the risk of a future premature delivery. An "incompetent cervix" raises cerebral palsy risk, as do maternal infections. Consequently, it is fair to say that induced abortion is producing a medical and social disaster in those countries where it is freely available. Writing in the *Journal of Reproductive Medicine*, a group of researchers has estimated that in the United States in one year alone, prior induced abortions caused at least 1096 cases of cerebral palsy in very low birth weight newborns.[29] Globally this translates into well over 15,000 cases of cerebral palsy annually attributable to prior induced abortions. It is interesting to compare this with the birth of an estimated 10,000 babies with serious defects in the late 1950s as a consequence of thalidomide

---

28 See nn. 7 and 8.
29 Calhoun BC, Shadigian E, Rooney B. Cost consequences of induced abortion as an attributable risk for preterm birth and impact on informed consent. Journal of Reproductive Medicine 2007; 52(10): pp. 929-37.

use.[30] This personal and collective tragedy was then greeted with universal horror.

A glimpse of the benefits that might accrue from reducing the number of induced abortions is furnished by the experience of Poland. Twenty-three years ago the new democratic regime took the drastic step of banning almost all induced abortions in that country. As we have seen, and as illustrated in Figures 15.1 and 15.2 below, this action was followed by a more than 70 per cent drop in the deaths of children under the age of five from cerebral palsy in the succeeding fifteen years.[31] Moreover, in the three-year period from 1995 to 1997 Poland's extreme preterm birthrate dropped by 21 per cent, while the total of all births declined by only five per cent.[32]

Figure 15.1 Poland: Cerebral Palsy deaths, 1985–2006

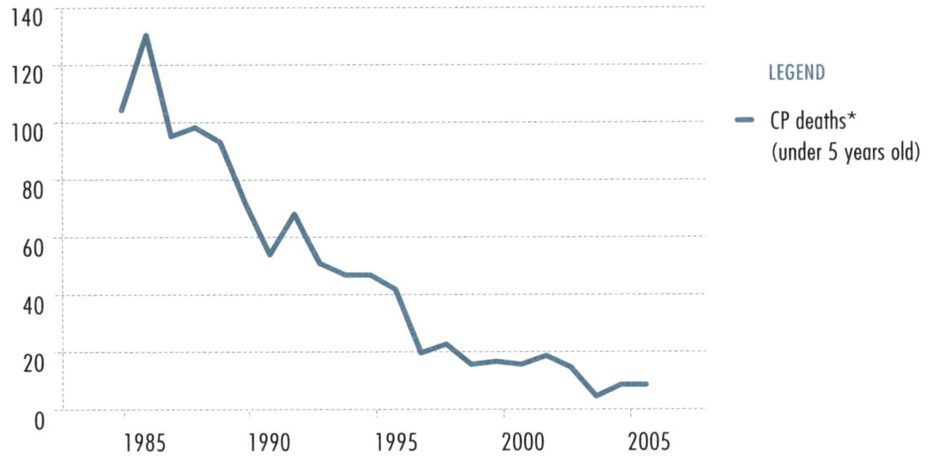

LEGEND
— CP deaths* (under 5 years old)

Source: Cerebral Palsy deaths in Poland, 1985-2006, Poland Central Statistical Office.

---

30   Stephens T, Brynner R. *Dark Remedy: The Impact of Thalidomide and Its Revival as a Vital Medicine.* Cambridge, MA: Perseus, 2001, p. 37.
31   Cerebral Palsy deaths in Poland, 1985-2006, Poland Central Statistical Office (2008). See also Chapter 2, Table 2.1 and Table 2.2, pp. 40-1.
32   *United Nations demographic yearbook: focusing on natality* (1999), p. 4: Table 12, Live births by gestational age: 1990-1998. [Note: this is the most recent UN Yearbook focusing on natality](accessed: 19 Aug. 2011). http://unstats.un.org/unsd/demographic/products/dyb/DYBNat/NatStatTab12.pdf http://www.unicef-irc.org/databases/transmonee/2007/Country_profiles.xls

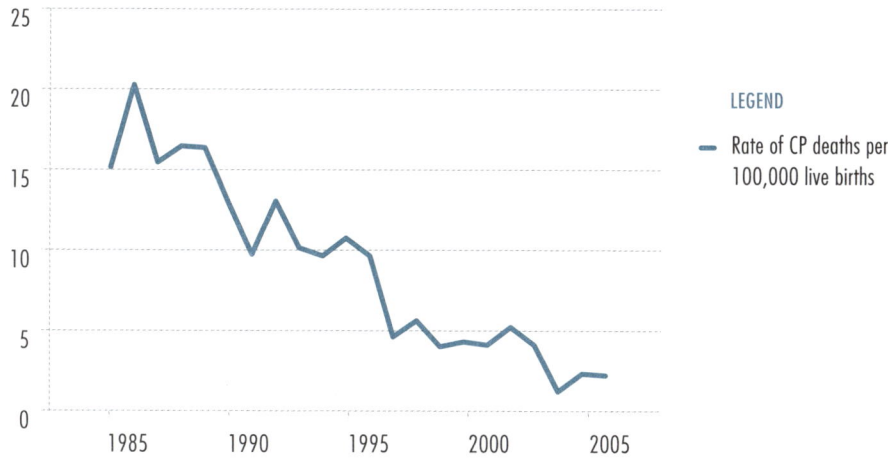

Figure 15.2 **Poland: Rate of Cerebral Palsy deaths per 100,000 live births**

* **For years 1985-1996 - the ICD 9 (code 343); since 1997 - the ICD 10 (code G80) has been implemented.**
Source: Communication from the Poland Central Statistical Office, 2008.

No other country has achieved such a dramatic reduction in extremely preterm births in such a short time. By contrast, both the US and Canada, where abortion is freely available, experienced a rise in preterm births during the same period. On the principle of informed consent, countries that are unable or unwilling to take steps to reduce the incidence of induced abortion, ought at the very least to require abortion providers to inform their clients of the direct connection between induced abortion, subsequent premature births, and the elevated risks of infant mortality, cerebral palsy, autism, intellectual impairment, and other medical or psychological disabilities.

Chapter 16

Pain during and after abortion

KEY POINTS

- Abortion generally causes mild to moderate pain in the majority of women, with some women experiencing severe pain.

- Even widely-used pain reduction methods are not always effective.

- Pain perception can be increased by pre-operative anxiety and a host of other factors, some of them specific to abortion.

- Doctors and abortion providers seem to underestimate the amount of pain that women experience.

Introduction

There is general agreement among medical experts, both that abortion can cause pain in women, and that the methods used to treat this pain are not always beneficial or sufficient. In a review of five studies Penney noted that "many women undergoing early medical abortion experience pain of a severity that requires narcotic analgesia; almost a quarter of women experience pain that they rate as almost being as bad as it can be."[1] Renner and colleagues noted that "[anesthesia] is important for women undergoing an abortion since most will experience pain with the procedure."[2] Despite advances in pain control, between 78 and 97 per cent of women say they experience at least moderate pain during a surgical abortion.[3]

Pain would seem to vary according to the procedure used. Abortions done by suction evacuation seem to be the most painful.[4] Most women fall within the mild to moderate range, but a few women experience severe pain.[5]

Many widely-used techniques for pain reduction may not actually work. A paper published in *Human Reproduction* found no lessening of

---

1   Penney G. Treatment of pain during medical abortion. Contraception 2006 July; 74(1): 45-7, p. 47.
2   Renner RM, Jensen JT, Nichols MD, Edelman AB. Pain control in first-trimester surgical abortion: a systematic review of randomized controlled trials. Contraception 2010 May; 81(5): 372-88, p. 372.
3   Ibid., p. 373.
4   Singh RH, Ghanem KG, Burke AE, Nichols MD, Rogers K, Blumenthal PD. Predictors and perception of pain in women undergoing first trimester surgical abortion. Contraception 2008 August; 78(2): 155-61.
5   For studies that correlate pain levels with the procedures used see Sik Yau Kan A, Hung Yu Ng E, Chung Ho P. The role and comparison of two techniques of paracervical block for pain relief during suction evacuation for first-trimester pregnancy termination. Contraception 2004 August; 70(2): pp. 159-63; Sik Yau Kan A, Caves N, Yuen Wai Wong S, Hung Yu Ng E, Chung Ho P. A double-blind, randomized controlled trial on the use of a 50:50 mixture of nitrous oxide/oxygen in pain relief during suction evacuation for the first trimester pregnancy termination. Human Reproduction 2006 October; 21(10): pp. 2606-11; Wong CYG, Ng EHY, Ngai SW, Ho PC. A randomized, double blind, placebo-controlled study to investigate the use of conscious sedation in conjunction with paracervical block for reducing pain in termination of first trimester pregnancy by suction evacuation. Human Reproduction 2002 May; 17(5): pp. 1222-5; Dean G, Cardenas L, Darney P, Goldberg A. Acceptability of manual versus electric aspiration for first trimester abortion: a randomized trial. Contraception 2003 March; 67(3): pp. 201-6; Singh RH, Ghanem KG, Burke AE, Nichols MD, Rogers K, Blumenthal PD. Predictors and perception of pain in women undergoing first trimester surgical abortion. Contraception 2008 August; 78(2): pp.155-61.

pain from conscious sedation during suction evacuation abortion;[6] another study found limited pain reduction from two different types of paracervical block;[7] two South African researchers determined that diclofenac by itself provides limited pain relief and thus works better in conjunction with a local anaesthetic.[8] A review of 40 studies found that conscious sedation, general anaesthetic and some non-pharmacological interventions were effective in reducing pain, but that "data were insufficient to show a clear benefit of a paracervical block (PCB) compared to no PCB" — a conclusion they found surprising, given that PCB is used widely for abortion pain relief.[9]

When women were asked whether they felt that the pain relief offered was satisfactory, 40.4 per cent in one study scored the effectiveness of the pain relief as ranging from 0 to 25 on a scale out of 100, where 0 indicated no pain relief and 100 indicated complete relief.[10]

A major difficulty in all pain research is the complicated nature of pain perception, which encompasses physical, psychological and social elements. The physical causes of pain during abortion are fairly well known. During suction evacuation abortion, "pain mainly comes from two components: cervical dilatation and uterine contractions during the suction procedure."[11] A recent study tells us that "during dilation and curettage, pain commonly occurs during the procedure with injection of the cervical block, cervical dilation, suction aspiration, and postoperatively with uterine cramping. In some cases, placement of a speculum causes significant pain."[12] There are many other factors that also influence pain perception. In its review of analgesia and pain management in first-trimester surgical abortion, the same study lists factors linked to increased pain perception in women undergoing surgical abortion: fewer past pregnancies, younger age, history of dysmenorrhea, pre-procedure anxiety and depression, length of the

---

6   Wong et al. See n. 5.
7   SikYau Kan et al. See n. 5.
8   Owolabi OT, Moodley J. A randomized trial of pain relief in termination of pregnancy in South Africa. Tropical Doctor 2005 July; 35: pp. 136-9.
9   Renner et al. See n. 2, p. 372.
10 Hamoda H, Flett GMM, Ashok PW, Templeton A. Surgical abortion using manual vacuum aspiration under local anaesthesia: a pilot study of feasibility and women's acceptability. Journal of Family Planning and Reproductive Health Care 2005 July; 31(3): pp.185-8.
11 Sik Yau Kan et al. See n. 5, p. 2606. Similar comment in Singh et al. See n. 5.
12 Meckstroth KR, Mishra K. Analgesia/pain management in first trimester surgical abortion. Clinical Obstetrics and Gynecology 2009 June; 52(2): 160-70, p. 160.

procedure, the abortion provider, and even the atmosphere in the clinic.[13]

Pre-operative anxiety seems to have a significant role in pain perception.[14] A particular aspect that induces pre-operative anxiety is that the procedure is "unique because of the psychological and emotional factors involved in terminating a pregnancy, including ambivalence about the decision and concern about the future impact on fertility."[15] This is in keeping with the comment by Renner and colleagues, that "moral problems" with abortion have been linked to higher pain perception.[16] Sik Yau Kan and colleagues also found anxiety levels to be correlated positively with pain during suction evacuation abortion.[17]

Women have a right to specific, accurate information about how much pain they may expect during an abortion. The reality is that they are often given only the sketchiest notion of what lies ahead. Canadian abortion clinics sometimes compare abortion pain with menstrual cramps. Yet at least one study suggests that women find the pain during abortion to be more severe than having a period.[18] Another study compared the uterine cramps experienced during suction evacuation abortion to labour pain, although no evidence or source for this comparison was cited.[19]

The websites of some Canadian abortion providers downplay abortion pain. The Morgentaler Clinic paints the following picture of a surgical abortion experience:

> Your doctor will place a speculum into your vagina in order to access and cleanse your cervix... Over the next couple of minutes, your doctor will gently widen your cervix by carefully inserting a series of small tapered rods... During this stage of the procedure you may experience slight pressure or mild cramping, much like menstrual cramps.

Then, describing the removal of the fetus, it continues, "as your uterus

---

13   Ibid.
14   Pud, D, Amit A. Anxiety as a Predictor of Pain Magnitude Following Termination of First-trimester Pregnancy. Pain Medicine 2005 March; 6(2): 143-8, p. 146.
15   Ibid., p. 144.
16   Renner et al. See n. 2.
17   Sik Yau Kan et al. See n. 5.
18   Hamoda et al. See n. 10.
19   Sik Yau Kan et al. See n. 5.

contracts, you may experience some period-like cramping."[20] Nowhere is there an admission that these steps can cause pain, ranging from moderate to severe. Indeed, the word pain is never mentioned.

Women and physicians also seem to differ in their perceptions of pain. Two recent studies assess physicians' perceptions of women's pain during abortion and compare them with the assessments of the women themselves. Both studies find that physicians tend to rate women's pain lower than the women themselves rate it, although not vastly lower. Dean and colleagues, in comparing manual aspiration (MVA) and electric aspiration (EVA), report that the physicians indicated that 26 MVA patients had "little or no pain", twelve had "some or moderate pain", and three had "a lot or severe pain"—however, according to the women's scores, sixteen had "little or no pain", nineteen had "some or moderate pain", and six had "a lot or severe pain." There were similar discrepancies in the EVA group.[21] Singh and colleagues discover a similar contrast between physicians' perception their patients' pain, and that of the patients themselves.[22]

Is there a link between physical pain and psychological problems after abortion? Suliman and colleagues attempted to compare the effects of abortion on mental and physical health according to whether conscious/ intravenous sedation (IS) or local anaesthesia (LA) was used. Specifically, the study "aimed to determine if either LA or IS predicted post-traumatic stress disorder, depression, anxiety or physical ill-health in women at one-month and three-month follow-up."[23] Those who received IS reported less pain during surgery than those receiving LA. This is interesting, because LA patients also experienced higher levels of dissociation immediately after the procedure, higher levels of post-traumatic stress syndrome (PTSD),[24] higher levels of depressive symptoms,[25] and higher levels of anxiety (60 per cent versus 51.7 per cent). More telling, however, is that LA patients seemed to have had a harder time as the months passed. Those with PTSD

---

20   The Morgentaler Clinic, *The Procedure*, http://www.morgentaler.ca/procedure.html (2008).
21   Dean et al. See n. 5.
22   Singh et al. See n. 5.
23   Suliman S, Ericksen T, Labuschgne P, de Wit R, Stein DJ, Seedat S. Comparison of pain, cortisol levels, and psychological distress in women undergoing surgical termination of pregnancy under local anaesthesia versus intravenous sedation. BMC Psychiatry 2007 June; 7(24): 24-32, p. 25.
24   28 per cent at both one and three months, as opposed to 9.4 per cent and ten per cent for IS.
25   25.7 per cent versus 13.8 per cent.

symptoms almost doubled.[26] In addition, 21.8 per cent of IS patients had scores suggestive of clinical depression prior to the abortion, as opposed to 23.1 per cent of LA patients. However, at both one and three months, the percentage of IS patients with such scores had dropped dramatically to 13.8 per cent, but the percentage of LA patients had *increased* to 25.7 per cent. Similarly, 66 per cent of IS patients had "high" anxiety prior to the abortion, as opposed to 62.6 per cent of LA patients: both percentages dropped in the ensuing months, but while the IS percentage dropped to 51.7 per cent, the LA percentage declined only slightly, to 60 per cent. Thus, LA patients not only experienced more pain during the abortion, but also more and longer lasting PTSD, depression, and anxiety.[27]

Conclusion

The recent literature on pain during abortion indicates little progress in the understanding of pain and how to reduce it during abortion. The complex nature of pain perception is widely recognized, as well as the fact that most women will experience some pain during abortion, mainly in the moderate range, but with a certain percentage undergoing severe pain. Finally, there is a variety of questions about the patient/physician relationship concerning abortion—physicians seem to perceive the women's pain during abortion as less than the women do themselves, and there is little indication of how much women are told about pain prior to abortion, or whether what they are told corresponds to the pain they actually feel. Indeed, one study seems to suggest that comparing abortion pain to that of menstruation may actually undervalue and trivialize the amount of pain abortion causes.

In sum, a large number of issues surrounding abortion pain still need to be studied. More work needs to be done on determining the validity of the menstrual cramps/abortion pain comparison, the effectiveness of preoperative information on pain, and the assessment of women's satisfaction with pain relief. Despite a lot of research in the past decade, little new information has come to light and few improvements made in controlling the pain women actually experience during an induced abortion.

---

26   28 per cent at both 1 and 3 months.
27   Suliman et al. See n. 23, p. 25.

Section III: The Psychological and Social Impact

Abstract

Chapter 17 deals with family formation. Contrary to expectation, abortion has contributed to the rise in single-parent families. This is apparently because men are now much less likely to take responsibility for the child their partner conceives if she refuses to have an abortion. At the same time men who *want* the child they have fathered find that they have no say in the matter if their partner chooses abortion.

Chapter 17:

Psychological outcomes: Abortion and family formation

In the last half-century we have witnessed a transformation of the family, brought about in part by the advent of abortion on request. Single women who have an induced abortion are more likely never to marry. Married women who have an abortion experience a much higher rate of divorce than those who do not have abortions. Paradoxically, abortion may also have contributed to the increasing feminization of poverty. This may be traceable to the fact that many men are no longer willing to take responsibility for supporting the child that their partner has refused to abort.

Before legalization of abortion the promise was confidently made that if every child was a wanted child there would be much less child abuse. That promise has not been kept; on the contrary the incidence of child abuse has risen in the US and Canada. Why is this? It may be because of the emotional or psychological strain that abortion puts on a woman. It may be because of an inability to bond with a child born subsequent to an abortion. It may be because of unresolved bereavement or feelings of guilt and shame associated with a past abortion. On the other hand, several studies of children born to women who applied for but were denied legal abortion found that they fared no differently than children whose mothers had *not* sought to abort them. Wantedness is an ambiguous and changeable concept.

Chapter 18:

Depression, suicide, substance abuse: Contested research

Chapter 18 addresses the great debate on whether induced abortion has any significant, measurable impact on women's mental health. The debate is so politically charged that it is difficult to weigh evidence and draw conclusions objectively. People cannot even agree on the best research methodologies. In some circles prospective studies are the gold standard. Prospective studies begin with the woman at the time of her abortion, and study her for months or years after that event.

The rarely-acknowledged problem with prospective studies is the high rate of dropout they encounter — known as "sample attrition". The question is not addressed as to why so many drop out.

Retrospective research looks back and considers women's abortion experiences after the fact. Even though these types of studies reflect women's actual stories, they are often criticized for a lack of scientific rigour. Record linkage studies assemble numerical data from large national samples or questionnaires. They are objective in that the identity of the subjects being studied is unknown. They too have been rejected for not being prospective. Meta-analyses look at large numbers of already-published studies, seeking to find an overall pattern. Controversy rages over which studies qualify for meta-analysis, and which do not.

Two years ago Patricia Coleman published a meta-analysis in the *British Journal of Psychiatry* documenting an 81 per cent greater risk of mental health problems for women who had an abortion compared to those who did not. These mental health problems included anxiety, depression, alcohol and marijuana use and suicide behaviours. Others who deny any link between abortion and later mental health disorders usually confine their attention to the first few months after the abortion. Such is the case with the Danish study by Munk-Olsen, and also the report by the American Psychological Association (APA). On the other hand, numerous other studies by researchers with no ideological axe to grind lend credence to Coleman's findings.

Those who would deny a link between abortion and later mental health disorders almost never refer to the rate of suicide and suicide ideation (thinking about suicide) among women who have had abortions. Four large-scale studies from Scandinavia, the US and Britain have documented a sharply higher rate of suicide among women who have had abortions compared to women who have completed their pregnancies. Giving birth has an indisputable protective effect for women against suicide and suicide ideation.

In summary, the increase in the rate of depression, anxiety, substance abuse and suicide among women who have had abortions is drastic and incontrovertible.

Each year in the United States, intimate partner violence results in an estimated 1200 deaths and two million injuries among women. Do women who have abortions experience a disproportionate share of this violence, and if so is there a link between the two phenomena? This is the question explored in Chapter 19. The findings are very clear. Studies from across the world report a correlation between intimate partner violence (IPV) and abortion. Women who suffer intimate partner violence are more likely to have abortions—both induced and spontaneous—than those who do not. Conversely, women who seek induced abortion are more likely to be victims of coercion and/or intimate partner violence. For these women it is therefore illusory to characterize abortion as a woman's choice. Moreover, for a woman, obtaining an abortion, far from eliminating abuse by her partner, can actually serve to increase such harm.

Chapter 19:

Intimate partner violence and abortion

Chapter 17

Psychological outcomes: Abortion and family formation

KEY POINTS

- In North America, the and an increase in the number of single-parent families can be correlated to the legalization of abortion and its impact on premarital sexual relations.

- Fewer marriages are occurring when unmarried couples become pregnant. This suggests that single men are taking less responsibility as fathers.

- On the other hand, men who would like to keep the child that their partner wishes to abort have no legal say in the matter.

- Although abortion is said to alleviate child abuse and neglect studies have shown that child abuse has risen with the legalization of abortion.

- In what has been called the "feminization of poverty", an increasing number of the poor are women; this may be associated with the practice of abortion.

- The social impact of abortion is, as yet, mostly unexplored and merits further research.

INTRODUCTION

One aspect of legalized abortion that has received surprisingly little attention both in the mainstream media and among academics is the impact it has had on the formation of family. No doubt, the family has undergone significant changes over the last five decades. In accounting for this change, research has focused on such areas as the widespread use of contraceptives, a change in society's understanding of gender roles and the increase in divorce rates. Very little research has been done, however, on what may be one of the most influential factors altering family formation. This chapter offers a summary of work that has been done on the subject of legalized abortion's impact on family formation.

SINGLE-PARENT FAMILIES AND BIRTHS TO SINGLE MOTHERS

Far from abortion reducing the number of children born to single-parents, since its legalization in the early 1970s there has been a significant rise in the numbers of single-parent families and children born to single mothers. An American study puts this change into historical perspective by comparing rates of births to single women over several decades: "In 1950 only four per cent of all births occurred outside marriage. By 1970, the figure was up to eleven per cent; by 1990, 28 per cent; and by 2003, 35 per cent."[1] Although there may be several factors contributing to this increase, Cherlin, the distinguished sociologist who authored this study, notes the significant role legalized abortion played in bringing about a rise in single-parenting. Although legalized abortion may have caused birth rates to fall for all unmarried women, there has been an increase in births outside of marriage "because birth rates have fallen faster for married women than for unmarried women."[2] Therefore, "a larger share of women who give birth are unmarried."[3] "Of further concern to many," Cherlin continues, "...is that about half of all unmarried first-time mothers are adolescents."[4]

Research conducted at the University of California, Berkeley, also revealed that legalized abortion may have contributed to the increase in single-parent families and births outside of marriage. Abortions to unmarried women before complete legalization in 1973 were fewer than

---

1   Cherlin AJ. American marriage in the early twenty-first century. marriage and child wellbeing 2005 October; 15(2): 33-55, p. 35.
2   Ibid., p. 35.
3   Ibid., p. 35.
4   Ibid., p. 35.

100,000 per year. In roughly the same period (1965-9) there were about 322,000 births to unmarried women. The numbers of induced abortions increased rapidly in the 1970s. By the early 1980s legal abortions to unmarried women averaged more than 1.25 million annually, while births outside of marriage rose to 715,000 per year.[5] Whether or not the rapid increase in abortions contributed directly to the rise in births to unmarried women, it certainly did nothing to reduce them.

EXPLAINING THE RISE IN SINGLE-PARENT FAMILIES

Since the rapid rise in legalized abortion has been paralleled by a similar increase in the number of children born into single-parent families, how are we to understand this correlation? The Berkeley economists' theory is that the legalization of abortion, as well as the sudden widespread use of contraceptives, created a "technology shock," which dramatically altered the way in which premarital sexual relations and marriage were perceived. With any technology shock, they suggest, there are winners who adopt the new technology, and losers who fail to adopt the new technology for whatever reason.[6] The legalization of abortion creates losers among women because "those women who want children, who do not want an abortion for moral or religious reasons, or who are unreliable in their use of contraception, may want marriage guarantees but find themselves pressured to participate in premarital sexual relations without any such assurance. They have been placed at a competitive disadvantage."[7] Thus, legalized abortion is correlated with an increase in the number of children born to unmarried women because it opened the way for widespread premarital sexual relations, both generally and among women who would not obtain an abortion in the event of an unplanned pregnancy.

In addition to the pressure of premarital sexual relations, legalized abortion changed the way in which men reacted to an out-of-wedlock pregnancy. The technology shock that occurred with the legalization of abortion led to a decline in marriages precipitated by pregnancy, where a man recognizes an obligation to marry a single woman if he makes her pregnant. The ratio of such marriages fell between 42.6 and 66 per cent from the late 1960s to the late 1980s.[8] Easy access to abortion made it much

---

5   Akerlof, Yellen and Katz. See Chapter 4, p. 63 n. 28, 277-317.
6   Ibid.
7   Ibid., p. 280.
8   Ibid., pp. 277-317.

less likely that a man would marry his pregnant girlfriend, thus leaving the woman to raise the child on her own, should she choose to bring it to term.

Hence, legalized abortion has led to a rise in single-parent families and births outside of marriage because men are much less likely to take responsibility for the child if the woman refused to have an abortion.

It is also noteworthy that with the advent of legalized abortion "…the norm of premarital sexual abstinence all but vanished."[9] As a result, "with premarital sex the rule, rather than the exception, childbirth outside of marriage could no longer serve as a sign that society's sexual taboos had been violated. The stigma attached to out-of-wedlock childbearing thus gradually but, ultimately greatly, eroded."[10]

With little or no stigma now being attached to single-parenthood, there was a decline in the number of children placed for adoption. "Prior to the 1970s, only a small fraction of children born out-of-wedlock were kept by mothers who never married. In contrast, today only a small fraction are put up for adoption or given to other relatives."[11] Since mothers are much less likely to place their child for adoption, there are more children being raised by a single-parent than there are being raised in a two-parent family.

THE ROLE AND RESPONSIBILITY OF FATHERS

Fathers Refusing to Accept Responsibility

As we have seen, the legalization of abortion has led to a change in the way many men respond to a premarital pregnancy. Although they no longer seem to feel pressured to take responsibility for the welfare of their pregnant partner by marrying her, they are still legally expected to give child support should she choose to bring their baby to term. But given the accessibility of abortion, this expectation has also been called into question. It has been asserted that, given the availability of legalized abortion, requiring a father to pay child support for a child he never intended or wanted to have is illogical. "If women's partial responsibility for pregnancy does not obligate them to support a fetus, then men's partial responsibility

---

9   Ibid., p. 309.
10 Ibid., p. 309.
11 Ibid., p. 289.

for pregnancy does not obligate them to support a resulting child."[12] If a woman is free to choose abortion, according to this line of reasoning, a father should not be forced to pay child support for a child he never wanted to have. If a woman chooses to carry a child to term without the father's agreement, the responsibility both financial and otherwise should rest with her. In other words, "if a man has used contraception, disagreed with the mother's decision to bear the child, and generally absents himself from the proceedings, it is difficult to see how he could be said to have assumed responsibility."[13] It has also been argued that *nothing*, not even financial support, should be expected of him if the mother chooses to bring the child to term against his wishes. This line of reasoning is only possible because not carrying a child to term is now a viable option.

The Rights of Fathers

Although legalized abortion has seemed, from one perspective, to offer fathers an escape from the responsibility of parenting a child they did not want or intend to have, it has also extinguished their right to an equal say in bringing a child to term that they *do* want to have. Given that abortion is a woman's choice, men's wishes may be overridden. This can result in a traumatic experience for a man who wants his child to be brought to term but is powerless to stop his partner from obtaining an abortion. Here is how a young medical student described his inability to stop his wife from aborting an unplanned pregnancy: "Even though I was the father and wanted to care for my child, I couldn't unless my wife wanted to have it. She controlled her life, our child's life and my life. I controlled nothing. I had no rights. I was just the father."[14]

LEGALIZED ABORTION AND MARRIAGE

Relationship Break Down

Although it may seem reasonable to assume that abortion has had a substantial impact on relationships between men and women, surprisingly little work has been done on this subject. One study looking at the effects of induced abortion on relationships compared a group of stably partnered

---

12   Brake E. Fatherhood and child support: do men have a right to choose? Journal of Applied Philosophy 2005 March; 22(1): 55-73, p. 56.
13   Ibid., p. 58.
14   Moore RC. Husband mourns outcome of wife's painful decision. American Medical News 1991: 14 October, p. 24.

women who chose to have an abortion to a matched control group of women in stable partnerships not desiring a child who had successfully avoided pregnancy.[15] Examining the relationships of women in both groups one year after the abortion had taken place, Barnett and colleagues found that "at the time of follow-up, twenty of the 92 study group couples and sixteen of the [92] control group couples had separated...All separations occurring in both groups were among the 62 unmarried couples. Married couples in neither the study group nor the control group had even considered separation."[16] With the exception of married couples, therefore, those in the study group had a higher incidence of relationship breakdown than those in the control group, though admittedly by a small (25 per cent) margin.

In addition, the researchers reported that "In the study group sixteen of the twenty, in the control group seven of the sixteen separations, were initiated by the female partner."[17] Thus, separations in the study group were overwhelmingly initiated by the female partners, "whereas in the control group separation was instigated [almost] equally by men and women."[18] Furthermore, the pre-abortion couples already showed signs of relationship breakdown or at least of unhealthy relationships: "The relationships of the future abortion patients were significantly worse on almost all dimensions. In times of conflict the male partners often showed behavior non-conducive to problem solving, such as shouting at the partner, insulting her, twisting her arguments, disparaging her opinion, or blaming her when something went wrong."[19]

Divorce

A more recent study on legalized abortion and marriage was conducted by Paul Sullins. Examining data from the 1995 National Survey of Family Growth (NSFG), "with some validating comparisons made to two national surveys of abortion patients conducted by the Alan Guttmacher Institute in 1987 and 1995," Sullins finds a positive connection between abortion and marriage breakdown.[20] Comparing the marriage history of women who

---

15   Barnett W, Freudenberg N, Willie R. Partnership after induced abortion: a prospective controlled study. Archives of Sexual Behavior 1992 October; 21(5): pp. 443-55.
16   Ibid., p. 450.
17   Ibid., p. 450.
18   Ibid., p. 455.
19   Ibid., p. 450.
20   Sullins P. Abortion and family formation: circumstance or culture? Life and Learning XIII 2003: 31-64, p. 34.

abort to those who do not, Sullins finds the following: "A quarter (25.1 per cent) of aborters over age 35 are currently divorced or separated, compared to only 19 per cent of non-aborters. The result is that only 60 per cent of aborters, but 72 per cent of non-aborters, over age 35 are currently married. Moreover, almost 40 per cent of aborters, but only 22 per cent of non-aborters this age who are married, have been married more than once... The cumulative effect of these marriage failures is that, by their late thirties, only a minority (37 per cent) of aborters remain in their first marriage, compared to over 56 per cent of non-aborters."[21] Thus, according to Sullins, a married woman with a history of abortion is more likely to experience divorce than a married woman who has never had an abortion.

Why should abortion increase the rate of divorce? The phenomenon appears paradoxical, since many women obtain an abortion precisely because they have hopes and plans for a future family. Marriage, therefore, is a strong factor that women consider when deciding whether to abort. However, rather than having a positive impact on a women's future marriage plans, an abortion in fact negatively affects a marriage, as many women with a history of abortion will find that their marriages end in divorce. Sullins writes: "As each pregnancy necessarily involves two persons, it is rare for an abortion decision to be made apart from the interpersonal context of conception. Social context, particularly education and work participation, are strong predictors of abortion. Furthermore, an abortion, like a child, is conceived as part of an implicit or explicit career plan or hopes for family formation. These expectations become more formalized, in most cases, in marriage; thus it is that marital status is the strongest single factor influencing the probability of aborting a pregnancy. The characterization, therefore, of abortion decisions as pre-eminently private and personal is too simple; the actual situation is much more complicated."[22] According to the 1995 National Survey of Family Growth, of ever-pregnant women over 35, 51.1 per cent of aborters had a failed marriage (divorced, separated or more than one marriage) compared to 37.3 per cent of non-aborters; 36.5 per cent of aborters had an intact single marriage compared to 56.2 per cent of non-aborters; and 12.4 per cent of aborters never married compared to 6.5 per cent of non-aborters.[23] Ironically, while women may consider abortion because they plan in the future to marry and have a family, having an abortion increases the likelihood that they will never marry, or that the marriage they had planned for will fail.

---

21 Ibid., p. 38.
22 Ibid., p. 33.
23 Ibid., p. 40.

Abortion and Marriage

Not only are women with a history of abortion more likely to divorce, but women who abort are more likely to marry older or never to marry at all, than women who have never aborted. While the fact that marriage inhibits abortion is well known, it is much less widely recognized that having an abortion also inhibits marriage. The National Survey of Family Growth (NSFG) indicates this reciprocal effect in a number of ways. First, women who abort delay marriage more than women who do not abort. The average age at marriage for aborters is 23.1 years; for non-aborters it is only 21.7 years. This is not surprising, since delayed marriage, like abortion, is a direct means of reducing fertility, and would be likely to result from many of the same motivations. However, aborters are also somewhat less likely ever to marry than non-aborters. By their late thirties almost all sexually-active women who will ever marry have done so; on the NSFG only eight per cent of all ever-pregnant women over age of 35 remain unmarried. But this proportion is almost twice as large for aborters (12.4 per cent) as for non-aborters (6.5 per cent).[24] To sum up, "women having abortions are twice as likely never to marry, 37 per cent more likely to divorce, have (on average) twice as many lifetime sexual partners and three times as many partners before marriage, have fewer children, and experience both earlier sexual onset and later marriage."[25]

ABORTION AND CHILD ABUSE

One surprising effect of legalized abortion is the positive correlation between a woman's history of abortion and abuse of her future children. Contrary to expectation, legalized abortion has not ensured that every child who is not aborted is a wanted one who will not be neglected. It appears instead to have contributed to an increase in child abuse.

A study by Dr. Philip Ney and colleagues in the *Pre- and Perinatal Psychology Journal* revealed that rather than being associated with a reduction in the incidence of child abuse, legalized abortion has been accompanied by an increase in the phenomenon. A number of factors may have contributed to this increase, such as better reporting mechanisms, but Ney and colleagues note that where a greater number of abortions are performed is also where a greater incidence of child abuse cases are

---

24   Ibid., p. 38.
25   Ibid., p. 31.

reported. Ney and colleagues state that

> Canadian provinces that have high rates of abortion also have high rates of child abuse. The rates have increased parallel with each other. In British Columbia the rates of deaths of children and adolescents from social causes seem to have increased shortly after the change in legislation liberalizing abortion. Although this association may be due to common causes such as socio-economic conditions or societal attitudes towards children, it is clear that there is no evidence that there has been a diminution in the rate of abuse.[26]

In an effort to explain the correlation between legalized abortion and child abuse, these researchers comment: "It is possible that a mother who has had an abortion is more anxious during the next pregnancy and more depressed post-partum. Consequently, she is less able to bond with her next child…It is possible that the abortion alters the mother's innate response to the infant's cry. Abortion may make it difficult for the mother to touch the baby, lessening the chance of breast-feeding and a healthy child."[27]

Expanding on the work of Ney and colleagues is a study by Coleman and colleagues. They examined 292 women from the Baltimore, Maryland area in the mid-1980s who were receiving Aid to Families with Dependent Children (AFDC).[28] All the study participants engaged in child maltreatment or allowed someone else to mistreat at least one of their children.[29] After instituting statistical controls, they discovered that "women who had an abortion history reported more frequent slapping, hitting, kicking or biting, beating, and use of physical punishment compared to women without an abortion history."[30]

Coleman and colleagues give several reasons for the positive correlation between abortion and child abuse. First, like miscarriage and

---

26   Ney PG, Fung T, Wickett AR. Relationship between induced abortion and child abuse and neglect: Four studies. Pre-and Peri-natal Psychology Journal 1993 October; 8(1): 43-63, p.44.
27   Ibid., p. 58.
28   Coleman PK, Rue VM, Coyle CT, Maxey CD. Induced abortion and child-directed aggression among mothers of maltreated children. Internet Journal of Pediatrics and Neonatology 2007; 6(2),http://www.ispub.com/journal/the-internet-journal-of-pediatrics-and-neonatology/volume-6-number-2/induced-abortion-and-child-directed-aggression-among-mothers-of-maltreated-children.html.
29   Ibid.
30   Ibid.

stillbirth, induced abortion may be experienced as a non-voluntary loss.[31] Consequently, "unresolved grief responses associated with perinatal loss… may increase the risk of parenting difficulties and increase the likelihood of child maltreatment."[32]

Secondly, abortion disrupts a natural bonding process that may begin for many women during pregnancy. As Coleman and colleagues explain,

> child maltreatment is essentially a physical or emotional manifestation of a disrupted parent-child relationship and although many variables undoubtedly factor into disturbed parent-child relationships, termination of a pregnancy may very well represent one key variable in some cases.[33]

Thirdly, abortion-related feelings of guilt or shame, which range from 30 to over 75 per cent, may hinder the development of feelings of closeness to later-born children. This in turn "may increase the likelihood of negative parenting attitudes and abusive or neglecting parenting behaviors."[34]

Fourthly, abortion is associated with a heightened risk for mental health problems, including anxiety, depression, and substance use, which in turn may heighten the risk of child maltreatment. "Substance abuse is a particularly strong risk factor as it is implicated in almost half of all substantiated cases of child maltreatment."[35]

DOES AN UNWANTED PREGNANCY MEAN AN UNWANTED CHILD?

Another striking, if counter-intuitive finding is that the children of women who applied for and were denied abortion fare almost as well those whose mothers wanted them. A Czech study reported that compared to the controls, "the care of these unwanted children, as far as feeding, general health and actual state of health [was] very good; they practically did not

---

31 Ibid.
32 Ibid.
33 Ibid.
34 Ibid.
35 Ibid.

differ from their siblings and other average children."[36] Summing up the results from five other studies, Del Campo reported that the great majority of women who were denied an abortion completed their pregnancy and experienced no greater incidence of complications than their paired controls. There was "good acceptance of the infant by the mother...and minimal to moderate psychosocial disadvantages for the child." There was no statistically significant difference in the rates of drunken misconduct, crime or "educational mental subnormality" between the two groups.[37] These findings also call into question the assumption that if women are prevented from having a legal abortion they will inevitably seek an illegal one. Another paper revealed that while the "unwanted" children scored higher in "maladaptation", the overall differences between them and the "accepted pregnancy" children were "not dramatic". [38] Moreover, the "unwanted" children were rated higher by their classmates for audacity and sense of humour, and slightly higher by their teachers for self-confidence.[39] Most authoritative was the Swedish study, which tracked from birth to age 35 a group of children born to women denied abortion. Measured against four major criteria, the differences between the "unwanted" children and the control children (whose mothers had not sought abortion), were statistically insignificant. The criteria were: psychiatric consultation and hospitalization, criminal record, drunken misconduct, and dependence on public assistance. The authors concluded that whatever social-psychiatric difficulties the "unwanted" children experienced were manifested for the most part early in life and became progressively smaller later on.[40]

THE FEMINIZATION OF POVERTY

Another way in which legalized abortion may have affected family formation is through what has been called the "feminization of poverty". Poverty has been and continues to become an increasing problem among women, and legalized abortion may have significantly contributed to this change. Diane Pearce, who first coined the term "feminization of poverty",

---

36   Schüller V, Stupkova E. The unwanted child in the family. International Mental Health Research Newsletter 1972; Fall 14 (3): 2-16, p. 8.
37   Del Campo C. Abortion denied—outcome of mothers and babies. CMAJ 1984 (Feb. 15); 130: 361-2.
38   Matejcek Z, Dytrych Z,Schüller V. Children from unwanted pregnancies. Acta Psychiatrica Scandinavica 1978; 57: 67-90, 81-2, p.86.
39   Dytrych Z, Matejcek Z, Schüller V, David HP, Friedman HL. Children born to women denied abortion. Family Planning Perspectives 1975; 7(4): 165-71, pp. 167, 168.
40   Forssman H, Thuwe I. Continued follow-up study of 120 persons born after refusal of application for therapeutic abortion. Acta Psychiatrica Scandinavica 1981; 64(2): 142-9, pp. 147-8.

commented on the dramatic increase of women living in poverty: "This dramatic change is not a reaction to recent fluctuations in the economy, but instead reflects long-term structural shifts both in the labor market and in marriage and childbearing practices. Today, three-quarters of the poor are women and children."[41] She further comments that, "the proportion of *poor* families that are maintained by women has risen in the 1970s from 36 per cent to more than 50 per cent. Moreover, there is evidence that this trend is accelerating."[42] Interestingly, this "feminization of poverty" coincides with the legalization of abortion, beginning in the early 1970s.[43] It may well be worth asking, then, how changes in marriage and childbearing practices, most notably the legalization of abortion, may have contributed to the feminization of poverty.

In the first place, abortion may have contributed because once it was legalized there was less pressure on a man to marry the woman he had made pregnant, since she now had easy access to abortion. Now, if she chooses to bring the child to term a man can reason that this was her choice and therefore not his responsibility. Consequently, more children are being raised by single mothers. In addition, the stigma of single-parenthood has gradually diminished, making it less likely that single mothers will give up their children for adoption.

Supporting the theory that a lack of support from fathers is a significant reason why women choose to abort is a study examining the motivations of women who gave birth to a first child but decided to abort a subsequent pregnancy. Women who chose to abort a second pregnancy did so because of a lack of support: "women who feel the first child's father has not assumed enough paternal responsibility and/or lacks the ability to contribute to their efforts to raise the child, are reluctant to bear another child."[44] It is suggested that such a finding should prompt professionals to seek "strategies for helping fathers assume a more active role in the lives of their children" or, in cases where a father in not able—for physical or emotional reasons—to assist with the child, professionals should offer practical assistance to the

---

41 Pearce DM. The feminization of ghetto poverty. Society 1983; 21(1): 70-4, p. 70.
42 Ibid., p. 70.
43 Strahan T. Studies suggesting that induced abortion may increase the feminization of poverty. Studies in Pro-Life Feminism 1995; 1(3): pp. 235-247.
44 Coleman PK, Maxey CD, Spence M, Nixon CL. Predictors and correlates of abortion in the fragile families and well-being study: Paternal behavior, substance abuse and partner violence. International Journal of Mental Health and Addiction 2009; 7(3): 405-22, p. 416.

mother so that she feels there are options available to her and is not forced to choose abortion as the only option.[45]

A second reason why legalized abortion may have contributed to increasing the number of women living in poverty is that women who have an abortion are more likely to develop psychological and emotional problems, such as depression and addictions. Coleman and colleagues found that women who chose abortion within eighteen months of a previous birth were more likely to report "recent heavy use of alcohol and cigarette smoking" than women who delivered a second child within eighteen months of a previous birth.[46] Of course, the researchers acknowledge that this does not necessarily mean that those who have undergone an abortion are more prone to substance abuse; however, "this interpretation is supported by the fact that substance use during the initial pregnancy (alcohol, tobacco) as well as ever having been treated for substance use were not systematically related to the choice to abort."[47] In other words, substance abuse may not have been an issue for many of these women until after their abortion. Substance abuse and emotional and mental health problems are widely recognized as factors that may contribute to or arise from poverty and substandard living conditions, but they may also be factors resulting from an induced abortion. More research needs to be done to determine whether this is the case.

Conclusion

The legalization of induced abortion together with the widespread availability of contraception has had a profound impact on family formation. Originally the legalization of abortion was expected to decrease the number of children born into single-parent families. In defiance of logic it has apparently done the opposite: contributed to the growing percentage of children raised by a single parent. Sociologists and economists speculate that single-parent families and births outside of marriage have become increasingly prevalent in the past half century because of an altered social norm: no longer are pre-marital sex, pre-marital pregnancy or single-parenthood stigmatized. Now that contraception and abortion are readily available, women are expected to have premarital sexual relations, yet single men are no longer expected to take responsibility as fathers.

---

45 Ibid., p. 418.
46 Ibid., p. 415.
47 Ibid., p. 416.

The legalization of abortion is also associated with relationship breakdown, female poverty and increased rates of child abuse. This may be due to the harmful impact of induced abortion on women. Even if a causal relationship between induced abortion and poor social outcomes may be questioned, it is hard to argue that the legalization of abortion has had any *positive* impact on the wellbeing of families.

Chapter 18

Depression, suicide, substance abuse: Contested research

KEY POINTS

- The question of abortion's psychological impact on women is highly contested in the social science literature.

- Research based on statistical measurements can never accurately reflect the full range and depth of women's post-abortion suffering.

- Much of the research on post-abortion mental health is intrinsically flawed on account of its politicization.

- The weight of evidence supports the conclusion that for a significant minority of women abortion has a devastating long-term psychological impact.

- The psychological impact of abortion includes much higher rates of depression, anxiety, substance abuse and suicide.

> "I remember laying down and wanting to die there. Never wanting to wake up. I stopped eating."
>
> "I feel like I'm dead inside."
>
> "Right after the abortion, I went into depression. I slept (more than normal, twelve hours per day) for two years."
>
> "I had nightmares for the first few years."
>
> "Looking back after having the benefit of education in Psychology and working as a social worker I realize that I was most likely seriously and clinically depressed. I have absolutely no doubt that the abortion triggered this episode even though I did not connect it at the time."[1]

---

[1] These quotations are from the deVeber Institute's Questionnaires of American and Canadian women about their abortion experiences, conducted between 2007 and 2012. The questionnaires from which the quotations are drawn are coded CSNM 31, CSNM 45, ID 11 and ID S6.

INTRODUCTION

Because of the highly controversial nature of the mental-health consequences of abortion, it is extremely difficult to carry out objective, scientific research in this area. Abortion's impact on women's mental health is simply too politically charged an issue. As in other areas, such as climate change or nutrition, once a politically correct position has been established, any publications that challenge that position tend to be ignored, dismissed or undermined. Sadly, the methodological differences in the study of post-abortion psychological problems make it difficult to weigh evidence and draw definitive conclusions.

The major approaches to research in this area fall into four distinct categories: prospective studies, retrospective studies, record linkage studies and meta-analysis.

Prospective research looks at women's status at the time of the abortion and afterwards—usually at six to twelve months following the event. Some of these studies have control groups of non-aborting women for comparative purposes, while others focus only on the abortion group. The results from those with control groups are considered to be the most rigorous types of research but as with all work in this area, the results usually reflect the criteria set out by the authors and the statistical approach used to analyze the data. These studies are marked by what is called "sample attrition," which means that many subjects drop out of the study following the abortion event. Rarely is there any discussion of why so many women drop out.

Retrospective research considers women's abortion experiences after the fact and allows for personal judgements of the participants rather than purely statistical analysis, though the information is coded and subjected to statistical analysis. Even though these types of studies reflect women's actual stories, they are often criticized for a lack of scientific rigour.

Record linkage studies look at longitudinal data collected from large national samples or questionnaires, often done by telephone. These tend to follow a particular cohort or group of people over time. They are designed to gather a large set of data about social or medical questions, and do not focus primarily on abortion.

Meta-analysis is a technique for analyzing already-published studies to determine an overall pattern. Authors apply statistical formulae to look for correlations that can be found in the previous data sets. Meta-analysis is based on the criteria for inclusion of studies set up by the researchers at the beginning of the process.

No matter what the format of the research used, those authors who publish results that challenge the prevailing position that abortion does not cause negative psychological impacts, are accused of having an anti-abortion agenda. Those whose research supports the status quo, on the other hand, are characterized as "independent" scientists. In the area of psychological outcomes after abortion, no pro-abortion bias is ever identified or even suggested in the mainstream literature. As a result, those working on this topic must carefully pick their way through the primary research and ask whether all the data have been accurately presented and whether the researchers' conclusions are valid.

COMPARISON OF RESEARCH

The British Journal of Psychiatry: Priscilla Coleman

The systemic bias in the abortion research comes most clearly to the fore when one considers the reaction to Priscilla Coleman's recent meta-analysis that uncovered a clear link between abortion and subsequent mental health problems. Her study, and several criticisms of it appeared in the *British Journal of Psychiatry* in its summer and fall issues of 2011.[2] Coleman's criteria for including a study in her meta-analysis were: a sample size of at least 100, the use of a comparison group, and controls for third variables—demographics, exposure to violence, prior history of mental health problems, among others. It identified 22 studies. Her review of these studies strongly supported an association between abortion and mental health problems. She discovered an overall 81 per cent greater risk of mental health problems for women who had an abortion compared to those who did not. When broken down by category, the mental health risks were as in Table 18.1

---

2   Coleman PK. Abortion and mental health: quantitative synthesis and analysis of research published 1995-2009. British Journal of Psychiatry 2011; 199(3): pp. 180-6; 200(1): pp. 77-80.

Table 18.1 **Increased mental health risks after induced abortion**

Type of Risk	Percentage Increased Risk
Anxiety disorders	34
Depression	37
Alcohol use/abuse	110
Marijuana use/abuse	220
Suicide behaviours	155
All mental health risks	81

Source: Coleman PK. Abortion and mental health: quantitative synthesis and analysis of research published 1995-2009. British Journal of Psychiatry 2011, 199: 3; 180-6.

She also calculated the overall population-attributable risk (PAR) to be 9.9 per cent. This means that *nearly ten per cent of all mental problems experienced by women are attributable to abortion alone, independent of any other factor.*

No abortion study can be perfect, since there is always another factor that might have been controlled for, but Coleman's methodology was sound enough for her paper to be accepted for publication in a prestigious, international, peer-reviewed journal. Once published, however, it attracted a barrage of criticism. Some critics accused her of not listing the studies she excluded, even though few other meta-analyses include such lists. In reality, no studies that met her eminently reasonable criteria were excluded. She was also attacked for having authored the study alone, for being biased, and for not adequately describing her research strategy. Such criticisms, however, failed to weaken the significance of her main findings.

Another criticism was that she had authored or co-authored eleven of the 22 studies included and was therefore biased; some even accused her of having an undeclared conflict of interest. In reply, Coleman pointed out that she is the most widely published researcher in this particular field, and so it is to be expected that many of the studies are hers. In addition, she could hardly exclude studies that met the selection criteria regarding size of sample, and having control groups, just because those studies happened to be hers. We may also note that the authors of several of the studies included in Coleman's meta-analysis—Fergusson,[3] Thorp,[4] Gissler[5] and others—are scientists of impeccable reputation who have not been accused of bias. Yet their findings are essentially similar to Coleman's.

Coleman also rejected the accusation of conflict of interest. The editors of the *British Journal of Psychiatry* supported her right to be published, maintaining that neither controversial subject matter nor failure to declare a conflict of interest—even if such existed—would be reason enough to retract Coleman's systematic review, as some of the angry critics demanded.

Another criticism levelled at Coleman's meta-analysis was that calculating population-attributable risk is misleading, because abortion can never be an independent factor that causes mental health problems. Her critics evidently consider it to be axiomatic that any causal relationship between abortion and mental health problems is an impossibility. While it is true that correlation does not necessarily imply causation, it is also true that a correlation repeated across many independent studies may be interpreted as a cause warranting further investigation. The correlation between abortion and poor mental health outcomes has been established, even if the nature of the correlation is still in dispute. Most researchers assume that poor mental health may cause a woman to seek an abortion, or that some third factor (typically unintended pregnancy or a history of violence) may cause both the abortion decision and poor mental health. However, Coleman is suggesting an alternative and perhaps more reasonable possibility—that abortion may itself be a cause of poor mental health. Similarly, the abortion-mental health correlation may be a self-reinforcing system, each increasing the likelihood of the other. Coleman cannot be faulted for making logical inferences concerning the correlations that emerge from her large-scale survey of the data.

In the introduction to her study, Coleman criticizes previous narrative reviews that concluded that abortion poses no greater risk to a woman's mental health than does carrying an unintended pregnancy to term. She provides three reasons for making this criticism: 1) some pertinent peer-reviewed literature was excluded from previous meta-analyses without

---

3   Fergusson DM, Horwood LJ, Boden JM. Abortion and mental health disorders: evidence from a 30-year longitudinal study. Br J Psychiatry 2008; 193: pp.444–51.
4   Thorp, Hartmann, Shadigan. See Chapter 9, n.38.
5   Gissler M, Hemminki E, Lonnqvist J. Suicides after pregnancy in Finland, 1987-94: register linkage study. BMJ 1996 December; 313(7070): pp. 1431-4.

explanation; 2) there was a lack of "sufficient methodologically based selection criteria;"[6] and 3) there was no quantification of effects. These are telling and accurate criticisms, as a reading of those reviews reveals.[7]

An additional point of contention between Coleman and her critics is the importance of pregnancy intention. Many researchers think that only if a pregnancy was intended would a woman react negatively to a pregnancy loss; therefore, they dismiss the findings of studies that do not control for pregnancy intention. However, as Coleman notes, few studies have controlled for pregnancy intention because the concept is not well-defined in the literature. It is treated as a dichotomous measure (intended vs. unintended), yet it actually falls on a continuum. For example, how would one classify a woman who welcomed a pregnancy that she had not consciously been seeking? Moreover, pregnancy intention can fluctuate over the course of the pregnancy: one minute a woman can be excited about motherhood and the next minute think she is not ready to be a mother. When women who aborted were compared with woman who did not abort, Coleman found a 59 per cent greater risk of experiencing mental health problems after an abortion; when women who aborted were compared with women who carried an unintended pregnancy to term, Coleman found a 55 per cent greater risk of experiencing mental health problems after an abortion. Since these results are similar, Coleman concluded that an "unintended pregnancy delivered" group is neither the only, nor the most appropriate, control group for studies of abortion and mental health.

Danish Study: Monk-Olsen

Nevertheless, Coleman's critics argued for the greater credibility of a Danish study by Munk-Olsen[8] and colleagues that used unintended pregnancy aborted and unintended pregnancy delivered as its comparison groups. By extension, its conclusion that there is no increase in mental disorders after

---

6   Coleman. See n. 2, p. 181.
7   American Psychological Association (APA) Task Force on Mental Health and Abortion. *Report of the American Psychological Association Task Force on Mental Health and Abortion.* Washington, DC: APA, 2008; Charles VE, Polis CB, Sridhara SK, Blum RW. Abortion and long-term mental health outcomes: a systematic review of the evidence. Contraception 2008; 78:, pp. 436-50; Robinson GE, Stotland NL, Russo NF, Lang JA, Occhiogrosso M. Is there an 'abortion trauma syndrome'? Critiquing the evidence. Harvard Rev Psychiatry 2009; 17: pp. 268-90.
8   Munk-Olsen T, et al. Induced first-trimester abortion and risk of mental disorder. NEJM 2011; 27: 332-9.

a first-trimester abortion is assumed by these critics to be more reliable than Coleman's entire meta-analysis. While the Munk-Olsen study is claimed to be methodologically sound, in fact it has glaring shortcomings. To begin with, mental problems were assessed by first psychiatric contact between the beginning of the pregnancy and one year later. Thus, women who may have experienced mental problems associated with their abortion later than 90 days (three months) after giving birth, as well as anyone who did not seek professional help, were completely overlooked by the researchers. Furthermore, besides pregnancy intention the only other variables Munk-Olsen and colleagues controlled for were age and parity (number of pregnancies). Finally, although over 40 years of Danish Civil Registration System data were available to them, they selected only twelve years, without offering any explanation as to why those particular years were chosen. If so many women were excluded from this study, how reliable can its conclusions be? Unless we are told why the other 28 years were excluded, how confident can we be of the reliability of the study's findings?

Coleman's results show emphatically that women who abort are more likely to experience poor mental health outcomes than those who carry their pregnancies to term. This finding is consonant with studies showing that pregnancy carried to term protects mental health.[9] Insisting that abortion is necessary to protect a woman from the negative sequelae of an unintended pregnancy carried to term has no factual grounding to support it. Furthermore, "procedure benefits of abortion have not been empirically established."[10] Therefore, Coleman concludes that women should be made aware of the risks before making an abortion decision.

Royal Medical Colleges

Shortly after the appearance of Coleman's meta-analysis the Academy of Royal Medical Colleges published its own systematic review.[11]

---

9   See for example Appleby L. Suicide during pregnancy and in the first postnatal year. BMJ 1991; 302: pp.137–40; Kleiner GJ, Greston WM (eds). *Suicide in Pregnancy*. Boston: John Wright, 1984; Lindahl V, Pearson JL, Colpe L. Prevalence of suicidality during pregnancy and the postpartum. Arch Womens Ment Health 2005; 8: pp. 77–87; Schiff MA, Grossman DC. Adverse perinatal outcomes and risk of postpartum suicide attempt in Washington State, 1987–2001. Pediatrics 2006; 118: e669–75.
10   Coleman. See n. 2, p. 185.
11   National Collaborating Centre for Mental Health (NCCMH). *Induced abortion and mental health: a systematic review of the mental health outcomes of induced abortion, including their prevalence and associated factors.* London: Academy of Medical Royal Colleges, December 2011.

Among its findings were, first, the rates of mental health problems for women with an unwanted pregnancy were the same whether they had an abortion or gave birth. Secondly, they said that the most reliable predictor of post-abortion mental health problems was having a history of mental health problems before the abortion.

The report also acknowledged that other factors could trigger mental health problems related to abortion, "such as pressure from a partner to have an abortion and negative attitudes towards abortions in general and towards a woman's personal experience of the abortion."[12]

Shortcomings in British Report

Unfortunately the report has a number of serious flaws that render its findings questionable. Many sound studies are ignored, while others are dismissed for vague or inappropriate reasons. Only three reviews of the literature are included, while nineteen are overlooked. Thirty-five peer-reviewed studies were eliminated because they only studied mental health consequences during the first three months after abortion.[13] It is ironic that the APA Report considered *only* studies that focused on the first three months after abortion. By the criteria of the Royal Medical Colleges, the APA Report is not worthy of consideration. The Academy Report also wrongly stated that Coleman's meta-analysis did not control for previous mental health problems.[14] Nor did the Report address the problem of the high attrition rates of participants in many of the studies it relied upon. Furthermore, its conclusions are based on a very small number of studies that are not properly rated for quality. In fact, its final conclusion that abortion is no riskier to women's mental health than unintended pregnancy brought to term, is based on only four studies.[15] Finally, the report ignores the massive evidence that women who have abortions have a suicide risk several times higher than women who bring their pregnancies to term (See below, pp. 281-2).

Systemic Bias

In response to the Academy and other critics of her meta-analysis Coleman wrote in the *British Journal of Psychiatry*:

---

12   Ibid., p. 10.
13   Ibid., p. 12.
14   Ibid., p. 21.
15   Ibid., p. 108. The four studies are Fergusson (2008), Cougle (2005), Gilchrist (1995), and Steinburg (2008) study 1.

> By raising concerns of publication bias and attempting to undermine the credibility of an individual researcher who managed to publish in a high-profile journal, several people have sought to shift attention from the truly shameful and systemic bias that permeates the psychology of abortion. Professional organisations in the USA and elsewhere have arrogantly sought to distort the scientific literature and paternalistically deny women the information they deserve to make fully informed healthcare choices and receive necessary mental health counselling when and if an abortion decision proves detrimental.[16]

In other words, so strong is the political agenda to preserve unrestricted access to induced abortion that in spite of abundant evidence to the contrary, abortion continues to be upheld as a "safe" procedure that is good for women. In addition, the many voices of women attesting to the negative impact abortion has had on their lives are ignored or suppressed because of this agenda.

From the testimonies of many women it is clear that whatever their reasons for having obtained an abortion, the experience, or their later interpretation of it, can cause grief as real as if the child had been wanted in the first place. For some women, induced abortion may trigger mental problems or exacerbate existing ones.

Strong support for Coleman's indictment of the American Psychological Association came from David Fergusson, John Horwood and Joseph Boden, medical researchers at the University of Otago, New Zealand. Having followed the restrictive guidelines laid down by Howard and colleagues, they conducted another meta-analysis limited to eight studies. Like Coleman they found that induced abortion was associated with a significantly increased risk of anxiety disorder, mood disorder, alcohol misuse, illicit drug misuse, and suicidal behaviours. There is therefore no justification for denying "that abortion has adverse mental health consequences."[17] Among the most strident defenders of the American Psychological Association's position are Gail Robinson, Professor of Psychiatry at the University of

---

16   Coleman PK. Author's reply. British Journal of Psychiatry 2012; 200(1): 79-80, p. 80.
17   Fergusson D, Horwood J, Boden , letter to the British Journal of Psychiatry online, Oct. 5,2011. The authors state that a detailed paper describing their findings is currently under review.

Toronto, and colleagues. Referring to, but not citing, "huge numbers of papers...that have not found negative mental health consequences", they are harshly dismissive of Coleman's meta-analysis, and excoriate the *British Journal of Psychiatry* for failing to recognize the "deficiencies" in it.[18] Yet they cannot gainsay that numerous studies by researchers with no ideological axe to grind lend credence to Coleman's findings.

Major Findings

Depression

In a recent study Mota and colleagues found that among 3310 American women, 48.8 per cent of those with both a lifetime psychiatric diagnosis and an abortion history had their first onset of depression *after* their first abortion.[19] However, the researchers were able virtually to eliminate the significance of this finding by "adjusting" for violence (including "physical abuse by parents and (or) guardians; physical abuse by partner; physical abuse by anybody else; rape; other sexual assault; and [being] mugged, held up, or threatened with a weapon").[20] In this way they were able to conclude that depression was not significantly associated with abortion.

By contrast, Coleman has found a 37 per cent greater risk of depression among women who had had an abortion. The population-attributable risk of depression was 8.5 per cent; in other words, 8.5 per cent of the entire incidence of depression in a given population could be attributed directly to abortion, independent of any other factor.

Post-abortive women have also indicated somatic problems related to depression, such as disturbed sleep. "Sleep disturbances are leading manifestations of major depression."[21]

Anxiety

Mota and colleages found that 45.3 per cent of those with both a lifetime

---

18 Robinson G, Stotland N, Nadelson C, letter to the British Journal of Psychiatry, published online, Sept. 22, 2011.
19 95% CI 40.1-57.5
20 Mota NP, Burnett M, Sareen J. Associations between abortion, mental disorders, and suicidal behaviour in a nationally representative sample. Canadian Journal of Psychiatry 2010; 55(5): 239-47, p. 241.
21 Brasic JR. Screening people with disturbed sleep for depression. Perception and Motor Skills 2006; 103: pp. 765-6.

psychiatric diagnosis and an abortion history had their first onset of generalized anxiety disorder *after* their first abortion.

Coleman calculated a 34 per cent greater risk of anxiety for women who had had an abortion. The population-attributable risk of anxiety was 8.1 per cent; in other words, 8.1 per cent of the incidence of anxiety can be attributed directly to abortion, independent of any other factor.

Substance Abuse

A study of 700 women in New York State found that the use of illicit drugs was 6.1 times higher among women with a history of induced abortion when compared to women without such a history.[22] In another study, those who aborted, even those with no prior history of substance abuse, were 4.5 times more likely to report subsequent substance abuse compared to those who continued their pregnancies to term.[23] In her meta-analysis Coleman discovered that after induced abortion the increased risk of a woman abusing alcohol was 110 per cent, while her increased risk of marijuana use or abuse was 220 per cent.[24]

Suicide

Those who would persuade us that abortion has no harmful effect on women's mental health almost never refer to the much higher suicide rate of women who have undergone abortion. The high rate of suicide among whom women with a history of induced abortion is documented in at least four major studies. We are not aware of any study that contradicts these findings from Scandinavia, Britain and the US.[25]

A large study of British women found that those who had induced abortions were 225 per cent more likely to attempt suicide than those admitted for normal delivery.[26] This study also found that the rate of attempted suicide *prior to pregnancy* was similar for both groups. In other

---

22   Yamaguchi D, Kandel D. Drug use and other determinants of premarital pregnancy and its outcome : a dynamic analysis of competing life events. Journal of Marriage and the Family 1987; 49: pp. 257-70.
23   Reardon DC, Ney P. Abortion and subsequent substance abuse. American Journal of Drug and Alcohol Abuse 2000; 26: pp. 61-75.
24   Coleman. See n. 2. See also Coleman PK. Induced abortion and increased risk of substance abuse: a review of the evidence. Current Women's Health Reviews 2005; 1: pp. 21-34.
25   For a more extensive treatment of the subject of suicide see chapter 10.
26   Morgan CL, Evans M, Peters JR. Suicides after pregnancy. Mental health may deteriorate as a direct effect of induced abortion. BMJ 1997 March; 314(7084): pp. 902-3.

words, women prone to attempt suicide were not more likely to have abortions and attempt suicide again.

Two Scandinavian studies have uncovered a much higher mortality after abortion than after childbirth. A large-scale, linkage study of Finnish women found that within one year of the end of pregnancy, the suicide rate associated with childbirth was *six times lower* than the suicide rate associated with abortion.[27]

A recently-published investigation of the impact of abortion in Denmark, while it does not specifically deal with suicide, has come up with similar findings.[28] This large-scale, 25-year study employed a rigorous methodology based on data linkage to completed pregnancy and abortion records. Surveying the entire female population born between 1962 and 1993, the authors compared mortality rates linked to induced abortion, miscarriage ("natural losses"), and live births. Covering the period from 1980 to 2004, the study included over a million women. Those who had experienced induced abortion and miscarriages suffered more than three times the risk of death of women who had only experienced birth. By contrast, giving birth had a protective effect, with the women who gave birth twice experiencing the greatest reduction in mortality—108 per cent reduced risk.[29]

The fourth large-scale study comes from California. It too is methodologically rigorous, based exclusively on data linkage.[30] Medical records were linked to death certificates for 173,279 low-income women who underwent a state-funded delivery or induced abortion in 1989. Four years later the annual suicide rate among the women who terminated their pregnancies was found to be 160 per cent higher than among the women who gave birth. When the effects of previous psychiatric history were removed, the relative risk for woman who had abortions actually increased, compared with that of delivering women.

---

27   Gissler et al. See n. 5, pp. 1431-4.
28   Coleman, Reardon, Calhoun. See Chapter 12, n. 6; Reardon DC, Coleman PK. Short and long term mortality rates associated with first pregnancy outcome: Population register based study for Denmark 1980-2004. Medical Science Monitor 2012; 18(9): PH71-76.
29   Ibid., p. 3.
30   Reardon DC, Ney PG, Scheurer FJ, Congle JR, Coleman PK. Suicide deaths associated with pregnancy outcome: A record linkage study of 172,279 low income American women. Archives of Women's Mental Health 2001; 3(4 Suppl.2): p. 104.

Conclusion

Abortion is a controversial topic, and the causal link between abortion and mental health sequelae is particularly contentious. Nevertheless, women deserve to know where the evidence points. It is all too clear that the experiences of many post-abortive women are currently ignored in most of the professional literature. It is surely incumbent on researchers to produce rigorous and objective studies as befits their science.

The testimonies of post-abortive women reveal their psychological pain in a variety of ways: a woman may become depressed or anxious; as we will see, she may also engage in harmful behaviours in an attempt to suppress the pain. Regardless of its expression, the psychological pain associated with elective abortion is inextricably linked with guilt. As noted at the beginning of this chapter, post-abortion studies can never accurately measure the experiences of many women. Many of those who struggle with mental health problems following abortion are not represented in the statistical studies of abortion and yet these women exist. We know about them through their stories, their affidavits and their testimonies. They have not always had mental health problems before their abortion as many researchers suggest. Finally, the increase in the rate of depression, anxiety, substance abuse and suicide among women who have had abortions is drastic and incontrovertible.

Chapter 19

Intimate partner violence and abortion

> "I told him I was pregnant at about two months gestation; he became physically violent and just about killed me. I jumped out of a moving vehicle to get away. He had his necktie around my neck…He chased me."[1]

> "My boyfriend was 19 and went into a rage. He insisted that I have an abortion to 'get rid of this stupid mistake!' I was terrified at his extreme fit of anger. He grabbed me by the throat and threatened to kill me if I didn't have an abortion."

> "He threatened to burn my house down and take the baby away after it was born."

> "He wanted me to get an abortion, and all, when I was pregnant…He was never around. When he was, he was hitting me and being abusive when I was pregnant."

> "My husband started threatening me with separation if I did not agree to have an abortion . . . While he was pulling my hair, he kept yelling at me to sign the papers or abort the baby; he said I only had two choices: abort the baby or return to India."

> "I wouldn't know how he would deal with it if I had the child; that's one of the reasons I would have the abortion…If I knew for sure that he would be away and he wouldn't bother me, then I wouldn't have a problem because I've always wanted another child."

---

1 This and the other boxed quotations in this chapter are taken from the deVeber Institute's Interviews and surveys of Canadian and American women regarding their experience of induced abortion. 2011 (unpublished).

> "My boyfriend was relentless. I am deliberately omitting the details of the violence, both real and threatened, but I finally caved in to my boyfriend's insistence not to have our baby."

> "He destroyed our apartment...and told me to get rid of it. Now! The whole time he cornered me...throwing things and killing me with his words... The abortion ripped me apart. Any strength I had to leave the abuse was torn away from me."

> "I was thirteen…the pursuit was constant by my boyfriend, and under the influence of alcohol I didn't stop the sexual advance. By today's standards that would have been called 'date rape'."

KEY POINTS

- Studies worldwide report a correlation between intimate partner violence (IPV) and abortion.

- Women who suffer intimate partner violence are more likely to have abortions—both induced and spontaneous—than those who do not.

- Women who seek induced abortion are more likely to be victims of coercion and/or intimate partner violence.

- Abortion-seeking women who have experienced intimate partner violence are more likely to have been coerced to terminate their pregnancy; it is therefore highly problematic to characterize induced abortion as a woman's choice.

- Women who have had an induced abortion may subsequently experience or exacerbate intimate partner violence.

- Researchers call for more screening for abuse during pregnancy; such screening is just as important among women seeking induced abortion.

Intimate Partner Violence Defined

Also known as Domestic Violence, "Intimate Partner Violence (IPV) is defined as threatened, attempted, or completed physical or sexual violence or emotional abuse by a current or former intimate partner."[2] Physical abuse includes acts such as hitting, kicking and beating. A psychologically abusive partner intimidates, belittles or humiliates. Sexual violence includes forced intercourse, incest, and sexual harassment and molestation. One form of intimate partner violence tends to accompany another. For example, a woman can face "severe physical or social consequences if she resists sexual advances."[3]

Consequences of Intimate Partner Violence

Each year in the United States, intimate partner violence "results in an estimated 1200 deaths and two million injuries among women."[4] Well-documented physical complications of intimate partner violence include pain, headaches, dizziness, fatigue, insomnia, nausea or vomiting, gastrointestinal problems and shortness of breath.[5] Incomplete strangulation or blows to the head can cause brain damage. Studies have also shown that intimate partner violence increases substance abuse, which can lead to later physical complications.[6] Furthermore, abused women may also be less likely to seek adequate health care.

As one researcher explains, "violence not only causes physical injury, it also undermines the social, economic, psychological, spiritual and emotional well-being of the victim."[7] Such consequences include grief, shame, depression, posttraumatic stress disorder (PTSD), suicide ideation, social isolation, and difficulty establishing intimacy and trust.[8]

---

2   Black MC and Breiding MJ. Adverse health conditions and health risk behaviors associated with intimate partner violence—United States, 2005. Morbidity and Mortality Weekly Report 2008; 57(5): p. 113.
3   Yimin C, Shouging L, Arzhu Q, et al. Sexual coercion among adolescent women seeking abortion in China. Journal of Adolescent Health 2002; 31(6): p. 485.
4   Black and Breiding. See n. 2, p. 113.
5   Cobia DC, Robinson K and Edwards L. Intimate partner violence and women's sexual health: implications for couples therapists. Family Journal: Counselling and Therapy for Couples and Families 2008; 16(3): 249-53.
6   Vos T, et al. Measuring the impact of intimate partner violence on the health of women in Victoria, Australia. Bulletin of the World Health Organization 2006; 84(9): 739-44.
7   Kaur R and Garg S. Addressing domestic violence against women: an unfinished agenda. Indian Journal of Community Medicine 2008; 33(2): p. 74.
8   Cobia, Robinson and Edwards. See n. 5, p. 250.

Sexual abuse, particularly forced sex, increases the likelihood of getting a sexually transmitted infection (STI) and experiencing gynaecological problems such as urethral, anal and vaginal trauma, fibroids,[9] menstrual irregularities, pain during intercourse, infertility, hysterectomy[10] and pelvic inflammatory disease.[11] Immediately after rape, women may experience such physical symptoms as "nausea, vomiting, headache, sweating, palpitations, and muscle pain."[12]

Sexually abused women also present mental health sequelae. In a study of in-depth interviews with 68 female victims of rape during the Bosnian war, "The most frequent psychological symptoms felt immediately after the rape were depressiveness (n = 58), avoidance of thoughts or conversations associated with the trauma (n = 40), and suicidal ideas (n = 25)... Although none of the women had a psychiatric history before the rape, at the time of study 52 suffered from depression, 51 from social phobia, 21 from posttraumatic stress disorder (PTSD), and seventeen had sexual dysfunctions [such as sexual arousal disorder or orgasmic disorder]. These disorders were often comorbid."[13]

Child sexual abuse (CSA) increases the risk of experiencing adult sexual violence.[14] Later in life, victims of child sexual abuse may experience sexual dysfunction, intimacy disorders, sleep disturbance, difficulty with concentration and memory, and irrational guilt.[15]

CONSEQUENCES OF INTIMATE PARTNER VIOLENCE ON PREGNANT WOMEN

Women who endure intimate partner violence while pregnant are at further risk for kidney infection, insufficient weight gain, operative delivery,

---

9   Campbell JC. Health consequences of intimate partner violence. The Lancet 2002; 359(9314): pp. 1331-6.
10   Coker AL. Does physical intimate partner violence affect sexual health? A systematic review. Trauma, Violence, & Abuse 2007; 8(2): pp. 149-77.
11   McFarlane J, et al. Intimate partner sexual assault against women: frequency, health consequences, and treatment outcomes. Obstetrics and Gynecology 2005; 105(1): pp. 99-108.
12   Lončar M, et al. Psychological consequences of rape on women in 1991-1995 war in Croatia and Bosnia and Herzegovina. Croatian Medical Journal 2006; 47: p. 71.
13   Ibid., p. 67.
14   Hamelin C, et al. Childhood sexual abuse and adult sexual health among indigenous Kanak women and non-Kanak women of New Caledonia. Child Abuse & Neglect 2010; 34: pp. 677-88.
15   Cobia, et al. See n. 5.

and reduced levels of breastfeeding;[16] besides, they often delay seeking obstetrical care.[17] A plethora of studies concurs that negative pregnancy outcomes, such as low birth weight, premature labour or delivery, small size for gestational age, stillbirth and late entry into prenatal care are more common among abused than non-abused women. In addition, sexual trauma increases "vulnerability to PTSD and depression in subsequent pregnancy."[18]

In the worst case scenario, intimate partner violence can cause death: "The risk for maternal mortality is three times as high for abused mothers."[19] Moreover, studies abound as evidence that intimate partner violence "increases the risk of injury or death to both mother and fetus."[20] A systematic review of hundreds of intimate partner violence and pregnancy outcomes found that intimate partner violence increased fetal deaths in affected pregnancies by about 16 per 1000.[21] For instance, a study conducted in India demonstrated that victims of intimate partner violence "were significantly more likely than other women to have experienced fetal wastage [including induced abortion] or infant deaths," even after logistic regression controlling for other factors.[22]

Intimate Partner Violence and Spontaneous Abortion (Miscarriage)

> "He got his friends to beat me up and throw me on the ground so I would miscarry."
>
> "When I got pregnant, he didn't want me to have the baby. But I did. He tried to kick the baby out of me when I was like five months along. But it didn't work."

---

16   Boy A and Salihu HM. Intimate partner violence and birth outcomes: a systematic review. International Journal of Fertility and Women's Medicine 2004; 49(4): pp. 159-64.
17   Devries KM, et al. Intimate partner violence during pregnancy: analysis of prevalence data from 19 countries. Reproductive Health Matters 2010; 18(36): pp. 158-70.
18   Hamama L, et al. Previous experience of spontaneous or elective abortion and risk for posttraumatic stress and depression during subsequent pregnancy. Depression and Anxiety 2010; 27(8): p. 706.
19   Boy and Salihu. See n. 16, p. 159.
20   Cobia, et al. See n. 5, p. 250.
21   Boy and Salihu. See n. 16, pp. 159-64.
22   $P \leq 0.01$: Jejeebhoy SJ. Associations between wife-beating and fetal and infant death: impressions from a survey in rural India. Studies in Family Planning 1998; 29(3): p. 305.

> "Before I had my last baby, I had a miscarriage, by him, from him fighting, jumping on me."
>
> "Suddenly, without any warning, he slammed me up against our dresser and then punched me in my belly and screamed, 'And I don't want that baby either!'... Around 10:30 or 11:00 pm that night, I noticed that I was bleeding."

Spontaneous abortion can be caused directly by violence, through the inability of an abused woman to seek adequate care during pregnancy, and/or through *embodiment*—the biological incorporation of the abused woman's social and material world, for example with a hyperactive physiological response to stress.[23]

Several studies have shown that some women are violently attacked by their partner "in attempts to cause spontaneous abortions."[24] In one African study, "eight women had been raped while they were pregnant, which resulted in either spontaneous abortion or preterm stillbirth. Two women had been raped when they were four and five months pregnant, respectively, and suffered spontaneous abortions within a few days of being attacked."[25] In a qualitative study of battered women conducted in the United States, "out of the ten women total, two had spontaneous abortions they attributed to attacks. Three others reported attacks aimed at causing miscarriage. One delivered a baby prematurely and attributed it to stress. Another delivered a large baby and believed the macrosomia [excessive birth weight] was caused by her partner force-feeding her."[26] In one final example, of 4750 British Columbia women who gave birth from January 1999 to December 2000, 22.7 per cent of those who experienced physical abuse or fear of their partner had had one or more previous spontaneous abortions, compared to 16.9 per cent of those who were not abused or fearful.[27]

---

23   Fanslow J, et al. Pregnancy outcomes and intimate partner violence in New Zealand. Australian and New Zealand Journal of Obstetrics and Gynaecology 2008; 48(4): pp. 391-7.
24   Coggins M and Bullock LFC. The wavering line in the sand: The effects of domestic violence and sexual coercion. Issues in Mental Health Nursing 2003; 24(6/7): 723-38, p. 734.
25   Onsrud M, et al. Sexual violence-related fistulas in the Democratic Republic of Congo. International Journal of Gynecology and Obstetrics 2008; 103(3): p. 266.
26   Coggins and Bullock. See n. 24, p. 728.
27   Janssen PA, et al. Intimate partner violence and adverse pregnancy outcomes: a population-based study. AJOG 2003; 188(5): pp. 1341-7.

VIOLENCE TRIGGERED OR EXACERBATED BY PREGNANCY

Pregnancy is a vulnerable time for women. Sadly, it can trigger or amplify abuse.[28] Women who experience intimate partner violence often report that the abuse becomes more frequent and severe after they become pregnant.[29] One researcher effectively explains why this is the case:

> Stress often accompanies even the happiest of pregnancies; however, it can exacerbate the tension between the couple, especially if there is ambivalence about wanting the pregnancy. If there already exists a pattern of abuse in addressing conflict, it is more likely that it will continue and escalate during and after pregnancy. Qualitative studies of women's perceptions regarding why partners are abusive during pregnancy included jealousy and resentment of the unborn child, anger at the pregnancy effects on the mother, continuance of ongoing abuse, the need for the partner to have control, the partner's definition of manhood, and alcohol abuse by the partner.[30]

Another researcher notes that the redirection of assault from a woman's face and breasts to her pregnant abdomen "implies hostility toward the woman's fertility."[31] Williams and Brackley particularly highlight this disturbing trend: One woman's partner threw a microwave at her stomach; another, who reported she had been beaten fifteen times while pregnant, also "reported punching and kicking and severe bruises to her abdomen and pelvis. This woman was eight weeks gestation at time of interview."[32]

An enhanced pregnancy mortality surveillance study in Maryland "led to the disturbing finding that a pregnant or recently pregnant woman is more likely to be a victim of homicide than to die of any other cause."[33] Supporting this finding, a study of 437 attempted or completed female homicide victims

---

28   Devries. See n. 17, pp. 158-70.
29   Williams GB and Brackley MH. Intimate partner violence, pregnancy and decision for abortion: Issues in Mental Health Nursing 2009 April; 30(4): 272-8.
30   Kramer A. Stages of change: surviving intimate partner violence during and after pregnancy. Journal of Perinatal & Neonatal Nursing 2007; 21(4): p. 286.
31   Reardon DC. Report misses association of violence with pregnancy. Letter: Violence as a public health problem. BMJ 2003; 326(7380): p. 104.
32   Williams and Brackley. See n. 29, p. 276.
33   Horon IL and Cheng D. Enhanced surveillance for pregnancy-associated mortality—Maryland, 1993-1998. JAMA 2001; 285(11): p. 1455.

and 384 abused women in ten major US cities concluded that the odds of a woman becoming a completed or attempted homicide victim increased between two- and threefold if she was abused during pregnancy.[34] An earlier study showed that in North Carolina alone from 1992 to 1996, "62 women died either while pregnant or within one year of pregnancy termination or delivery from external causes of injury" including four cut/pierce homicides, fifteen firearm homicides, one struck homicide, two suffocation homicides, five suicides, and six cocaine-related deaths.[35]

How common is abuse during pregnancy? In a study of intimate partner violence in nineteen countries across four continents using Demographic and Health Surveys and International Violence against Women Surveys, researchers observed that "intimate partner violence during pregnancy is more common than some maternal health conditions routinely screened for in antenatal care."[36]

INTIMATE PARTNER VIOLENCE AND UNWANTED PREGNANCY

Unintended pregnancies carry "an even greater risk of violence than intended pregnancies."[37] And, as Miller and colleagues acknowledge, there is "mounting evidence that unintended pregnancy occurs more commonly in abusive relationships."[38] Intimate partner violence is more likely to foster an unintended or unwanted pregnancy as a result of forced sex or an intimate partner's rejection of contraception.[39]

Abuse during childhood is linked to risky sexual behaviour later in life, which can cause an increase in unwanted pregnancy and abortion. One study found that the experience of child sexual abuse "was significantly associated with increased rates of pregnancy during ages fifteen to 25."[40]

---

[34] OR 3.70, 95% CI 2.33, 5.87; aOR 3.08, 95% aCI 1.86, 5.10; McFarlane J et al. Abuse during pregnancy and femicide: urgent implications for women's health. Obstetrics & Gynecology 2002; 100(1): pp. 27-36.
[35] Parsons LH and Harper MA. Violent maternal deaths in North Carolina. Obstetrics and Gynecology 1999; 94(6): p. 991.
[36] Devries. See n. 17, p. 158.
[37] Moore AM, Frohwirth L and Miller E. Male reproductive control of women who have experienced intimate partner violence in the United States. Social Science and Medicine 2010; 70(11): p. 1737.
[38] Miller E, et al. Reproductive coercion: connecting the dots between partner violence and unintended pregnancy. Contraception 2010; 81(6): p. 457.
[39] Moore et al. See n. 37, pp. 1737-44.
[40] $p < .0001$; Boden JM, Fergusson DM and Horwood LJ. Experience of sexual abuse in childhood and abortion in adolescence and early adulthood. Child Abuse & Neglect 2009; 33(12): p. 870.

Another study of 125 sexually abused adolescent girls aged between twelve and seventeen found that "adolescents with a history of sexual abuse involving penetration were thirteen times as likely to have been pregnant."[41] In a qualitative study of sixteen teenaged girls, "the increased rate of abortion was felt to be mainly due to initiation of sexual activity at a younger age."[42] Such findings "suggest a causal chain association in which experience of CSA [child sexual abuse] plays a causal role in increasing sexual risk-taking leading to pregnancy, and an increased risk of elective abortion."[43] Erdmans and Black noted the same "well-trod trajectory" from child sexual abuse to teen pregnancy.[44]

One study discovered that, compared to non-victims, victims of abuse are more likely to report "unhappy feelings about their current pregnancy (twenty vs. 33 per cent), perceiving their partners (eleven vs. 22 percent) and families (fourteen vs. 27 percent) as unhappy about their pregnancy, and feeling a lack of support during their pregnancy (thirteen vs. 36 percent)."[45] Understandably, if an abuse victim is unsupported, let alone mistreated during this time, she will be more likely to elect to terminate her pregnancy. Women who have experienced both an unintended pregnancy and prior abuse are more likely to seek induced abortion.

INTIMATE PARTNER VIOLENCE AND INDUCED ABORTION

A World Health Organization report found miscarriage to be associated with partner physical and/or sexual violence, but there was an even stronger association between abuse and induced abortion: "In the majority of settings, ever-pregnant women who had experienced partner physical or sexual violence, or both were significantly more likely to report having had at least one induced abortion than women who had never experienced

---

41   Cinq-Mars C, et al. Sexual at-risk behaviors of sexually abused adolescent girls. Journal of Child Sexual Abuse 2004; 12(2): p. 2.
42   Thorsén C, Aneblom G and Gemzell-Danielsson K. Perceptions of contraception, non-protection and induced abortion among a sample of urban Swedish teenage girls: Focus group discussions. European Journal of Contraception and Reproductive Health Care 2006; 11(4): p. 302.
43   Boden et al. See n. 40, p. 871.
44   Erdmans MP and Black T. What they tell you to forget: From childhood sexual abuse to adolescent motherhood. Qualitative Health Research 2008; 18(1): pp. 77-89.
45   Amaro H, Fried LE, Cabral H and Zuckerman B. Violence during pregnancy and substance use. American Journal of Public Health 1990 May; 80(5): 575-9, p. 577.

partner violence."⁴⁶ Many studies have shown that intimate partner violence is correlated with an increase in sexual risk-taking behaviour, adolescent, unplanned or unwanted pregnancy, and induced abortion.⁴⁷ In fact Taft and Watson found that "partner violence is the strongest predictive factor of pregnancy termination among young Australian women;"⁴⁸ and these researchers thought their study actually underestimated the impact of intimate partner violence on induced abortion because their population tended to be of higher socio-economic standing, the abuse had to be self-reported, and, finally, because of sample attrition.⁴⁹

In a study of 4750 Vancouver, BC residents who gave birth over a two-year period, 32.9 per cent of those who experienced physical abuse or feared their partner had one or more previous induced abortions in contrast with 20.9 per cent of those who were not abused or fearful.⁵⁰ Additionally, in a recent survey of 1318 men aged between eighteen and 35 in Boston, researchers found that 31.9 per cent self-reported perpetrating intimate partner violence and 33.2 per cent self-reported being involved in pregnancies that ended in induced abortion.⁵¹ "Experiences of abortion involvement were more common among men reporting IPV perpetration (48.9 per cent versus 25.9 per cent)."⁵² Some men admitted to having violently promoted the abortion, others to having violently opposed it.

Abusive intimate partners may also coerce a woman to become pregnant, perhaps by forcing sexual intercourse, making induced abortion seem like her only way out of a forced pregnancy. As Fanslow and colleagues note, "Generally speaking, [induced] abortions are a matter of choice, although the extent of a woman's alternative options may also be limited by experiencing violence in a relationship."⁵³

In some cases, the correlation between intimate partner violence and

---

46   Garcia-Moreno C, et al. Executive summary. *WHO multi-country study on women's health and domestic violence against women.* Geneva: World Health Organization, 2005: xv.
47   Cobia et al. See n. 5.
48   Taft AJ and Watson LF. Termination of pregnancy: associations with partner violence and other factors in a national cohort of young Australian women. Australian and New Zealand Journal of Public Health 2007; 31(2): p. 141.
49   Ibid.
50   Janssen et al. See n. 27, pp. 1341-7.
51   Silverman JG, et al. Male perpetration of intimate partner violence and involvement in abortions and abortion-related conflict. American Journal of Public Health 2010; 100(8): pp. 1415-17.
52   RR=1.79; 95% CI=1.54, 2.06; Ibid., p. 1416.
53   Fanslow, et al. See n. 23, p. 396.

induced abortion is one of coercion. Janssen and colleagues affirm that "some women are forced under threat of violence, even death, by their partners to terminate their pregnancy."[54] Seven of 38 women in an American study "reported being pressured or forced to have abortions."[55] In follow-up interviews with 23 of the intimate partner violence victims studied by Raj, "women also reported feeling forced by their abuser to undergo an abortion when they did not want it."[56]

Even in the absence of direct coercion, a woman who experiences intimate partner violence and wants to carry her pregnancy to term may nonetheless be deterred by fear for her child's future safety; she may also view having a child as an impediment preventing her from getting out of the relationship. Many studies have shown that a woman's decision to terminate her pregnancy is often due to relationship problems, pressure from her partner, or her experience of abuse. To illustrate: Boden, Fergusson and Horwood found that "there remained a marginal association between CSA [child sexual abuse] experiences and abortion after control for confounding factors."[57] Hamelin and colleagues found that "only abortion appears significantly associated with CSA [child sexual abuse]."[58] Finally, Ely and Otis found that "Women who experienced multiple abortions were more likely to indicate that the person responsible for the current pregnancy was abusive."[59]

Owing to the increased likelihood that those who have been abused will seek induced abortion, we must agree with intimate partner violence researchers who insist that "health professionals should be aware that a woman's attendance for a termination of pregnancy may not be her choice."[60]

---

54   Janssen, et al. See n. 27, p. 1346.
55   Hathaway JE, et al. Impact of partner abuse on women's reproductive lives. Journal of the American Medical Women's Association 2005; 60(1): p. 42.
56   Raj A, Liu R, McCleary-Sills J and Silverman JG. South Asian victims of intimate partner violence more likely than non-victims to report sexual health concerns. Journal of Immigrant Health 2005 April; 7(2): 85-91, p. 89.
57   Boden, et al. See n. 40, p. 875.
58   Hamelin, et al. See n. 14, p. 682.
59   Ely GE and Otis MD. An examination of intimate partner violence and psychological stressors in adult abortion patients. Journal of Interpersonal Violence 2011; 26(16): p. 3260.
60   Keeling J, Birch L and Green P. Pregnancy counselling clinic: a questionnaire survey of intimate partner abuse. Journal of Family Planning and Reproductive Health Care 2004; 30(3): p. 166.

Intimate Partner Violence and Nondisclosure

Suggestive of the link between induced abortion and intimate partner violence is the prevalence of non-disclosure among abused women seeking pregnancy termination. A recent US study confirmed that women who have experienced intimate partner violence "are significantly less likely than non-abused women to have informed their partner of the pregnancy or to report having partner support in the abortion decision."[61]

In the survey of Boston-area men aged between eighteen and 35, those who reported perpetrating IPV "were also more likely to report conflicts with pregnant female partners regarding decisions related to seeking abortion. This finding is consistent with studies demonstrating that women who experience IPV are less likely to discuss abortion decisions with a partner, often because of fear."[62]

In a study of women presenting for abortion in Houston, Texas, 139 (17.2 per cent) did not disclose the abortion to their partner; non-disclosers were twice as likely to report physical or sexual abuse than those who disclosed, and eleven (7.9 per cent) of the non-disclosers said the primary reason their partner was not informed was because disclosure would have resulted in physical harm.[63] Researchers found "the rate of recent abuse (abuse within the last year or while pregnant) among abortion clients at 13.8 per cent."[64]

Post-Abortion Intimate Partner Violence

Interestingly, some research has also been devoted to examining induced abortion as a cause or correlate of intimate partner violence, rather than the other way around. As early as 1997 Gissler and colleagues discovered that, compared to other female homicide victims, the odds ratio of homicide after abortion was 4.33, compared to 0.31 after birth and 1.82 after miscarriage among 281 Finnish women who died up to one year after the end of

---

61   Jones RK, Moore AM and Frohwirth L. Perceptions of male knowledge and support among U.S. women obtaining abortions. Women's Health Issues 2011; 21(2): p. 117.
62   Silverman. See n. 51, p. 1416.
63   Woo J, Fine P and Goetz L. Abortion disclosure and the association with domestic violence. Obstetrics and Gynecology 2005; 105(6): pp. 1329-34.
64   Ibid., pp. 1332-3.

pregnancy.[65] One of the participants in Leung's study was not abused while pregnant, but did experience physical abuse after her induced abortion.[66] In another study, "significant risk factors for any police-reported IPV during pregnancy [among Seattle residents] included...previous spontaneous or induced abortion."[67] In India, one researcher found that "as the proportion of intervals in which abortion occurred increases, the odds of experiencing violence increases significantly."[68] As recently as 2011, researchers admitted that "a temporal relationship between IPV and induced abortion could not be established; therefore, [they] cannot discount the possibility of reverse causality: that is, induced abortion causing acts of IPV."[69]

Why might a woman's induced abortion make her intimate partner violent? Coleman, Rue and Coyle offer the idea that "associations between abortion and relationship conflict and intimate partner violence are logical based on research indicating that anger is a common post-abortion emotional response."[70] Another study by Coleman and colleagues suggests that "a man may become very upset that his 'baby' was aborted against his will. Alternatively, the woman may suffer from depression if she chose abortion for situational as opposed to personal reasons and she may become withdrawn, triggering anger in a man prone to violent behaviour."[71] While offering similar explanations, Lee-Rife presents the "possibility of a feedback loop—a woman in a violent marriage may be more likely to seek an abortion, but also more likely to experience violence upon the discovery of her abortion, as well as more likely to experience violence at a later period, and so on."[72]

---

65   Age-adjusted OR 95% CI 1.03-18.2, p 0.02-4.42 and 0.36-9.10 respectively; Gissler M et al. Pregnancy-associated deaths in Finland 1987-1994—definition problems and benefits of record linkage. Acta Obstetricia et Gynecologica Scandinavica 1997; 76(7): pp. 651-7.
66   Leung TW et al. A comparison of the prevalence of domestic violence between patients seeking termination of pregnancy and other general gynecology patients. International Journal of Gynecology & Obstetrics 2002; 77(1): pp. 47-54.
67   aORs 1.39 and 1.34, respectively; Lipsky S. et al. Police-reported intimate partner violence during pregnancy: who is at risk? Violence and Victims 2005; 20(1): p. 69.
68   OR 3.74: Lee-Rife SM. Women's empowerment and reproductive experiences over the lifecourse. Social Science & Medicine 2010; 71(3): p. 639.
69   Alio AP, Salihu HM, Nana PN, et al. Association between intimate partner violence and induced abortion in Cameroon. International Journal of Gynecology & Obstetrics 2011 February; 112(2): 83-7, p. 86.
70   Coleman PK, Rue VM, Coyle CT. Induced abortion and intimate relationship quality in the Chicago Health and Social Life Survey. Public Health 2009; 123(4): p. 332.
71   Coleman PK, et al. Predictors and correlates of abortion in the Fragile Families and Well-Being Study: paternal behaviour, substance use, and partner violence. International Journal of Mental Health & Addiction 2009; 7(3): p. 417.
72   Lee-Rife. See n. 68, p. 640.

IS CONTRACEPTION THE SOLUTION?

The tendency of those who investigate the abuse-abortion link is to assume that much of intimate partner violence has to do with withholding contraception. As one researcher notes, "intimate partner violence may influence...use of contraceptives, which has implications for the high risk of unintended pregnancies among abused women."[73] Granted, women in abusive relationships may lack reproductive control or simply have too chaotic a lifestyle to use contraception.[74] As we have seen, however, the correlation between intimate partner violence and induced abortion is more complex than the explanation that men force unwanted babies on women suggests; women are also prevented from becoming pregnant, even to the point of forced sterilization.[75]

In developing countries, abortion is often limited, but contraception encouraged. Yet, in Cameroon, "in unadjusted analyses, women with access to contraception were 2.5 times more likely to have had an induced abortion. These results were almost identical for women reporting knowledge of family planning."[76] Increasing contraception does not automatically decrease unwanted pregnancy. Although artificial contraception is commonly used to prevent pregnancy, it is not fail safe. Phillips has pointed out that some women seeking induced abortion were on the birth control pill and may have missed taking only a couple pills before conceiving.[77] Condoms break, IUDs and diaphragms fail, and even hormonal treatments are not 100 per cent effective. The link between abortion and intimate partner violence can by no means be attributed solely to a forced disuse of contraception.

---

73   Williams CM, Larson U and McCloskey LA. Intimate partner violence and women's contraceptive use. Violence Against Women 2008; 14(12): p. 1382.
74   Wiebe ER and Janssen P. Universal screening for domestic violence in abortion. Women's Health Issues 2001; 11(5): pp. 436-41.
75   Coggins and Bullock. See n. 24, p. 729.
76   OR 2.51; 95% CI, 1.74—3.60 and OR 2.52; 95% CI, 1.74—3.65, respectively; Alio, Salihu, Nana, et al. See n. 69, p. 85.
77   Phillips SP. Violence and abortions: what's a doctor to do? CMAJ 2005; 172(5): pp. 653-4.

CONCLUSION

There is a clear link between intimate partner violence and abortion in scientific literature. Women who suffer intimate partner violence are more likely to experience miscarriage. Moreover, women who present for induced abortion are more likely to have endured abuse, and women who endure abuse are more likely to seek induced abortion; perhaps because of coercion, perhaps fearing for herself or her child if he or she were to be born, perhaps feeling so unsupported that she believes herself to have no other choice. Health-care professionals should be aware of the correlation between abuse and abortion and strategize to provide suffering women with the best possible care. Increasing a woman's access to birth control, while perhaps helping to limit unwanted pregnancy, does nothing to address the underlying problem of intimate partner violence. And far from eliminating abuse, obtaining an induced abortion can actually increase intimate partner violence, besides possibly damaging women in the other ways explored in this book.

Section IV: Women's Voices

Abstract

The last two chapters are concerned with what women themselves have said about their experience of abortion. This includes original research of the firsthand accounts of over 100 women. The importance of narrative evidence is more and more recognized in the fields of psychology and medicine. Yet abortion researchers have been slow to make use of the narratives of post-abortive women. The authors of a report to the American Psychological Association (APA) deny the existence of psychological distress after abortion. They do this in the face of the published narratives of thousands of women. They also appear unaware of the acceptance by many courts in the US of women's affidavits testifying to the great distress they experienced after their abortions. The women who recounted their stories to the de Veber Institute researchers all testified to the devastating impact of abortion in terms of depression, broken partner relationships, and the resort to alcohol and other substances. Fully two-thirds of them said that they were pressured or coerced into having the abortion. Coercion could be exercised by the woman's partner, her mother, her employer, her friends, or by medical professionals. Over 70 per cent reported that the abortion procedure was not properly explained to them by medical professionals. Not infrequently they were misled about the procedure and the nature of the life that was growing inside them.

Hardly any of the 101 women in the study reported psychological problems that existed before their abortion. Immediately following the abortion many felt relief, but this was soon followed by regret and self-blame. Only a minority had physical complications, which for the most part were short-lived. Within weeks, almost all of the women experienced depression. Three-fifths reported that the abortion had a destructive impact on their intimate relationships. Two-fifths reported resorting to alcohol and other drugs as a means of coping with

Chapter 20:

Who are the experts? What 101 women told us

feelings of regret and depression. More than two-fifths considered suicide, while 35 per cent reported at least one attempt at suicide. A surprising 23 per cent reported being unable to have children after the abortion. Very few doctors or clinics followed up with their patients after the abortion.

Some of the women were able to find emotional and spiritual healing after the abortion, often after going through a religious conversion experience. However, all the women, without exception, continued to be troubled by the memory of their abortion, eight of them up to the time of their own death.

To sum up, the APA's denial of psychological sequelae to induced abortion is eloquently refuted by the thousands of women who have testified to the devastating impact of abortion in their lives.

Chapter 21:

Women's voices: Narratives of the abortion experience

Chapter 20

Who are the experts? What 101 women told us

KEY POINTS

- The importance of narrative is more and more recognized in the fields of psychology and medicine.

- Yet in the professional literature there is apparently no room for the narratives of post-abortive women.

- This is because their narratives contradict the widespread assumption that abortion is safe, easy and uncomplicated.

- Fully two-thirds of the women who shared their stories with us were pressured or coerced into having the abortion.

- Over 70 per cent report that the abortion procedure was not properly explained to them by medical professionals.

- While the American Psychological Association (APA) continues to deny the existence of psychological distress after abortion, courts in the US have accepted the validity of affidavits from women testifying to the great distress they experienced after their abortions.

- In addition, the women who told their stories to us all testified to the devastating impact of abortion in terms of depression, broken partner relationships, and the resort to alcohol and other substances.

COUNTER NARRATIVE

Research in narrative ethnology has produced the concept of counter narrative to explain the stories and interpretations that stand in opposition to the prevailing cultural, narrative norm. When it comes to abortion the narrative norm stipulates that abortion has few negative consequences for women.

Feminist narrative analyst Patricia Stevens confirms the importance of narrative in research on marginalized women and concludes that:

> significant life events are commonly communicated in story form, so narrative inquiry taps into people's everyday ways of expressing themselves...As feminist research, it was done in the interest of women, about phenomena of concern to them. Women's own stories and interpretations were afforded primacy.[1]

Likewise in Social Work, narrative understanding plays a vital role, for as Reissman notes,

> stories more than other forms of discourse, effectively pull the listener into the teller's point of view. They represent a slice of life, often by dramatizing and re-enacting a particular interaction, thereby providing 'proof' of how it was.[2]

NARRATIVE IN MEDICAL RESEARCH

There is a large body of research on narrative and counter narrative in the social sciences that has moved into the sciences with the advent of Narrative Medicine. Narrative Medicine is defined by Charon[3] as "medicine practiced with the narrative competencies to recognize, absorb, interpret and be moved by the stories of illness." This new initiative recognizes the

---

1   Stevens P. Marginalized women's access to health care: a feminist narrative analysis. Nursing Science 1993 December; 16(2): p. 41.
2   Reissman CK. Strategic uses of narrative in the presentation of self and illness: a research note. Social Science & Medicine 1990; 30(11): 1195—1200.
3   Charon R. Narrative medicine: attention, representation, affiliation. Narrative 2005 October; 13(3): 261-70.

essential nature of the doctor-patient relationship and the integral part the patient's story plays in facilitating appropriate diagnoses and is done using interview methodology, which includes a "battery of questions".[4] By definition the narrative in this case is holistic, considering the full individual as not just a collection of body parts, and is becoming important in understanding patients and their needs.

In this same context the counter narratives of post-abortive women speak to both the medical and psychological aspects of their lives and yet in the "scientific" literature there is apparently no room for their stories. The pain and suffering they report cannot be easily contextualized into a narrative concept that abortion is safe, easy and uncomplicated. Consequently they are ignored and marginalized while individuals with other medical or psychological stories are seen as vital. In the work of abortion research these women do not exist or the few who do are women who were disturbed before the abortion so what could we expect?

A NEW STUDY BASED ON WOMEN'S NARRATIVES OF THEIR ABORTION EXPERIENCE

Thirty-three interviews by deVeber Researchers, eight interviews of dying women conducted by a palliative care nurse, and 60 affidavits collected by Silent No More Canada were analyzed based on the issues around informed consent and post-abortion outcomes. This is an opportunistic sample of women wishing to come forward to tell their story. The time since each woman's abortion varied from one to 38 years, but each narrative speaks to one woman's struggle to deal with consequences that were not supposed to happen. Is this a representative sample? Yes and no. The 101 women represent all of those who feel that they have been in some way harmed by the abortion experience but not those for whom their experience continues to be framed within the context of feminist rhetoric about choice or who have compartmentalized the event into a life experience and interpreted it as necessary and no longer central to their lives. These 101 women's stories also reach out to those who have experienced similar feelings, but who have not yet connected them to their earlier abortion.

Many of the respondents express a strong religious faith that has helped them to cope with and share their experiences. Is religious conversion one of the keys to healing? Only one of the of the women report pre-existing psychological problems, which are often identified as a precursor for post-

---

4   Ibid.

abortion distress, although some note that they came from chaotic, broken or dysfunctional families and were shaped by their family of origin.

COERCION AND PRESSURE

Our findings include:

- 69 incidents of pressure from partners[5], parents or medical staff to abort where the pressure included an implied negative outcome for their relationship coupled with a pedagogical approach to coercion.
- At least thirteen clear incidents of direct threats or predatory coercion.

Current sociological and political literature defines three main types of coercion:

1. predatory
2. pedagogical
3. ideological[6]

1. Predatory coercion
The purely selfish kinds of coercion are a form of predatory behaviour by the coercing party, whose aim is to narrow down the scope of other people's actions so as to make them instrumental to their own personal interests. This form of coercion is particularly apparent in the stories of post-abortive women who repeatedly report being "threatened" by their partner with the loss of the relationship if they continue their pregnancy.

2. Pedagogical coercion
At the other end of the spectrum one finds attempts to use coercion altruistically, as a pedagogical device to improve—in some supposedly objective sense—the way other people *think*, with particular regard to their

---

5   Broen A, Torbjor M, et al. Reasons for induced abortion and their relation to women's emotional distress: a prospective, two-year follow-up study. General Hospital Psychiatry 2005 (27): 36-43: "Male pressure on women to have an induced abortion has a significant, negative influence on women's psychological responses in the 2 years following the event." The authors found few other negative results but only 46% of the women who were asked to participate agreed to be included in this study.

6   The basic definitions of the types of coercion are so ubiquitous that they are found online in Wikipedia while the application to the abortion discussion is based on the research of the deVeber Institute.

basic attitudes and values. Pedagogical coercion may be applied within a strictly educational context as *thought coercion*, i.e. the coercive attempt to affect the basic values of a population. This type occurs most frequently in the abortion context in counselling for families with prenatally diagnosed conditions when they are given only negative or inaccurate information that will guide them to the abortion decision.

3.   *Ideological coercion*

Ideological coercion is the use of thought coercion to modify people's social and political philosophy. Quite different from plain propaganda, or even the simple persecution of political opponents, its objective is to force individual ideological conversions.

INFORMED CONSENT AND FETAL DEVELOPMENT

There is increasing cause for concern about the nature of informed consent in beginning and-end-of-life issues—both abortion and euthanasia/assisted suicide. As we have noted in Chapter 5, the Canadian Medical Association has published a code of ethics, which includes the requirement that physicians provide patients with the information that allows informed decisions, and which responds to any patient questions. The physician must ensure that the communication is clear enough that the patient comprehends the information. Only diagnostic and therapeutic interventions that "you consider to be beneficial to your patients" are permitted. Consent must be obtained for any public health reporting.

While the CMA principles of informed consent are designed to provide clear guidelines for doctors, it is clear that the subjective interpretation of the concept of "benefit" is central to this ethic. Other information is provided to meet the legal requirements of informed consent but in the end it is the doctor's personal judgment of efficacy that matters.

How this applies to decision-making around abortion is even more subjective. When the pregnancy does not carry specific medical risks then the doctor's recommendation to abort is based on her or his perceptions and personal interpretations of the likely psycho-social impacts. Her determination of benefit is based on socially, not medically constructed information. Thus some of the women in the present study stated that their doctor used sociological statistics to encourage them to abort. The usual approach was to insist that the woman would never be successful, would be doomed to a life of poverty, and would be unable to support her child properly. In general her life would be worse if she did not abort.

As well as those who reported that they were given sociological not medical information as a rationale for the abortion, analysis of the responses from post abortive women in this study indicates that 72 per cent specifically note that the abortion procedure was not properly explained to them, nondirective pre-abortion counselling was not provided, and if any advice was given it was that the abortion was the best thing. All comments by medical staff were directed to allay any thought that there could be complications:

- "It's easy, fast and uncomplicated"
- "Safe, no long-term effects"
- "It's like pulling a tooth"

Sixty-four per cent addressed the issue of fetal development and reported that any information they were given was at best inaccurate, at worst a direct lie, and often paternalistic. For the vast majority the abortion ended their first pregnancy and they were unaware of prenatal developmental stages and in some cases the attending physicians wished to keep it that way:

> He did not discuss pregnancy or childbirth beyond the basic fact that I was physically pregnant. However, he did say that he could book me an appointment to perform the abortion… and then I saw on the wall a poster of the development of a baby. I stepped in to take a closer look and the gynaecologist stepped in front of me and said, "You don't want to look at that, it will only make you confused and your decision harder."

Those who were given information about the fetus told us that it was most often characterized by a minimizing of fetal development with dismissive phrases such as "it's just ….a group of cells", "a blob of tissue", "products of conception", "a mere lump of tissue", "dense tissue spots." What is interesting is that such erroneous and minimizing phrases were pronounced regardless of the gestational age of the fetus. The women in this sample were most often from ten to sixteen weeks pregnant. Pathology reports of abortions at that stage must consider the presence of fetal parts to determine the success of the procedure and yet these women were not made aware that the entity they were carrying had such distinct parts. How could "a blob of tissue" have arms and legs that needed to be accounted for after the procedure?

In 2008 the American Psychological Association (APA) Committee on abortion disseminated a report on the psychological impacts of abortion on women.[7] The task force came to the same conclusion as the APA's 1990 review of abortion research—that the research still did not support the presence of negative post-abortion psychological distress. Recently published papers that found linkages between abortion and future psychological problems were dismissed as unscientific. Only studies that were prospective in design and/or undertaken by members of the task force were deemed to meet the highest standard of scientific enquiry and therefore valid.

In September 2008 the American Association of Pro-Life Obstetricians and Gynecologists (AAPLOG) issued a Response to the APA Task Force Report. They addressed the APA's assertion that:

> ...the most methodologically sound research concludes that among women who have a single, legal, first-trimester abortion of an unplanned pregnancy for nontherapeutic reasons, the relative risk of mental health problems are no greater than the risks among women who deliver an unplanned pregnancy.[8]

The first author of the APA report, Brenda Major, is one of the few researchers whose work was found to be appropriately "scientific" but nowhere in the report does she recuse herself due to conflict of interest. AAPLOG identifies the methodological flaws in the studies used by the APA and notes that the Task Force did not account for the fact that nearly

---

7   American Psychological Association Task Force on Mental Health and Abortion. See Chapter 18, n. 7: Adler NE, David HP, Major BN, Roth S, Russo N and Wyatt G. Psychological responses after abortion. Science 1990 April 6; 248 (4951): 41-4.
8   American Assocation of Pro-life Obstetricians & Gynecologists (AAPLOG). AAPLOG response to the APA Task Force Report on Mental Health and Abortion. September 2008.
http://aaplog.octoberblue.com/wp-content/uploads/2010/02/AAPLOG_Response_To_APA_Task_210109.pdf.. On line 216 the APA report notes that "there is unlikely to be a single definitive research study that will determine the mental health implications of abortion 'once and for all' given the diversity and complexity of women and their circumstances." In the AAPLOG Response, Patricia Coleman asks "Why does the APA promote the blanket conclusion that having an abortion carries the same mental health risks as having a baby? She concludes that this statement is ultimately "based on one study by Gilchrist which has a number of ignored flaws."

50 per cent of all abortions in the United States are repeat abortions and that a significant number are done at later stages in pregnancy. They say, "thus, this sweeping conclusion only addresses half the women affected. So the report's conclusion (whether accurate or inaccurate), at best pertains to only 50 per cent of women who chose abortion. This select sample is hardly representative of all the women who have had the abortion experience."[9] Nowhere in the Task Force Report was there a discussion of narrative experiences or counter narrative, even though the authors were members of the APA Women's Programs Office and in their acknowledgements thanked the staff of that unit. Where is the concern for the voices of women in this?

NARRRATIVE AND JUDICIARY

At the very time the APA was conducting its investigation, courts and state legislatures in the United States were considering the medical and psychological consequences of abortion. Courts were accepting Amicus Curiae briefs that included the very research material dismissed by the APA. Thus we find the government of South Dakota citing this research in its legislative initiatives around abortion. One such Amicus Curiae brief in *Gonzalez vs Carhart*[10] was submitted by The Justice Foundation of San Antonio, Texas. This brief contained sworn affidavits from 178 post-abortive women all attesting to the negative consequences of their abortions. The Foundation had collected 3000 such counter narrative statements from women in 39 American states.

At the same time the state of South Dakota had also established a Task Force charged with studying abortion. That final report included the research dismissed by APA and found it to be pertinent to its deliberations. They concluded:

> The Task Force finds that it is simply unrealistic to expect that a pregnant mother is capable of being involved in the termination of the life of her own child without risk of suffering significant psychological trauma and distress.[11]

---

9   Ibid.
10   127 S. Ct. 1610 (2007) Alberto R. GONZALES, Attorney General, Petitioner v. Leroy CARHART el al. Alberto R. Gonzales, Attorney General, Petitioner v. Planned Parenthood.
11   South Dakota Task Force to Study Abortion. *Report of the South Dakota Task Force to Study Abortion*. Submitted to the Governor and Legislature of South Dakota, December 2005: 1-71, pp. 47-8. http://www.dakotavoice.com/Docs/South%20Dakota%20Abortion%20Task%20Force%20Report.pdf.

It should be noted that the submissions that the Task Force found particularly compelling were the counter narrative affidavits of over 1940 women who related the negative consequences of abortion in their lives. The Report speaks of these submissions in the following terms:

> We received and reviewed the testimony of more than 1940 women who have had abortions. This stunning and heart-wrenching testimony reveals that there are common experiences with abortion. Women were not told the truth about abortion, were misled into thinking that nothing but 'tissue' was being removed and relate that they would not have had an abortion if they were told the truth.[12]

The report goes on to note that they are:

> aware that the APA has submitted various amicus briefs before the US Supreme Court supporting abortion rights and in opposition to any abortion regulations including parental involvement in a minor child's abortion decision-making. Further the APA's position does not represent the majority of their own membership, but rather, the opinions of a group of members of various committees of interest.[13]

Thus, because the APA dismisses research that shows an association between abortion and future mental health impacts and also devalues women's stories, the South Dakota Task Force did not recognize them as the ultimate authoritative experts. They instead honoured the legal understanding of the affidavit, which has a long history in American Jurisprudence as factual, valid evidence. As sworn statements affidavits are given authority within the judicial system.

> most personal affidavits are related to court matters, particularly in civil trials, but can be used whenever truthful dealing is

---

12   Ibid., p. 2.
13   Ibid., p. 46.

> required. Personal affidavits exist as a means of verifying the truth, and false statements made within them can subject the signatories to court sanctions for perjury and other offenses.[14]

The narrative and counter-narrative are considered an important aspect of modern feminist scholarship. As K.R. Gilbert puts it, "story-telling is integral to research."[15] Yet we have the strange phenomenon of competing experts: a judiciary that supports narrative as important, and the APA —who *should* be concerned with women's mental health—dismissing research because it includes retrospective narratives about abortion. For the APA, it seems that the narrative is only valued when the story being shared supports the "correct" conclusion, namely that abortion is a benign experience, and only women who have previous mental health problems will exhibit negative sequelae.

Psychological Outcomes And Publication Bias

While the American Psychological Association denies the presence of psychological damage following abortion, the women we interviewed themselves paint a different picture. Other research that has included the perspectives of post-abortive women has often been debunked on the grounds that it is retrospective and open to recall bias. Few of the studies that show links between psychological sequelae and abortion are ever published in the numerous APA-sponsored journals.[16]

In order for a research report to be published in a refereed journal it must be approved by the editor of that journal as meeting the criteria for inclusion and then be recommended for publication by a process of "peer review". Peer review is done by "experts" in the field being studied, and they are by definition academics who have already been published in mainline journals. As a result there is a tendency for material to be scrutinized with a bias reflecting the "expert's" own research and conclusions as well as the scientific validity of the article. "Bias may be defined as systematic prejudice that prevents the accurate and objective interpretation of scientific results."[17]

---

14   http://www.wisegeek.com/what-is-a-personal-affidavit.htm.
15   Gilbert KR. Taking a narrative approach to grief research: finding meaning in stories. Death Studies 2002; 26: 223-9.
16   The APA publishes more than 55 journals.
17   Benos D, et al. Ups and downs of peer review. Adv Physiol Educ 2007 June; 31(2): 145-52.

In less controversial areas than life-issues research there has been a growing concern about the potential biases that reviewers bring to their critiques of new manuscripts. Biases can occur on the basis of gender, status and research attitudes. For instance, papers published in an issue of the *Journal of the American Medical Association* in 2002 devoted to peer review presented evidence for nationality bias, language bias, specialty bias, and perhaps even gender bias, as well as the recognised bias towards the publication of positive results."[18] In 1990 Lloyd sent identical manuscripts with male and female names to reviews for comment. Female reviewers were more likely to accept female-written manuscripts (62 per cent) than were male reviewers willing to accept male-written manuscripts (21 per cent).[19]

In the context of the abortion discussion the biases reflect what could be described as an internalized and therefore undisclosed conflict of interest. This is not conflict based on personal gain but a conflict of interest rooted in the assumption that abortion is benign and a woman's right. Studies that contradict this "fact" or assumption are often viewed as flawed in design, conclusion or scope. This is particularly true for material by authors who are deemed to be anti-abortion, as their material is retrospective and based on large national data sets and often composed of opportunistic or convenience samples. Opportunistic or convenience samples are those in which the individuals who participate do so willingly and are not recruited before their abortion occurred. What is interesting about the dismissal of such studies is that given the large rate of sample attrition in many prospective studies, their findings are ultimately derived from equally opportunistic cohorts. Only those who are willing to respond after the abortion are represented in the research. Yet a great many women are unwilling to respond.

A 2003 editorial in the *British Medical Journal* discussed the issue of peer review and concluded that there was little hard evidence to suggest that peer review improves the quality of published biomedical research. A 2002 study published in the *Journal of the American Medical Association* concluded that "editorial peer review, although widely used, is largely untested and its effects are uncertain."[20] In fact, the problems with having research accepted

---

18   Ware M. Peer review: benefits, perspectives and alternatives. http://www.publishingresearch.net/documents/PRCsummary4Warefinal.pdf.
19   Lloyd M. Gender factors in reviewer recommendation for manuscript publication. J. Applied Behavior & Analysis 1990; 23(4): 539-43.
20   Jefferson T, Alderson P, Wager E and Davidoff F. Effects of editorial peer review: a systematic review. JAMA 2002; 287(21): 2784-6.

by peer review is not only limited to the study of abortion and other life issues. In a more recent article Campanario lists more than twenty Nobel Prize winners who experienced rejection of their papers by many journals, as well as others whose quest for publication was resisted by other scientists.[21]

Depression

Recently a team of Canadian researchers used the National Morbidity Survey for a retrospective study of 3310 women. They found that "after adjusting for socio-demographics, abortion was associated with an increased risk of several mental disorders—mood disorders, anxiety disorders, substance use disorders as well as suicide ideation and suicide attempts."[22] This result is corroborated by the post-abortive women in our sample, 96 per cent of whom reported that they have experienced significant and ongoing depression as a consequence of their abortion. Several discuss their experiences with counselling, but the majority have quietly dealt with this problem on their own. Many of those critical of narrative experience research point to the need for clinical labelling of disorders in order to guarantee that the criteria for depression found in the Diagnostic and Statistical Manual of Mental Disorders (DSM) are met and that the emotional problems can be directly linked to the abortion. However, it is clear from these women that they know what they feel and are able to describe it in very concise, even clinical terms. They are equally clear that the cause of their distress is lodged in the aftermath of the abortion not in other factors in their lives. Have they all had this diagnosis confirmed by a psychiatrist or psychologist? Usually not, but does that mean their symptoms are to be discounted? Expecting professional confirmation of a diagnosis has been an intrinsic flaw in post-abortion research. The application of strict scientific and clinical standards removes the human story and devalues these women's abortion experiences.

Support for this comes from a recent report on post-abortion psychopathology in Denmark. The data from which the authors drew their conclusions, that women who present with problems post abortion already experienced pre-abortion levels of disorder was derived from psychiatric

---

21   Campanario JM and Acedo E. Rejecting highly cited papers: the views of scientists who encounter resistance to their discoveries from other scientists. Journal of the American Society for Information Science and Technology 2007; 58(5): 734-43.
22   Mota N, Burnett M and Sareen J. Associations between abortion, mental disorders and suicidal behaviour in a nationally representative sample. Canadian Journal of Psychiatry 2010 April; 55(4): 239-47.

visits within *only* a year of the abortion event. They suggest that women who blame their abortions for their problems may have had previous psychiatric conditions that they are ignoring. At the same time however, the authors note that:

> it is important to highlight that we studied severe mental disorders necessitating treatment either at in- or outpatient facilities. This means we did not study symptoms of depression or feelings of sadness or regret and consequently cannot conclude anything regarding those aspects.[23]

A response to the Danish study was given by the AAPLOG who clearly pointed out the deficiencies in their research.[24] Likewise, it is important to stress that, unlike the women in the Munk-Olsen study, the majority of the respondents in our present sample have not shared their abortion experience with others, even close family members and therefore would not be found in a cohort that could be studied.

Here are typical statements by several of the women:

> "I couldn't get out of bed and cried constantly."
>
> "During those dark months after my abortion I had bouts of sadness, depression and increased anxiety marked with low self-esteem and anger."

---

[23] Munk-Olsen T. Induced first-trimester abortion and risk of mental disorder. NEJM 2011 Jan 27; 364(4): 332-9.

[24] "Regarding the "original article" found in the Jan 27, 2011 issue [of NJEM, pages 332-339] entitled Induced First-Trimester Abortion and Risk of Mental Disorder, by Trine Munk-Olsen, Ph.D, et. al.: This study concludes that the evidence does not support the hypothesis that there is an increased risk of mental disorders after a first-trimester induced abortion. It is interesting that the NEJM, given its prestigious reputation, would choose to publish a study with so definitive a conclusion, based (as it is) on less than 39% of women having an abortion. And from that number, the authors "cherry pick" the more healthy ones (ie, they excluded many women with a previous psychiatric history, and women with previous psychiatric history are known to have a higher incidence of post-abortion mental health problems.) We try hard to adhere to "evidence based medicine." This article is a fine example of "conclusion-based medicine," i.e., one establishes a conclusion, and then makes the "evidence" fit that conclusion." http://www.aaplog.org/get-involved/letters-to-members/danish-nejm-study/.

> "[I] have suffered from long-term depression, suffered nightmares and flashbacks. It has affected every relationship in my life."
>
> "I immediately spun into an eventual deep suicidal depression."
>
> "Severe depression for many years, cannot get better."

Technically well-controlled scientific studies cannot encompass the lived experiences of these women. Their testimonies indicate that for them depression and the failure of intimate relationships had the greatest impact in their lives following their abortion.

Partner Relationships

Sixty per cent of our sample reported that their abortion experience had a profound impact on their intimate relationships. The ways in which this occurred were identified as: promiscuity or multiple partners, marriage dissolution, and sexual dysfunction within relationships. The abortion event seemed to compromise their capacity to deal with sexuality and communications within marriage. Some felt betrayed by the men who pressured them to have the abortion or who were ambivalent and did not stand up for the life of their child. Few have found the healing that would allow them to describe their marital lives as fulfilling.

Also identified were the fracturing of parent-child attachments when the women felt that they had been pressured into the abortion by their parents. Along with difficulties in adult relationships 40 per cent reported that their abortion had an impact on their relationship with later children. Some indicated a complete incapacity to bond, while others explained that, as a result of their fear, they became overprotective and stifling of their children, always afraid that these children might be taken away as punishment for their abortion.

Life Style Impacts

Along with these factors the women in our cohort spoke of descent into alcoholism, with 40 per cent revealing that alcohol became a method to avoid dealing with the feelings of regret and depression.

> I preferred alcohol as a preferred method of numbing the pain. I went numb. It wasn't life it wasn't death. I didn't care one way or the other whether I lived or died.

Concomitant with the alcohol use was the fact that twenty per cent also reported that they used drugs in conjunction with alcohol or alcohol by itself as a soporific.

- Just about every day I struggled with depression, suicide, drugs, smoking pot and I even tried crystal-meth to try and kill the pain inside.

- I began drinking, smoking and experimenting with drugs.

More than 40 per cent of the women in this group considered suicide, with 35 per cent reporting at least one suicide attempt that they linked directly to their psycho-emotional state following the abortion. Some respondents reported multiple attempts. While all individuals who attempt suicide have ideation and often come to the attention of medical authorities, those who indicate that they experience suicidal ideation have usually not sought medical and intervention as they have not acted on these feelings. Ideation is therefore very hard to investigate and quantify, since by definition it implies no concrete action. Suicidal thoughts only come to light if the individual enters counselling, and many of these women did not seek help. Since they believed their problems were a result of their abortion, there was no opportunity for them to explore their feelings and share their fears in a supportive environment. After all, abortion is advertised as a "simple, safe procedure," "like pulling a tooth," so only those who are already disturbed would have problems afterwards.

Conclusion

As we have documented in chapter 17, a recent meta-analysis points to a variety of psychological problems associated with the aftermath of abortion. Yet, in the face of all this research the American Psychological Association (APA) continues to deny that a first-trimester induced abortion has significant psychological consequences for women. It does this by very narrowly defining what constitute acceptable research methodologies. The gold standard is apparently the prospective study. Retrospective studies, even when based on very large numbers of anonymous records, are dismissed as unscientific. Yet, the enormous problem associated with prospective research on abortion is the disturbingly high rate of attrition. It has apparently not occurred to APA researchers to ask why so many women who agree in advance to participate in a study on abortion then quit the study once they have undergone their abortion. Finally, the APA's denial of psychological sequelae to induced abortion is eloquently refuted by the thousands of women who have testified to the devastating impact of abortion in their lives.

Chapter 21

Women's voices: Narratives of the abortion experience

KEY POINTS

- Most of the 101 women who told their stories found having an abortion an emotionally devastating experience.

- Over two-thirds were pressured or coerced into having the abortion.

- All regretted having the abortion.

- A significant number were later helped to find psychological healing and spiritual renewal.

- All the women, even those who have had an experience of spiritual transformation after the abortion, continue to be troubled by the memory of it.

INTRODUCTION

Most of our book is devoted to reporting what scientific journals—medical and psychological—have discovered about the impact of induced abortion on women. We thought it would also be useful to hear what women themselves have to say, to listen as they speak directly of abortion's impact in their lives. This wish to hear women's stories first-hand led us to conduct a major piece of original research. We interviewed 101 women about their memories of their abortion experience. The resulting stories are organized into three parts. First, we have a detailed account from a woman in the Third World of her recent abortion. A professional, highly-educated person with a command of several languages, she found herself helpless before the combined pressures imposed on her by family, friends, employer, and medical personnel. Second, we have a group of 92 women who were interviewed in the United States and Canada, whose abortions occurred anywhere from three to 60 years ago. Finally, we have eight stories collected by a palliative-care nurse in Ontario from women approaching the end of life. Every story is in its own way powerful, penetrating and eloquent. Each one challenges the view often found in the scientific literature, that induced abortion is a minor operation for women, with few serious physical or emotional consequences, and that the memory of it soon fades away. Names have been changed in order to safeguard the privacy of those who entrusted their stories to us.

I

SHALEENA'S STORY

A middleclass, educated woman in South Asia shares her story:

> I was a happy woman, and we were a happy family, but I had grown up listening to radio commercials in our country telling us to keep the number of children at not more than two. Most women I knew said "even two is too much."

Surprisingly, when she visited Europe, most of the couples she met were not afraid of having more than two children; in fact, society seemed to encourage it. For various reasons, Shaleena had to wait almost twelve years for the birth of her second child, a son.

> [His birth] brought unbelievable joy to our rather monotonous lives. We were extremely happy. As I had had both my kids through caesarean section, the obstetrician wanted to sterilize me at the same time. She said, "You are a career woman and you have two kids. Let me ligate you dear." I said, "No, I want at least one more kid." She said, "You are not thinking properly; you have a job, you've had two caesarians, why take a risk?" I replied that I did not want sterilization. I still wanted at least one more child. To me the most beautiful thing is "unweaned babies' smile...during their sleep."[1] Can it be surpassed by anything in beauty? Not for me.

But then her second child, Ali, and her husband, Abdel, both developed serious health problems, almost simultaneously. Ali came down with asthma and Abdel was afflicted by hypertension caused by severely blocked arteries. Abdel became depressed. Around that very time, she conceived. When she told Abdel that she thought she might be pregnant, he became apprehensive and insisted that they go at once to the nearest pharmacy for "emergency contraception."

> I did not want to take the pill, but he was insistent, and sort of pushed me into the pharmacy... Tired and discouraged, he then sat down on a bench outside. When I requested emergency contraception from the pharmacist, he asked me a few questions and had me fill in a form. He said that since it was within 24 hours, the probability of conception was less than two per cent. My husband made me swallow the tablet then and there in the mall. He set the alarm clock so that I did not forget to take the second dose.

---

1   Browning EB. First book. *Aurora Leigh*. London: J. Miller, 1864. Reprinted: Chicago: Academy Chicago Printers (Cassandra Editions), 1979: 1-36.

Still not persuaded that she was actually pregnant, she took the pills "to calm my husband, who was sick with worry." But she missed her next period, and Abdel, who was now recovering from a recent heart operation, became very anxious again. They drove together to the doctor's office, where:

> [The doctor] bullied me...She told me that the emergency contraceptive pill is only 97 per cent effective and ordered me to have a blood test. We went to the city hospital for the test. After that I sort of forgot about my delayed period on account of our financial crisis, the multifarious demands of my boss, my husband's slow recovery, and my little son's severe continuing asthma attack.
>
> Our country has a population policy of no more than two children per family, and most women of my generation have only one or two. My job description stipulates that if I have more than two children, the third will not receive any benefit from my employer and I shall be denied any promotions.

Shaleena ignored all the evidence of her advancing pregnancy until finally Abdel insisted that she go for blood tests. The next day, she spoke to the doctor on the phone:

> **Doctor:** "Shaleena? I have a terrible news. Your blood tests are here. You are positive. What will you do now?"
>
> In one breath she told me all this. *Instead, could she not have congratulated me?*
>
> **Doctor:** "Halloo... are you listening Shaleena? You have to come and see me."

After hanging up, Shaleena took a deep breath and phoned Abdel. He was still recovering from his operation. His hospital bills were unpaid, and now she had to inform him that the blood test was positive. "He told me to come home. When I got there he hugged me," she recalled. But he insisted on accompanying his wife to the doctor. It was a dull drizzly day, and a cold fierce wind was blowing.

> ...a nipping day, a biting day;
> In which one wants a shawl,
> A veil, a cloak, and other wraps:[2]

"Why could not my husband have been a shawl to keep me warm?"

They waited patiently in the doctor's waiting room until she motioned them in. She had no sooner ordered Shaleena to sit down than she launched into a tirade and in a shrill voice demanded:

> "How can you be pregnant? What are you going to do now? You already have two kids and Abdel is sick."
>
> I told her in a little voice that I would like to have the baby. She did not listen, but continued her attack. She told my husband that he had not been careful, and anyway, our country did not allow more than two children. She lamented that she was not empowered to prescribe RU 486, the drug that induces abortion. She did not let either of us talk.
>
> **Doctor:** "You are over 35...there will be defects...you already have a sick kid..."
>
> I was exhausted, emotionally drained out; at that time I needed the smiling face of a kindly physician. Here she was, alleging that our child would have birth defects, and my husband believed her. I could not believe that he would. My husband whom I loved and adored. For him I could do anything. The doctor wrote a quick referral and gave us a phone number.

---

2   From "Winter My Secret" by Christina Rossetti.

When they got home, Abdel refused to discuss the matter beyond saying that the doctor was right, and that he would leave her if she insisted on continuing the pregnancy, because he did not want any more sick children. Shaleena was still determined that she was not going to have the abortion. If only her husband would give her just a little help, she thought, she could manage.

> I was confident that I could cope, I *could* carry out the responsibility entrusted to me by Allah. My child would see the beautiful world!
>
> Since I knew when I had conceived, I counted the weeks till his birth, and calculated that he would arrive in early April.

The next morning, she tried again to talk to Abdel but he would not listen: "I tried to make him understand that it was a human life we were talking about, but he was not feeling well and I gave up." There was a lot of pressure at work, and she had to put in nine-hour days, coping with terrible nausea all the while. "But I loved the baby. Not for a second did I think of killing my baby…I prayed and prayed to God to make me stronger and [to make] my husband understand. 'Allah, I am failing to convince my husband; he is influenced by the doctor; please make him understand'. I hugged my little son and cried."

Two days later, Shaleena called the doctor again and asked her to inform Abdel that she wanted to have the baby. The doctor replied that it wasn't a baby, it was a blob, and considering their family condition it would be better to "terminate the pregnancy." Finally, the implacable pressure from her husband and the doctor, and the lack of support from anybody else, drove her to make an appointment at an abortion clinic. But then she missed the appointment. Abdel was so upset that Shaleena immediately called for another appointment. The new clinic assured her that there would be counselling for her husband if she didn't want to terminate. The person at the other end of the line was very sympathetic when Shaleena told her that she wanted to have the baby. There was to be an ultrasound. "I thought, if only my husband can see the ultrasonogram, he might relent."

At noon on the appointed day, Shaleena and Abdel went to the clinic, behind an unmarked door on the second floor of a nondescript building.

She filled in the form handed to her by the staff. She was saying prayers and weeping silently. Seeing her tears, the nurse asked whether she wanted to go ahead with the termination. "I said NO. My husband said YES." The nurse tried to heal the disagreement with the observation that sometimes termination could save a family from breaking up, "and babbled on about how she could see there would be problems in our case. She added that termination was the right decision for me." The nurse took Shaleena into another room for the ultrasound, but did not invite Abdel to join them. Nor did she show Shaleena the results of the ultrasound, but instead brought her back to the counter and presented her with the consent form. Exhausted and crying, she tried to resist, but the nurse kept pressing her to sign. Under this unrelenting pressure, dizzy and worn out, she finally gave in and signed. Seeing her distress, the girl who took her money whispered, "If you do not want to terminate, I will refund your payment." The nurse overheard this, and at once shepherded Shaleena into another room, where she announced,

> "Doctor will do your pelvic exam and if you do not want to terminate you can tell him"
>
> I believed her. I looked at my husband appealing to him with my eyes. Tears rolled down my cheek. Could my husband ever really have loved me? If he did, my tears would surely have made him hold me and save my poor baby.

The pelvic examination did not take place. Instead the doctor ushered her into yet another room, told her to sit down, and then wrote a prescription and told her that he would come back. He did not come back. Instead, after a fifteen-minute wait another doctor arrived,

> and instructed me to follow him to a room where he would examine me. I did as he instructed, and he then ordered me to climb into a reclining chair so that he could examine me, and after the exam I would be able to decide. Then he informed me that the exam would be painful, so he would first give me a painkiller. Before I could reply he gave me an injection, and I think I fell asleep.

> When I woke up I was suffering terrible pain. I realized that they had just terminated my baby. I started crying loudly and they moved me to another room. They asked me whether I wanted my husband… I said NO. They brought him anyway, but I could not look at him. A nurse was sweetly talking with him, telling him that he should do the cooking tonight! He agreed. Another half-hour later they discharged me with a lot of soothing words. They told me I was crying because of hormones. The doctor shook hands with all the smiling women who had assisted at the termination, but ignored me. Two nurses sweet-talked me. They even gave me chocolates for my little boy.
>
> Then they handed me a feed-back form, which I filled in, requesting that they should help women who want to continue their pregnancy.

Abdel brought her home, still crying, bleeding and in agony from severe cramps. She phoned the abortion clinic that night, but they only counselled her to call her own doctor the next day.

> I writhed in pain and agony all night. I felt terrible anguish the next day and left a message in the clinic's voice mail. I missed my child. I would have been happy with the child. After all, I know when life starts! I could not cope any more. I called the clinic again, and again could not get through. I left a message on the answering machine indicating my anguish: I called them killers. Next day, a woman named Jill called me and offered counselling for a fee. I demanded why they did it to me. She became unsympathetic and abusive. I could not stop crying. I wanted to crash my car the next working day.

Finally, Shaleena went to her own physician, who put her on antibiotics and anti-depressants for a month. Despite the medication, she attempted suicide on at least two occasions. Her elder son intervened and restrained her during those attempts.

Only seven days had elapsed between finding out that she was pregnant and undergoing the abortion.

> I did not even have time to look into our Holy Book [the *Qur'an*] for guidance. The pressure of my job, our financial difficulties, the asthma attacks of my little boy, domestic chores and my husband's ill health occupied my time. As for friends, we were new in the country and I had nobody to talk to. I did not turn to my mother or sister, as they believe two children are enough…My mother is all for abortion if you have two kids. I am sure she would have aborted **me** if she could have figured out at the time that she was about to have one more daughter. Throughout my childhood, I heard her sighing for not having a son. When she conceived the baby who turned out to be my brother, she was unsure whether to risk having one more daughter [because at that time there was no way of finding out the baby's sex before birth]…
>
> The only person I thought could help me was the doctor. Doctors I believe take an oath to save lives, not to take them. What did my doctor do?
>
> In desperation, I started talking to Lifeline … and the Abortion Grief Counselling Association, who kept me going; they talked to me, told me to pray, and to live for my sons.

It did not help that Shaleena also experienced physical complications after the abortion. Her hemorrhaging continued, and her left breast was very sore. A new doctor determined that she was suffering from a ruptured ovary and lumps in her breast, which had not been there prior to the abortion. Indeed, she had previously received a clean bill of health after a thorough physical examination prior to immigrating to the new country where her job took her. When she phoned the abortion clinic to report these physical complications, she was again subjected to verbal abuse. Now the sight of any pregnant woman made her feel heartbroken.

> Again I tried to commit suicide, this time on 16 November 2006. *I feel violated, I feel extreme shame and guilt for not being able to protect my baby.*
>
> Before, I was a healthy woman with a nice career and an adorable family. Now I feel unable to go on. I am not the only victim; my family is as well. What will happen to my children? I can't sleep, can't eat. I lost ten kg (22 lbs) after the termination. My doctor told me to take legal action. Yet I am a powerless woman from a developing country that has a two-child policy for public servants. I will lose my job if I get entangled in legal action while abroad. My husband is ready to divorce me as I am too depressed and sick to live with. I am in constant agony....
>
> Religiously speaking I am excluded from salvation. I am a Muslim and for us abortion is an unforgivable sin. My children are also suffering as I am no longer the Mummy they knew.

After the abortion, Shaleena desperately wanted to become pregnant again. Even though a doctor advised Abdel to let her have one more child for the sake of her mental health, Abdel declined. She cannot stop thinking of her aborted baby or babies (since they might have been twins), and imagines them with her father, who died in 1996. She is sure that they are

> *...Safe where I hope to lie too,*
> *Safe from the fume and the fret;*
> *You, and you,*
> *Whom I never forget.*
> *Safe from the frost and the snow,*
> *Safe from the storm and the sun,*
> *Safe where the seeds wait to grow...*[3]

Thirty-three months after the abortion she writes, "I wake up each day with a feeling that I am pregnant, only to find my belly lifeless."

---

[3] From Christina Rossetti, "Is it Well With the Child?"

II

THE STORIES OF 92 AMERICAN AND CANADIAN WOMEN

Is Shaleena's an extreme, untypical case? Can she be dismissed as mentally ill, or a borderline hysteric who has overdramatized her plight? Hardly, since she continues to hold down a highly demanding job, and has recently been promoted to a position of even greater responsibility, all the while hiding her grief from everyone but her immediate family. That Shaleena's experience is not that unusual or restricted to the developing world is suggested by the testimonies of the other 100 women who have told their stories to us. They are divided into two groups. The first, numbering 92, consists of women who had one or more abortions anywhere from three to 60 years ago, the majority within the last twenty years. Many women do not want to talk about their abortions. The ones in our cohort wanted to, mainly because they regretted what they had done and wished to communicate to others the reasons why. The second group includes eight women on their deathbeds whose stories were taken down just before they died, by a palliative-care nurse working in Ontario. Though not a random sample, these eight constitute an important group. All the stories are compelling, and demand attention from anyone who is genuinely interested in the psychological, emotional and spiritual impact of abortion on women.

WHY DID THEY HAVE THEIR ABORTION?

Some of the women we are dealing with in this section faced excruciatingly difficult and often desperate circumstances: illness, living in poverty, addicted to drugs or alcohol, or (in three instances) had been raped; some were very young; their partner threatened to leave them, beat them up, or even kill them if they continued with their pregnancy; they would lose their job, or have to abandon their education; their parents would be mortified if the fact of their pregnancy became known; they already had several children and could not afford to raise another; in one instance the pregnancy resulted from adultery.

In short, every member of our cohort felt trapped when she learned she was pregnant. Yet every one of these women now tells us that if she had it to do over again she would go through with her pregnancy. When asked what advice they would give to other women considering abortion, all but one of them replied, 'Don't do it!' Why did they unanimously regret their abortion, and almost unanimously advise other women at all costs to avoid having one? Because, apart from moral considerations, the emotional and spiritual price that they paid after their own abortion was unacceptably high. Even those who subsequently found healing and forgiveness cannot forget what they did and are haunted by the memory. To the question "Would you have an abortion again if you found yourself pregnant?" here is how they typically responded:

> "I would complete the pregnancy and give up the child for adoption."
>
> "I would never have another abortion, it was so traumatic."
>
> "It's not worth all the negative feelings, zero self-respect, self-hatred, regret and all the self-hating on myself. It's not worth losing a child's life."
>
> "No no no *no*!"
>
> "I know now I was manipulated…into what they thought was best for me."
>
> "Imagine me as a young woman who loved life and nature and sunsets and all the wonderful things in life. Then imagine the day that I came to after my abortion and all those things were taken away—in their place was regret, grief, and guilt and self-hatred. I couldn't look at a sunset or a puppy again and just love life. The abortion took that away. If I could do it again I would have that baby and love it."

When it comes to offering advice to women considering abortion, they say things like:

> "Don't do it, because you'll regret it."
>
> "It's a fast fix at the time, but it has tremendous long-term consequences."
>
> "I want all women to know they shouldn't do it…It is insulting to vacuum out the life of your baby."

> "It will destroy your life. Whatever you're going through now can be overcome. You can never abort the knowledge of that abortion or that baby, or the memories of what you've done. There is no magic eraser."
>
> "Get counselling; get help; turn to someone you can trust."
>
> "It's not worth the extreme negative emotions, the self-torture, the self-hatred. You end up being an emotional basket case. You lose trust in yourself and in others. Your view on life is skewed because of the negative emotions and self-hatred and lack of self-respect."
>
> "Don't do it, you will have no peace later."
>
> "Abortion may seem like the only solution at the time, but as maturity comes in the future the thing keeps festering and festering."

HOW DID OTHERS REACT TO THEIR PREGNANCY?

As we have noted, virtually all the women were dismayed to discover that they were pregnant. What was the reaction of the people close to them, and the medical personnel and others to whom they confided their dilemma? A few were supportive and declared that they would stick by them no matter what they decided. A handful, mainly parents, opposed the abortion, and were distressed when it happened. A greater number neither supported nor opposed the abortion, but—doubtless thinking themselves to be tolerant and fair minded—told the woman that the decision was up to her. It might surprise these people to learn that their tolerance was interpreted as indifference and lack of support. Several women testify that had they received so much as a hug, or a word of encouragement when they announced their pregnancy, they would not have gone through with the abortion.

> "If the GP had taken five minutes to talk about other options, I may have reconsidered."
>
> "My father was not there to support me. I couldn't find him."

> "If someone had been sympathetic to my situation, if my mother had said 'we will love that baby,' I would not have had the abortion."
>
> "I so desperately wanted someone to hug me and tell me that everything would be okay. I wanted someone to offer reassurance that I was capable of being a mother and that it would be all right. Instead, I tearfully requested an abortion."
>
> "If [the nurse practitioner] had referred me to a pregnancy crisis counsellor and followed up with me, I believe I would have made a different decision. I succumbed to all my fears and the fears of those around me and not one person I confided with told me, 'Don't Do It!'"
>
> "[The father] said, 'I will support you in whatever choice you make'… I became very angry and asked him why he would think I wanted an abortion."
>
> "When I was just about to be put out, the thought went through my mind that if just one person at the hospital had asked me if this is what I really wanted, you know, 'are you sure you want to go through with this?', I would have jumped off the table and gone home and not gone through with the procedure."
>
> "I wish my girlfriend, the GP, and the gynecologist who did the abortion—*someone!*—would have taken five minutes to 'give a shit' about me."

How Many were Pressured into Having an Abortion?

More typical than indifference or lack of support was active opposition to the pregnancy. Of the 68 women who answered the question, "were you pressured or coerced into having the abortion?" 46 (68 per cent) answered "yes". Sometimes the pressure took the form of threatened or actual violence.

> "When I told my boyfriend I was pregnant he became violent and just about killed me. I jumped out of a moving vehicle to get away from him. He had his tie around my neck. I jumped out, hit my head on a mailbox post (we were out on a country road). I ran across a field to the closest farmhouse. He chased me. Later I had him charged...He was remanded to stay away from me."
>
> "My fiancé was mad at me for being pregnant."
>
> "I was afraid they [my partner and my parents] would kick the crap out of me."

It was not only Shaleena (Section I) who was violently coerced by medical personnel. Another woman on the operating table informed the doctor and nurses that she had suddenly changed her mind.

> "When I could finally speak and think clearly again the doctor had arrived and they were putting the gas mask on me. I began to fight. I tried to get out from under it. I was thrashing about so they had to try to hold me down, but I kept moving my head too much and they had to take the mask away to see what all the thrashing was about. I was trying to tell people again that I didn't want the abortion. Instead of honouring my choice they held me back and turned the mask up to sedate me. I heard someone say 'cold feet' as I went unconscious. I woke up out of the anaesthetic screaming and crying out, 'I just want to be a mom!'"

While other experiences of coercion were less brutal and less dramatic, they were no less effective. The father of the child frequently said that he could not support his partner going through with the pregnancy. Sometimes he cited money problems; other times he threatened to leave.

> "Bob was angry when I told him I was pregnant. I let his anger intimidate me."
>
> "Don said if I got pregnant, I'd have to have an abortion."
>
> "My boyfriend dumped me once I was pregnant."
>
> "My fiancé was mad at me for being pregnant. I felt unsupported and scared."
>
> "An e-mail from the father changed my mind. He said he couldn't support me."
>
> "When I said no [to an abortion] he said he would have to think about this and would call back. It was after the birthdate that he called again."
>
> "My husband … did not have a steady job and did not want to … depend on his family members for help."
>
> "My boyfriend told me to get the abortion."

Remarkably, it was sometimes the woman's mother who pressured her to abort, especially if she was single, or in her teens. Sometimes it emerged that her mother had also had an abortion. Only occasionally did the woman's mother oppose the abortion.

> "Mom told me if I kept the baby likely nobody would want me, and I wouldn't be able to get an education…Mom arranged the abortion."
>
> "My mother treated me very badly before the abortion."
>
> "… fear of my parents. They were going through a divorce. They weren't there before; how could they be there now?"
>
> "Mom said, 'What are the neighbours going to think?'"

> "There was genetic retardation in my family… My mother was scared about the genetic thing and didn't want me to continue the pregnancy."
>
> "My mom wanted me to keep the baby. She was upset and still suffers long-term effects from my abortion."

Sometimes the woman's father played a role, although in at least one instance the father opposed the abortion. Women who have been unloved by their father seem particularly vulnerable to abortion.

> "I was afraid of my dad. I could never do anything right."
>
> "I was looking for love in all the wrong places. Dad was abusive, physically once and mostly verbally and emotionally."
>
> "… my non-relationship with my father. I would take risks or trade my body just to be loved. I felt unloved by my father; something was inherently defective in me because my father didn't love me."

If it wasn't parents and partners who pressured the women to abort, it was often those who ought to have listened and offered support: friends, counsellors and physicians.

> "A feminist friend influenced me to have the abortion."
>
> "I was pressured by… my girlfriend. 'You're single, this guy will leave you, a baby will ruin your life.' Zero support."
>
> "The school counsellor told me I was too young, 'you need to get rid of it.'"

> "Planned Parenthood... told me the baby was unrecognizable as a human. It was a blob of cells, a blood clot... After this, I went to the doctor who told me I should have an abortion as soon as possible."
>
> "The doctor said, 'In Russia women do this all the time.' He was an authority figure and it was out of character for me to speak back, but I did and said 'I'm not Russian.'"

How Were They Treated By the Abortion Providers?

As if to soothe their anxiety about what lay ahead, medical experts and others often kept the women in a state of ignorance, or misled them as to the nature of the abortion procedure. They were told variously that what they were carrying was "just a clump of tissue"; "like a tissue, unformed"; "it was not a baby, it was a blob", or "the doctor called it a D & C", or "they said I would be cleaned inside and there would be nothing left." No one bothered to disabuse the women themselves of mistaken notions, such as "I thought the baby would be deformed because its father was my second cousin", or "I thought of it as a group of unformed cells", "a blob of cells", "just a bunch of cells"; "I didn't really know what it was"; "I didn't think of it as anything. It was something that was making me sick and interfering with my lifestyle."

It is a normal assumption that the people who work in abortion clinics and in hospital obstetrics departments where abortions are performed, wish to be of service to women distressed by an unwanted pregnancy. We would expect such clinic and hospital personnel to be respectful and supportive of the troubled patients who pass through their hands. Sometimes they are. A few of our cohort confirm that they were treated with sympathy, kindness and respect. The great majority, however, tell a different story. They report that when they went for the abortion they encountered no compassion, no warmth, and little regard for their dignity.

> "The intake nurse warned me not to show any emotion."

> "They were sweet to me at first—then they turned into mean horrid people treating me like cattle. I got in trouble for vomiting on the floor because I couldn't make it to a garbage can. I felt they were disgusted by me and that they had to clean up after me. I was in a lawn chair and they said, 'Get up, someone else needs this space.'"

> "The first doctor was yelling at me. It felt like rape. There was fear, pain, shame with all my [three] abortions."

> "The doctor was cold. I remember thinking he had the face of an assassin. But the staff were sympathetic."

> "The doctor patted my buttock saying, 'There, there.' I remember a horrible yuck feeling when he did that."

> "I cried 'I've changed my mind.' The nurse said, 'You've come this far…' Then I woke up crying. The doctor came over and said, 'It wasn't really a baby' and I said, 'What do you think it was, a cabbage?' I was furious."

> "It was an assembly line; they did so many abortions in one day."

> "I felt like they were there to make money off of me… Everyone seemed blank. No feeling."

> "I was afraid. I felt alone. The room was very cold; no one talked. I felt I had no humanity, like a non-person, a job to get done, an annoyance. When I woke up I cried, saying 'Where is my baby? I want my baby.' The intern told me to be quiet, 'You are upsetting the others.' I didn't like the abortionist…no one would show compassion. They couldn't."

It is striking how often the medical personnel displayed a punitive, uncaring attitude towards their abortion patients, many of whom were paying them a high fee to be treated. It is hard to escape the impression that these doctors, nurses and receptionists were unconsciously expressing their own disgust and self-loathing at the work they were involved in.

ON THE OPERATING TABLE

What about the physical experience of the abortion itself? Was it painful? Here the answers were straightforward. When the abortion was performed in a hospital the patient was put under general anaesthetic and usually experienced no pain. In clinics only local anaesthetics were administered, with the consequence that pain was experienced; sometimes it was extreme.

> "…excruciating pain. I was crying, screaming, begging the doctor to stop."
>
> "I felt pain; I vomited from the anaesthetic."
>
> "Yes, I had cramping."

The question of pain apart, how did the women experience their abortion, during the procedure and immediately after? It is commonly reported that women feel immense relief after their abortion, as if a terrible worry has been lifted from their shoulders. Of the 38 women who responded to our question about their immediate reaction to the abortion just over a third (37 per cent) reported a feeling of relief, while 67 per cent reported feelings ranging from regret to terrible sorrow.[4] Some actually changed their mind on the operating table, and two attempted unsuccessfully to stop the operation.

When they told the medical personnel that they had changed their mind they were either deceived, as Shaleena was, or ignored, or physically forced. Some were sterilized against their will. One said that the doctor removed her fallopian tubes, and that it was "done with a vengeance and without my knowledge. He took advantage of my weakness." Another cried that she had changed her mind, but the staff paid no attention.

---

[4] Two women reported feeling both relief and sorrow, which is why the percentages add up to more than 100.

Here is a sample of the comments of those who found the abortion experience one that they never wish to repeat:

> "I felt relief when it was done, kind of like an empty calm…"
>
> "I felt a little sadness…"
>
> "I felt emotionally traumatized during the procedure."
>
> "I felt dirty, empty, emotionally drained, brain dead, tired."
>
> "Self-loathing, disgust with myself."
>
> "I felt relief, shock, anger at myself and my boyfriend; how could I be so stupid?"
>
> "I just accepted it and felt nothing."
>
> "I made a conscious decision to become cold, hard and callous because the world was cold."
>
> "I knew I should have had the baby; I knew I did the wrong thing."
>
> "I felt like the scum of the earth."
>
> "I was crying inside and asked the baby to forgive me. I felt sick because they poured out the baby in front of me."
>
> "I felt like a sewer, disgusted by the sound of suction. I felt grief; I was crying; I felt self-hatred; I hated everybody."
>
> "When I woke up I cried, saying, 'Where is my baby? I want my baby.'"
>
> "I remember wishing and praying I would die so I wouldn't have to face my parents after killing my baby."

> "I woke up screaming. The burning I felt between my legs was unbearable. My tummy was hollow and my eyes felt as though they had sunken into my head. Like I was looking through long dark tunnels. It was as if my soul had dried up and shrunk into my inner core. My mother was there; I cursed her away and asked for my aunt. The nurses were unsympathetic and told me to calm down, I was making a scene. I remember wanting to scream, 'A scene! I just committed murder and you helped me, encouraged me! You're damn right I'm making a scene, I want my baby back!!'"

THE AFTERMATH: RELIEF, REGRET, SELF-BLAME

For most of the women, the experience in the clinic or the operating room was one of horror. How did they feel about it in the succeeding weeks and months? For a very few, their immediate feeling of relief persisted, and they were able to get on with their lives, grateful for the burden that had been lifted from their shoulders. The emotional and spiritual complications came later. For the vast majority, the enormity of what they had done hit them almost immediately like a ton of bricks. In the privacy of their own mind they grasped, with piercing moral clarity, that the rejection of their pregnancy would be a source of never-ending regret. While abortion is freely available in North America - indeed, in many jurisdictions it is paid for with public money—it nevertheless remains a shameful thing that cannot be discussed with others. Most of the women felt cut off and isolated on account of that shame. Many felt low self-esteem and depression, or engaged in self-destructive behavior.

Suicide was frequently on their mind. When asked whether they had had suicidal thoughts or attempted suicide, were depressed, or visited a psychiatrist, or mental hospital 70 of the 71 women who answered the question said yes. This finding sharply contrasts with those studies that have found minimal or no emotional distress among women who have undergone abortion. Many of our cohort were incapable of regarding the "product of abortion" as an undeveloped fetus, much less a "blob of tissue"; rather, it was a baby with whom they carried on an interior dialogue. A number asked the baby to forgive them.

> "I grieved for the loss of my baby. I wondered what gender it was. I wrote a special poem."
>
> "I miss them,[5] even though I physically never got to meet them."
>
> "I wonder, what would he be like? He would have been born at Christmas time. He'd be 37 now."
>
> "I'd see other mothers and babies, and cry. I think of my lost child and I grieve… I think what he or she might look like."
>
> "I think what he would be like. I went to a personal retreat in April 2007 and wrote a letter to my baby."
>
> "I think of what he would have looked like…I named the baby."
>
> "I grieved their loss. I named all three of them and I think of them. I look forward to meeting them in heaven."
>
> "I know that she is with God and that we will have a meeting one day."

Immediate regret was soon followed by self-recrimination and self-loathing in many cases. Several had flashbacks of the procedure. Hardly any were able to put the experience behind them.

> "After it was over I just went on with my life."
>
> "I didn't think about it, [yet] I attempted suicide eight or nine months after."
>
> "I felt great remorse, regret, guilt, disgust with myself."
>
> "Anger toward myself and the doctor when I realized the depth of what I'd done."

---

5   She had three abortions.

"My grandmother had fixed up the back room for me to recuperate. I remember laying down and wanting to die there. Never wanting to wake up. I stopped eating."

"Low self-esteem, promiscuity, anger, flashbacks of the procedure, fear of having the secret found out."

"I hated myself for putting myself before the child."

"Relief for two weeks, then depression."

"Right after the abortion, I went into depression. I slept more than normal, twelve hours a day for two years."

"Flashbacks: being on the table for the abortion."

"My heart hurts. I feel weird around the 19th of February [the date of the abortion]. I wish I could tell people about my secret."

"I drank, smoked, did drugs and was more promiscuous after the abortion."

"When others had their babies my pain was excruciating. I worked in a factory that made baby clothes—it was like a big punishment day after day."

"Whatever little bit of self-worth I had was gone. I was the worst human being on the face of the earth…I hated everybody."

"Whenever someone talked about abortion it was like sticking a knife into me. If people really knew who I was they would hate me."

"I could not forgive myself. I didn't think about it; I just drank."

"For about six months after the abortion I was OK. Then I had a nervous breakdown and was forced into quitting my job. I prayed for death to ease the pain."

"I'd see other mothers and babies and cry."

Time, it is said, heals all wounds. How did the passage of time alter women's perceptions of their abortion experience? We asked them about their reaction after one year, after five years, and "today", meaning anything up to 37 years later. One year later the memory of the abortion was still vivid, and emotions still raw.

> "It was like yesterday."
>
> "Self-loathing; I felt like I'd failed; I felt like a loser."
>
> "My low self-esteem led to alcohol and substance abuse, promiscuity, car accidents and an inability to forgive myself."
>
> "The same: regret, denial, resentment, self-condemnation, shame, fear of being found out... don't talk about it."
>
> "I was depressed, a zombie."

Five years later, emotions had begun to soften and self-blame was less acute for most, but the recollection of the abortion still loomed very large for the majority of women. Some had found spiritual healing and reconciliation. Others still could not face what they had done.

> "I was still in denial, blocking it."
>
> "I felt guilt around Mother's Day and Christmas."
>
> "I'll never forget."
>
> "Hurting, covering up the pain, alienated."
>
> "Less intense, but triggered by the Labour Day weekend (when I had the abortion)."
>
> "I weep less frequently in the last four years, especially since I now have a son."

> "The same—regret, denial, resentment, self-condemnation, shame, fear of having the secret found out…[but still] don't talk about it."
>
> "I was functioning very well, but there was a sadness, an incompleteness…"

Today, even those who have found forgiveness remember their abortion every day, and many are haunted by the memory.

> "I'll never forget my child, or the abortion, or the tube, the nurses, the 'man'[the abortionist], the table, the baby in the bottle…the South African accents."
>
> "Major regret [32 years later]."
>
> "Regret [fourteen years later]."
>
> "Today, twenty years later? Regret; I've never forgotten it."
>
> "I have been reconciled, though from time to time it will hit me hard."
>
> "Regret, but acceptance now."
>
> "Today I feel it was an event that changed my life, and me—who I am. I tell my story, and I have helped to stop others from doing the same."
>
> "I have achieved great healing."
>
> "I've been set free by God through Jesus. He's turned my sins to 'white as snow.'"
>
> "I want to be totally healed. I want to talk to my husband about it."

> "I'm angry, very angry… I'm angry that there were options never given to me. I'm angry at the lie at Planned Parenthood, angry that I was weak, angry at the abortionist, angry that people won't listen. I'm angry at Catholics or others who say it is 'a woman's choice.' I'm angry at the intern for telling me to be quiet."
>
> "Today (nineteen years after), I'm ok. This past Christmas I didn't get very emotional."
>
> "Today I'm a much stronger person."
>
> "Today I feel at peace. I have told the truth of my experience. I am more me than I have ever been… I am working more toward the will of God."
>
> "I had a recurring nightmare during my pregnancy with my first-born. A baby was crying behind the door of the bathroom in my apartment. I'd get up, open the door and find a low bassinet covered by a blanket. I'd pull back the blanket. The baby would stop crying, but it was a skeleton."
>
> "From about the age of 60 I have come to see this pregnancy as a baby that I grieve… My mind is always there. One day, while I was sitting in the rocking chair, I could swear I saw a child running out of the house. It was Sofia, the little girl who only lived a week because of complications,[6] the result of an attempted and failed abortion."

PHYSICAL AND PSYCHOLOGICAL COMPLICATIONS

So far in this chapter we have been dealing mostly with women's subjective reactions to their abortion. What of the objective evidence about physical and psychological complications? Because we only have evidence supplied by the women themselves, quantification is of limited utility. But what the women tell us is interesting nevertheless. Most of them emerged

---

6   She was born prematurely.

physically unscathed from the abortion. Only a minority experienced physical complications, and for the most part these were temporary. Normal health seems to have been restored after a few months of the operation. Hemorrhaging immediately after the procedure was the most common complication. It ranged from persistent bleeding that lasted as long as several weeks, to a sudden, immediate, frightening, seemingly torrential rush of blood: "I remember standing to go to the bathroom and blood gushed to the floor". There were also a few cases of infection. In the longer term, some women reported one or more miscarriages, which they attributed to the earlier abortion, or infertility from a damaged cervix or badly scarred uterus. Nine out of 40 (23 per cent) who answered the question, reported that despite their best efforts they were unable to have children after the abortion. One woman had to have a hysterectomy at age 45 owing to fibroids and scar tissue. Three others were certain that the endometriosis, breast cancer and cervical cancer from which they suffered respectively, were due to the abortion. It is sobering to reflect that none of the clinics, and very few of the hospitals evinced any interest in their patients once the abortion was over. Follow-up was at best minimal, and usually non existent. "Follow-up?!" exclaimed one. "No. You pay and leave. It was cut and dried."

Apart from depression and suicidal ideation, a few women had to see a psychiatrist, or were admitted to a mental hospital in the months or years after their abortion. Besides extreme anxiety, promiscuous sexual activity, and other self-destructive behaviours, including suicide ideation, a small number reported obsessive compulsive disorders. Several found they had difficulty bonding or relating to their own children born subsequent to the abortion(s), or to children in general. "I found it very difficult to be in the presence of children, babies, pregnant women, because they were conscious and sub-conscious reminders of the abortion and the incredible loss that I know and feel." A significant number also found it much more difficult to relate to men or trust men than before. Marriages and relationships fell apart after the abortion. It was common to resort to drugs, alcohol and tobacco as a way of coping with the psychological fall-out from the abortion. "I didn't care whether I lived or died" was typical of the large minority who suffered major depression. While some women had low self-esteem or were depressed *before* the abortion, by far the greater number encountered these psychological afflictions *after* the abortion, having previously enjoyed good mental health.

All these findings are consonant with the quantified results found by

Reardon and Cougle in their much larger objective study.[7]

THE SPIRITUAL LEGACY

Difficult as it is to quantify the psychological impact of abortion, it is almost impossible to measure its spiritual impact. In fact, the attempt has almost never been made. Still, we asked our subjects to write or talk about the spiritual change that abortion wrought in their lives. Some of the answers they gave make riveting reading. In a few instances, they confessed that abortion had caused them to build a shell around themselves, and to become permanently mistrustful of humanity. A handful, like Shaleena, were convinced that they had committed a sin that could never be forgiven, and therefore existed in a permanent state of despair. For the majority it was different. Abortion, while it dragged them down into an abyss of spiritual darkness, was in the end, the stepping stone to spiritual healing and renewal. This was not quick or easy. Sometimes it took nine, ten or even more years for healing to occur. It was brought about through searching self-honesty, or the help supplied by another caring person. In several cases it involved a conversion experience.

> "I was in a dark tunnel. The tunnel ended when I got into a close relationship with God."
>
> "Five years after the third abortion I became a born-again Christian... [Finally] knowing I was forgiven by God was a huge relief."
>
> "I received Jesus as my saviour ...in 1993."
>
> "This personal encounter with God...has changed my life 180 degrees."
>
> "He [Jesus] separated me from my sin—so I could love my child. I received healing and forgiveness and freedom—from God's Word."

---

7   Reardon DC and Cougle JR. Depression and unintended pregnancy in the national longitudinal survey of youth: a cohort study. BMJ 2002 January; 324 (7330): 151-2.

> "My morals...have become stronger. God will take care of me and my needs. I'm not in control. I trust in life, not in death. [Nine years after the abortion] slowly I went back to church. About 1999, I had a real conversion experience."
>
> "I didn't have a spiritual life at the time...Now I am certainly aware of life after death....I know I'm forgiven."
>
> "My church community is a very important part of my life."

As a result of the healing they experienced, and in gratitude towards those who had helped them achieve it, some of the women expressed the hope that they could assist others in the same situation to "overcome and get set free from the negative effects of abortion."

> "At the time of the abortion I was distant from God...Now the most important relationship in my life is Jesus."
>
> "It was the love and prayer of others who helped bring me back to the Lord."
>
> "Without the abortion, I might not have come to a personal relationship with Jesus."

III

CODA

There would be no public knowledge of the thoughts of women who have had abortions as they approach the end of life had it not been for the foresight of a palliative-care nurse in Canada who took down several of their stories shortly after she heard them. Trained at the Master's level as a nurse consultant in palliative care, **Jean Echlin** worked for many years in hospitals in two Ontario cities. The stories date from different periods in her professional career but they all have a common thread. Each of the eight women was tortured by the memory of an abortion, which had happened anywhere from a few years to many decades before. Some were able to achieve spiritual peace before they died; others were not.

Betty

Betty was 32, happily married, with two small children, aged two and four. Her family life was idyllic until she came down with an aggressive case of breast cancer, which chemotherapy and radiation therapy failed to halt. She was put on morphine to control the steadily increasing pain. But when she developed a pleural effusion—a fluid accumulation around the lungs—she had to be readmitted to hospital because the existing medication was no longer adequate for the pain. Various drastic steps at length controlled the pain, but not her steadily increasing anxiety. Just days before she died she broke down and told Jean that when she was seventeen she had become pregnant. Her boyfriend flew into a rage and threatened to kill her if she did not get rid of the baby. Terrified and without resources, she went and had the abortion. But she wrote a letter, which she always kept with her.

> *Dearest Baby:*
>
> *I am so sorry that I had to do this to you. Please know that this isn't my choice but this is just not the right time for us. I could never give you the life you need because I am too young and have no money... I will always love you. I will always remember you. I will light a candle for you every year on this terrible day. Please forgive me dearest baby.*
>
> *Love always,*
> *Your mother.*

Betty was convinced that "I'll never see my baby in Heaven because I'll never get there." She and Jean talked a great deal about forgiveness and God's love. Betty seemed less anxious and appeared to be comforted by their mutual sharing. Two weeks later she died peacefully.

Reflecting on Betty's death, Jean writes, "this experience clearly showed me again how earlier-in-life induced abortion causes psycho-spiritual pain and suffering near or at the end of life."

Caroline

Caroline was 92 years old and approaching the end of life. She was suffering unremitting abdominal pain along with extreme restlessness and anxiety. Her pain was brought under control with dilaudid, but her restlessness and anxiety persisted. Jean's palliative care team worked on the model taught by Cicely Saunders, the English founder of hospice care. When addressing the pain of the human spirit, care providers are to "watch with me."[8] When no medication could manage Caroline's anxiety, Jean gently prompted her to talk about her spiritual pain. Her eyes overflowing with tears, she recounted how after bearing two sons she became pregnant a third time, and was quite happily looking forward to the birth of another child. Her husband, however, was not happy; he hit the roof, said he could not tolerate another baby, and insisted that she go for an abortion. He found a clinic out of town and drove her to it, where the doctor and his nurse put her through an extremely painful procedure. She got pregnant again three years later, and went through the same scenario, except that this time she was five months pregnant. The operation was even more painful than the first, and when she got home she suffered massive haemorrhaging. "Somehow I survived," she told Jean, "but never in my life did I feel right again. Life felt sad and lonely all the time." When she was 40, she got pregnant a fifth time, but this time bore the child, a girl, who quickly became the light of their life. But still, "I could not stop thinking about my abortions."

When she was 48 she saw a TV show about a baby growing inside the mother. "It was then that I truly realized that... I had killed my babies." From that day on she was certain that "God could never forgive me, I am a murderer." Nor had she been able to forgive her husband, now dead, and

---

8   "The phrase 'watch with me' comes from the story of Jesus facing death in the Garden of Gesthemane (St Matthew's Gospel, 26:38) and sums up the deepest need of any person facing death or desolation." Quoted in Saunders C, ed., *The Management of Malignant Disease Series*. London: Edward Arnold, 1978, p. 8.

remained angry with him. On another occasion she broke down again as she relived the horror of her abortions. Jean prayed with her, picked up her Bible and read to her the comforting words of salvation and forgiveness. Caroline then relaxed and fell asleep. A short time later she died.

Catherine

Catherine, aged 90, was dying. She had come into hospice care because her anxiety, restlessness and sleeplessness had become too much for her daughter's family, with whom she was living, to cope with. Some days after being admitted she confided in Jean, "I cannot die…I can never be forgiven…I've never told anyone…I didn't even tell my darling husband!" At this point tears were flooding her pillow. In a soft voice she told Jean, "I killed my baby…I had an abortion." She explained that at the time—more than half a century before—she already had two children, and her mother was living with them in a small house. Her mother kept saying to her, "there is no room for you to have another one…What will happen to me?…I'll be out on the street…You must get rid of it! You have to do this at least for your mother!" Finally she went and had the abortion, and for the rest of her life suffered "disenfranchised grief", meaning grief that cannot be acknowledged or shared. "I wanted that baby…and Alex [her husband] loved the children so much…I could never tell him!" She perceived a loss of love from her two living children, while her mother took over the raising of them. Catherine had been active in her church, so Jean talked with her about the meaning of communion and what belief in the death and resurrection of Christ means to believers. That day she asked her daughter to bring her her Bible. The next morning, her pulse was weak, but she opened her eyes when Jean came to her bed and said, "I don't feel scared anymore. … I do believe that I can be forgiven. Isn't that great? A miracle at last!" Then, a few hours later, after saying good-bye to her family, Catherine took her last small breath and died.

Irene

Irene, 42 years old, was terminally ill from cancer of the cervix and uterus that had spread throughout her abdomen. Her husband was having an affair at the time, and was about to leave her because of her inability to have children. When Jean sat down at her bedside, Irene seemed to have lost all will to live, and was burdened with an overwhelming sense of guilt. She revealed that before meeting her husband she had had an abortion when she was eighteen. Early in her marriage her gynaecologist diagnosed

Asherman's syndrome, an irritation of the inner lining (endometrium) of the uterus that causes scar tissue. Her doctor asked her if she had ever had an abortion. More than two decades later, Irene felt that her cancer was the punishment for that earlier abortion. Now that her husband was leaving her, she had given up on life. "I don't have a family, I don't really have a husband anymore, so there is no reason for me to live." One of the hospice volunteers ascertained that Irene did not wish to discuss matters of faith. That wish was honoured; she died quietly and with dignity.

Jane

Jane had four children, all under the age of fifteen, to whom she was deeply devoted. But her husband was in the process of divorcing her, and had already won a court order giving him custody of the children. What made the situation exceptionally cruel was that Jane was suffering from an inoperable brain tumour and did not have long to live. She remained in her home, desperately trying to hang on to her children. Yet the only person she blamed was herself. In the midst of making complicated arrangements to manage Jane's pain and assist her breathing, Jean was entrusted with her story, but asked not to reveal it to anyone at the time. "This is my punishment. I have done something just horrible. I ruined my family, my marriage, and myself. And this is the price that I'm paying. I had an affair with my boss." The affair had to be kept top secret, so when she became pregnant the only answer was an abortion. Jane described her abortion as "one of the cruelest experiences of my entire life, far worse than any part of this cancer experience." She went on to describe the machine that was used to "suck" out the contents of her uterus. "To this day, and every day of my life I hear that sucking noise. All I can think of is that it sucked a living human being out of my body."

Jane did not want to discuss her belief system, nor was there anything that gave her comfort. She could not forgive herself or accept any concept of being forgiven. "I am a destroyer of life. I destroyed my baby's life, I destroyed my marriage, I destroyed my children's lives. And I won't be available to them…. I don't deserve forgiveness." It was in that spiritual state that she died.

Kara

Kara was in her second year of university, studying social work because she wanted to help people. She had recently developed an unusual, aggressive form of ovarian cancer that had quickly metasticized to her whole body.

Steadily higher doses of morphine were administered, yet she continued to be in pain. Her strong faith helped to carry her through, yet she questioned why this was all happening to her. Before long she came up with the answer: "I'm sure I'm being punished." One day as she neared the end of her life she called Jean to sit with her, and asked that her parents be out of the room. "As I sat with her, she cried and cried. I cried with her. Kara believed that this punishment was related to an induced abortion that she had at the age of sixteen." She wanted to carry the baby, but her boyfriend wanted to get rid of "it". Eventually she crumpled under his pressure. She said that after that "awful experience" in the abortion clinic, and the way she was humiliated, she felt less than human. Six years later, at the age of 22, she was still oppressed by that memory. Before the end came she committed her soul to God, and was able to die at home, but her parents never knew of the spiritual burden that had weighed her down.

Teresa

Teresa was only 26; already she had had six children. When admitted to the hospital she was in a wheelchair, doubled over in pain; the diagnosis being suspected abortion. Two RCMP officers sat outside her room. Their purpose was to listen for any indication from her that could possibly identify her suspected abortionist. At that time, the 1970s, pain management was not recognized as a part of necessary patient care, and palliative care had not yet been heard of. Her only treatment was intravenous fluid and good nursing care. Teresa worried about her family, but despite her steady decline her husband never came to visit her. She called for her parish priest, who came several times to her bedside, but she remained in too much anguish and physical pain to respond to his spiritual care. A week before her death, she revealed to Jean that her husband had forced her to have an abortion after her seventh pregnancy. Although legal abortions were available, they had opted for a criminal abortion in order to preserve secrecy. When asked if she would like her priest to administer the last rites she answered, "yes...Please ask Father to hurry." A day or two later as she came on shift, Jean heard Teresa's screams coming from down the hall. She ran to her room. "When she saw me, she mustered the last ounce of strength in her weary body and jumped over the side-rails of the bed, ripping out her intravenous needle. Teresa threw herself into my arms. She died standing on her feet with her arms around me, her head on my shoulder and my arms around her." As Jean later reflected, there had been no husband, no family, no friends to say goodbye to her, "just one terrified young nurse and one morally frustrated priest, who both felt that we had failed Teresa in so many ways."

Victoria

Victoria was a banking executive, who had been referred to palliative care for management of her pain. Only 56 years of age, she had been diagnosed with aggressive carcinoma of the breast three years before. Despite a mastectomy and removal of lymph nodes followed by chemotherapy, the cancer had come back, and now involved her lungs, liver and bone. Only massive, continuous dosages of morphine could bring the pain under control. She was also deeply anxious and depressed, with a feeling of worthlessness. She received minimal emotional support from her family, who missed her substantial pay cheque, and asked aggressively, "how can we possibly manage without your money coming in?" She blamed herself for their dilemma.

Given Victoria's mounting death anxiety, Jean delicately broached the question of her spiritual state. Victoria began to cry, "I can never be forgiven for what I've done...I have done an unpardonable thing...I have committed murder...I killed my own baby." Sobbing loudly, she went on, "Now look at me.... I'm wizened and dying.... This is my punishment.... God will never forgive me.... I can never forgive myself. Help me, help me.... I can't go on this way!" She then revealed that nearly 23 years before, she had an abortion. Her husband had insisted that "we needed my income and couldn't afford another child." The abortion clinic turned out to be "the worst experience of my life. The pain was ...even worse than what I'm having now! ...They wouldn't let me see my baby because it's skull was crushed or something." Victoria continued talking and weeping for more than two hours. She was finally giving voice to the psychospiritual pain that had afflicted her over many years. From the time of her abortion on, she felt estranged from her two children. She also harboured great resentment towards her husband, whom she held partly responsible. At length she asked Jean to "pray for me and my little lost baby." Previously, she had had little religious involvement but, with her consent, a pastor began visiting her daily. They prayed, read the Bible together, and spoke of forgiveness. She never discussed her abortion with him. "Six days later,' Jean recounts, "I was present when Victoria made a confession of her faith, through tears of joy!"

Astonishingly, her morphine requirements dropped steadily during this time. Victoria died gently, three days after taking Communion.

Conclusion

The testimonies we have read demonstrate that the notion of abortion as 'a woman's choice' is illusory for many. Every one of the women who shared her story with us says that if she had it to do over again she would go through with the pregnancy, and all but one would counsel others not to have an abortion, no matter how difficult the circumstances.

> Over two-thirds of the women who answered the question said that if they had not been pressured or coerced, and if they had received at least minimal support from medical personnel or significant others, they would not have had the abortion. The pressure was exerted not only by the male partner; it also came from parents (mothers in particular), employers, friends and medical personnel.

The experience of many of these women when they were in the hospital or clinic, and on the operating table, was nothing short of nightmarish. Their treatment ranged from cool indifference, to disrespect, to callous unconcern, to anger, even to violent refusal to follow their expressed wishes. In only a few cases did they encounter courtesy, concern and respect. At least two of them were brutally forced to endure the abortion after announcing that they did not want it. From their stories, one gets the definite impression that people who do abortions are not proud of their work, and express this feeling by behaving disrespectfully or punitively towards their patients.

Medical personnel and agencies such as Planned Parenthood often fail to tell pregnant women the straight facts about abortion. Abortion will solve all your problems, they imply. It is a minor medical procedure to "clean out" the uterus, or remove "a blob of tissue" or a "clump of cells". It is not about getting rid of a baby. Many of the women knew at the time that this is precisely what it was, or if they learned later that the fetus is not just an unformed group of cells, they were overcome with grief and self-reproach.

Over a third of the women found that the abortion brought them immediate relief, even if it resulted in long-term regret. Most of the women, however, were traumatized and filled with self-reproach, reporting that they felt dirty, ashamed, "like the scum of the earth," angry with everyone, or wishing they could die. In the coming weeks and months these feelings did not subside but if anything grew more insistent. Soon they came to realize with piercing clarity the moral significance of what they had done, and that the memory of it would never leave them. Many found themselves in the grip of a serious depression, and were plagued by thoughts of suicide. A few did attempt to kill themselves. A number of them carried on an interior dialogue with their aborted child, writing them poems and letters, naming them, and asking their forgiveness.

For some, the feelings of self-reproach gradually ebbed away, especially if they were able to have other children, and absorb themselves in raising a family. For others, the feelings persisted unabated for half a century and more. As Jean Echlin has documented, a significant number of women experienced the most acute spiritual pain on their deathbed stemming from an earlier abortion.

Most hospitals and clinics did not follow-up their patients after the procedure. Fortunately, most women—apart from a significant minority—did not have physical complications. Complications ranged from bleeding or infection, to subsequent miscarriages or inability to conceive. Graver still were the emotional and spiritual complications. Depression and suicidal ideation were common, with a few women having to seek psychiatric treatment, or admission to a mental hospital. Several found all their human relationships affected, experiencing particular difficulty bonding with their existing children or with the ones they subsequently bore.

Spiritually, many women reported that while the abortion "dragged them down into an abyss," it often proved to be the stepping stone to healing and renewal. Several underwent overpowering conversion experiences in which they felt redeemed and forgiven. In gratitude for their forgiveness, they expressed the hope that they could assist other women who were tormented by their abortions to be spiritually liberated as they had been.

What all of these narratives bring home to us is that abortion, far from being a trivial experience, shakes those who have experienced it to the core of their being. They are not able to forget the fateful day when they went on the operating table to terminate the life that was growing inside them. The stories of these women have been offered to help others who have experienced abortion or who may consider it.

Conclusion: Abortion's impact on women

The research for this book has led us to a number of unexpected, even counter-intuitive conclusions. For example, countries where abortion is freely available, such the US, the UK, Russia and Hungary, have a generally worse record on infant and maternal health than countries where abortion has long been unavailable such or Ireland, Egypt, Uganda, or where it has been recently banned, such as Poland, Chile, El Salvador and Nicaragua. The key to reducing maternal mortality is not to make abortion available on request, but to provide improved services for pregnant women, including:

- Skilled attendance at birth
- Community outreach
- Emergency obstetric care (caesarean sections in particular)
- Transportation for emergency obstetric care
- Improved education for women
- Improved referral systems

Another counterintuitive finding is that freely-available abortion has turned into a deeply ironic triumph of "a woman's right to choose", since it has led to the intentional deaths of millions of female unborn children. The world's two most populous countries, China and India, now have seriously skewed sex ratios, and a drastic shortage of women, with incalculable social harm.

Another counterintuitive finding: while it is highly doubtful whether the legalization of abortion in the US can be credited with lowering the crime rate in the 1990s, it is incontrovertible that legal abortion has been accompanied by a dramatic rise in single parenthood and child poverty.

There has been a long struggle on the part of women to win the right to sue abortion providers for failing to inform them of the risks of abortion. In the past few years several abortion providers have been successfully sued on these grounds, in particular for failing to inform their patients of the increased risk of breast cancer after abortion. We can be sure that women who believe they have been victimized by abortion will from now on show themselves less willing to accept any failure on the part of abortion providers to inform them of the risks of the procedure before they perform it.

Recent research demonstrates that physical complications are more common than is often thought, because of a general failure to track them, especially on the part of clinics. Before it stopped publishing them, the Royal College of Obstetricians and Gynaecologists reported an immediate complication rate of eleven per cent for surgical abortions.[1] The complication rate for medical or drug-induced abortion is up to four times higher.

Pain is a minor consideration compared to the other complications of induced abortion. Yet it is worth at least a mention that research shows how doctors and abortion providers seem to underestimate and downplay the amount of pain that women experience.

Among long-term complications the most important, and controversial, is breast cancer. Chapter 7 explains in biological terms why the human breast is more susceptible to developing cancer after induced abortion than after a completed pregnancy. The author of this chapter is a highly-qualified American breast surgeon. She shows that the great majority of studies on the subject have found a significantly increased risk of breast cancer among women who abort their first pregnancy. Yet this overwhelming weight of evidence is ignored by the National Cancer Institute in the US, which continues to maintain that there is no proven connection between induced abortion and breast cancer. What is remarkable is that they persist in this denial despite findings by their own researchers affirming the link.[2] The fiercely controversial nature of the question of the abortion-breast-cancer link has even corrupted the respect for truth that would be expected in a major text book. Thus, the 1991 edition of *The Breast: Comprehensive Management of Benign and Malignant Disease* clearly stated that induced abortion was a risk factor for breast cancer in the chapter concerning molecular biology, but the 1997 edition removed that information. In its place was a misleading table of breast cancer risks. Induced abortion is listed in the table as having "no effect" on breast cancer risk. This statement is contradicted by the accompanying text, which states that abortion after

---

1 Royal College of Obstetricians and Gynaecologists. *The Care of Women Requesting Induced Abortion*: 4. Information for women. 2000.
2 The researchers are Louise Brinton and Janet Daling. See: Dolle JM, Daling JR, White E, Brinton LA, Doody DR, Porter PL and Malone KE. Risk factors for triple-negative breast cancer in women under the age of 45 years. Cancer Epidemiology, Biomarkers and Prevention 2009 April; 18(4): 1157-66; Daling JR, Malone KE, Voigt LF, White E, and Weiss NS. Risk of breast cancer among young women: relationship to induced abortions. Journal of the National Cancer Institute Cancer Spectrum 86, 1994; 21: 1584-92.

twelve weeks carries a relative risk of 1.38, meaning a 38 per cent increase.[3] In the 2004 edition of this same textbook, induced abortion was not listed in any of the tables that tabulated risk factors, yet the same paragraph from the 1997 edition about the relative risk was repeated.[4]

This textbook is symptomatic of researchers drawing conclusions against the trend of their data, or concealing findings about abortion risks. Perhaps the most remarkable example of this phenomenon is found in the paper by Melbye and colleagues on the risk of breast cancer. Their study showed a statistically significant increase of 89 per cent in breast cancer risk in abortions performed over eighteen weeks' gestation. This fact was not mentioned in the conclusion of the paper, which merely stated that there was no link at all between abortion and breast cancer. The Melbye study is often cited in major textbooks to show there is no link between abortion and breast cancer.[5]

Another study, by Eaton and colleagues found that the unadjusted risk for autism among mothers who had experienced a previous abortion was 1.35 and the adjusted risk was 1.10. The unadjusted risk for intellectual impairment was 1.86, while the adjusted risk was 1.72. In one part of their report they acknowledged that "a history of provoked abortion increases risk for mental retardation and learning disorders." Yet later in the same report they drew back, stating, "it would be an improper extrapolation from the data, for example, to conclude that provoked [i.e. induced] abortions were causing mental retardation or learning disorders in later pregnancies."[6]

In a recent study Mota and colleagues found that among 3310 American women, 48.8 per cent of those with both a lifetime psychiatric diagnosis and an abortion history, had experienced their first onset of depression *after* their first abortion.[7] However, the researchers were able virtually to eliminate the significance of this finding by "adjusting" for violence,

---

3   Bland and Copeland. 2009. See Chapter 7, n. 1.
4   Vogel. See Chapter 7, n. 92.
5   Melbye M, Wohlfahrt J, Olsen JH, Frisch M, Westergaard T, Helweg-Larsen K and Andersen PK. Induced abortion and the risk of breast cancer. NEJM 1997 January; 336: 81-5.
6   Eaton, WW, Mortensen, PB, Thomsen, PH and Frydenberg M. Obstetric complications and risk for severe psychopathology in childhood. Journal of Autism and Developmental Disorders 2001; 31(3): 279-285.
7   95% CI 40.1-57.5.

including "physical abuse by parents and (or) guardians; physical abuse by partner; physical abuse by anybody else; rape; other sexual assault; and [being] mugged, held up, or threatened with a weapon."[8] In other words these various forms of violence before the abortion were to blame for the depression. In this way they were able to conclude that depression was not significantly associated with abortion. It did not occur to them to ask whether the pre-abortion violence was part of a concerted attempt to force the woman to have an abortion, and was thus directly connected to the abortion experience, and hence the post-abortion depression.

The last example is from a paper on Romania's experience with unwanted pregnancy after it made abortion illegal in 1967. The researcher reported that children born just after abortion became illegal "display *significantly better* educational and labor market achievements than children born just prior to the change" (emphasis added). In other words the many supposedly unwanted children did not suffer any disadvantages from the fact that their mothers had been unable to obtain abortions. Yet he overturns his own finding by explaining that a number of educated, wealthy women were now giving birth. This is important, he says, because "urban, educated women were more likely to have abortions prior to the policy change, so a higher proportion of children were born into urban, educated households after abortions became illegal." What he means is that more children of higher socio-economic status were being born as a result of the new law banning abortion. By this tortured reasoning Pop-Eleches is able to arrive at the opposite conclusion, namely that "children born after the abortion ban had *worse* schooling and labor market outcomes"[9] (emphasis added). Another remarkable instance of a researcher drawing a conclusion that contradicts their own findings.

Prenatal testing in the form of ultrasound sonography, amniocentesis and chorionic villi sampling (CVS) has become standard practice since the late 1970s. The purpose is to identify genetic and other disabilities in children before birth. Overwhelmingly the purpose has not been to correct these defects, or help parents to prepare to care for a child with disabilities, but to eliminate such children before birth. Women experience great pressure to undergo prenatal testing even if they are opposed on moral

---

8   Mota NP, Burnett M and Sareen J. Associations between abortion, mental disorders, and suicidal behaviour in a nationally representative sample. Canadian Journal of Psychiatry 2010; 55(5): 239-47, p. 241.
9   Pop-Eleches C. The impact of an abortion ban on socioeconomic outcomes of children: evidence from Romania. Journal of Political Economy. August 2006; 114(4): p. 745.

or personal grounds to terminating their pregnancy. Indeed, it has been determined that between 40 and 80 per cent of parents who are offered the option of perinatal palliative care—a supportive option for parents whose child has been diagnosed with a life-limiting anomaly—request this care, and choose to continue their pregnancy.[10]

Most studies of the physical impact of abortion pay little attention to long-term physical complications. Yet it has been established that dilation of the cervix during a surgical abortion can render the cervix incompetent, resulting in miscarriage or preterm births in subsequent pregnancies. The risk of placenta previa also rises after one or more induced abortions. It has also been well established that women who undergo an induced abortion later suffer a higher rate of Pelvic Inflammatory Disease (PID) than the general population. The evidence for this connection is overwhelming. The well-documented sequelae of PID include chronic pelvic pain, subfertility, infertility and ectopic pregnancy. Other sequelae include intraamniotic infection, neonatal sepsis, and stillbirth. A recent major English study determined that the risk of subfecundity increased by *no less than 620 per cent* after induced abortion.[11] Far from being attended by any fanfare, this alarming finding was buried in the depths of the paper and not referred to in the abstract.

There is a further physical complication, whose connection with induced abortion has only recently come to light: autoimmune diseases. Induced abortion is associated with a greater frequency of fetal microchimerism; in other words, a greater number of fetal cells are detected in women who have undergone induced abortion than in other women who have brought their pregnancy to term. Some researchers suggest that fetal microchimerism may cause, or contribute to, autoimmune diseases in women. In fact, one has flatly stated that "the consistently rising incidence of autoimmune diseases in women over the past four decades may be attributed to the increase in the utilization of abortion."[12]

---

10 Calhoun BC, Napolitano P, Terry M, Bussey C, and Hoeldtke NJ. Perinatal hospice: comprehensive care for the family of the fetus with a lethal condition. Journal of Reproductive Medicine 2003; 58(11): 718-19; Breeze ACG, Lees CC, Kumar A, Missfelder-Lobos HH and Murdoch EM. Palliative care for prenatally diagnosed lethal fetal abnormality. Archives of Disease in Childhood; Fetal and Neonatal 2007; 92(1): F56-8.
11 Hassan MAM and Killick SR. Is previous aberrant reproductive outcome predictive of subsequently reduced fecundity? Human Reproduction 2005; 20(3): 657-664. OR 7.2 (p 0.02): p. 662.
12 Miech RP. The role of fetal microchimerism in autoimmune disease. International Journal of Clinical and Experimental Medicine 2010; 3(2): 162-8; p. 162.

No one to date has questioned the research findings with reference to Pelvic Inflammatory Disease, subfecundity, infertility and autoimmune diseases. Highly contested, by contrast is the question of maternal mortality from abortion. Two US researchers have recently claimed that abortion is safer than childbirth. Unfortunately their paper is based on faulty methodology and incomplete data. It is contradicted by several large-scale, data-linkage studies from Scandinavia, Britain and the US that have documented a significantly higher maternal mortality from induced abortion than from childbirth.

When medical or drug-induced abortion was introduced more than twenty years ago it was hailed as a safe, efficient and discreet alternative to surgical abortion. However, it has since transpired that its failure rate ranges between four and sixteen per cent.[13] Medical abortion also has an alarmingly high rate of adverse side effects, ranging from nausea, to vomiting, severe stomach pain and bleeding, infection, uterine perforation, uterine rupture and death.

What about the impact of abortions on subsequent pregnancies? Two systematic reviews of the evidence have come up with very similar findings. After one induced abortion a woman's risk of giving birth to a preterm child rises by 25 to 27 per cent. After more than one abortion the risk rises by 51 to 62 per cent.[14] More recent studies have placed the risk even higher. Children who are born prematurely have many strikes against them. They die sooner, have a significantly higher rate of disabilities such as cerebral palsy, intellectual impairment, blindness, hearing loss, epilepsy and autism. They also suffer many social challenges, such as not attaining a high level of education, landing a well-paying job, or marrying and having children. In view of these findings it is no exaggeration to say that induced abortion is producing a social disaster of monumental proportions.

When it comes to the psychosocial impact of abortion on women the

---

13   Winikoff B, Sivin I, Coyaji K, et al. Safety, efficacy and acceptability of medical abortion in China, Cuba, and India: A comparative trial of mifepristone-misoprostol versus surgical abortion. AJOG 1996; 176(2): pp. 431-7; Kulier R, Gulmezoglu AM, Hofmeyr GJ, Cheng LN and Campana A. Medical methods for first trimester abortion. Cochrane Database of Systematic Reviews 2004; 1: CD002855.

14   Shah PS and Zao J. Induced termination of pregnancy and low birthweight and preterm birth: a systematic review and meta-analyses. BJOG: An International Journal of Obstetrics & Gynaecology May 2009; 116(11): 1425-42; Swingle HM, Colaizy TT, Zimmerman MB and Morriss FH. Abortion and the risk of subsequent preterm birth. Journal of Reproductive Medicine 2009 February; 54(2): 95-108.

consequences have been more difficult to measure, but perhaps no less momentous. Women who have an induced abortion are statistically more likely never to marry, to marry later, and to divorce or separate, than those who do not have an induced abortion.

Although abortion is said to have alleviated child abuse and neglect by making every child a wanted child, it is now known that child abuse has risen with the legalization of abortion. This may be due to the emotional and/or psychological strain abortion puts on a woman, her difficulty in bonding with a child born after an abortion, or unresolved bereavement or feelings of guilt and regret associated with a past abortion. It is evident too that widely available abortion has discouraged men from taking responsibility for their unintentionally pregnant partners. If the woman refuses to exercise the option to terminate the pregnancy then the child who is carried to term is exclusively her responsibility according to this reasoning. The unexpected consequence has been the increasing feminization of poverty: more and more of the poor are female, because more and more fathers have left mothers to care for their child alone.

Even if the link between abortion and these unfortunate social developments is questioned, it is abundantly clear that legalized abortion has had no discernible *positive* impact on the wellbeing of families.

It is a strange truth that, along with breast cancer, the most highly contested complication of abortion is its psychological impact. Twice the American Psychological Association has declared that there is no solid evidence that abortions do any psychological harm to women. Not only does this statement ignore testimonies to the contrary of countless women, it flies in the face of many scientifically impeccable studies. It is incontrovertible that women who undergo induced abortions have a much higher subsequent rate of suicide than women who complete their pregnancies. Large-scale, record-linkage studies from the US, the UK and Scandinavia have established this beyond the shadow of a doubt. Besides a higher suicide mortality, post-abortion women suffer much higher rates of depression, anxiety and substance abuse. A recent meta-analysis published in the *British Journal of Psychiatry* discovered an overall 81 per cent greater risk of mental health problems for women who had an abortion compared to those who did not. Even more arresting was the discovery that *nearly ten per cent of all mental problems experienced by women are attributable to abortion alone, independent of any other factor.*[15]

---

15 Coleman PK. Abortion and mental health: quantitative synthesis and analysis of research published 1995-2009. British Journal of Psychiatry 2011; 199(3): 180-6; 200(1): 77-80.

We now know of the curious connection between induced abortion and intimate partner violence (IPV). Women who experience intimate partner violence often report that the abuse becomes more frequent and severe after they become pregnant. The threat of violence can be used to force a woman to terminate her pregnancy. IPV also occurs at a much higher rate after abortion than after childbirth. Far from eliminating it, obtaining an induced abortion can actually increase intimate partner violence, besides possibly damaging women in the other ways explored in this book.

Forcing women to terminate their pregnancies is one of the leading themes of the last two chapters of our book. More than 100 women shared the stories of their abortion with us. Two-thirds of them were coerced or pressured into having the abortion. An even higher proportion were kept in the dark as to the real nature of the procedure they were about to undergo. Many were told that it was a minor, harmless operation that would remove "a blob of tissue" or the "products of conception" from their uterus. All of them testified to the devastating impact of abortion in terms of depression, broken partner relationships, and the resort to alcohol and other substances.

All the while that the American Psychological Association professed itself unable to uncover reliable evidence of the negative psychological impact of abortion, American courts were accepting the sworn testimonies of thousands of women as to its devastating impact in their lives. After reviewing this evidence one government task force concluded that

> it is simply unrealistic to expect that a pregnant mother is capable of being involved the termination of the life of her own child without risk of suffering significant psychological trauma and distress.[16]

Affidavits, as sworn statements, are treated with the utmost seriousness within the judicial system. False statements on affidavits are defined as perjury and can lead to severe punishment of the guilty party.

Many women report that the abortion event seemed to compromise their capacity to deal with sexuality and communication within their marriage. They found themselves in a vicious spiral of promiscuity or multiple partners, marriage dissolution, and sexual dysfunction. Relationships with

---

16   Report of the South Dakota Task Force to Study Abortion, submitted to the Governor and Legislature, December 2005 pp. 47-48. http://www.dakotavoice.com/Docs/South%20Dakota%20Abortion%20Task%20Force%20Report.pdf.

existing and subsequent children were negatively affected. They report that depression and alcoholism were frequent afflictions. Most of the women revealed their suffering to no one, not even close family members. Yet every one of them, even if she has found healing and forgiveness, continues to be troubled by her experience and would dissuade others from abortion.

> Although abortion is a grim topic, our book ends, just as it opened, on a note of encouragement. While abortion can be traumatic and feelings of grief can resurface after being buried for many years, some women are still able to experience healing after abortion. Forgiveness is an essential part of the healing process. There are agencies in every major city in North America ready to help women in their search for healing and forgiveness after abortion. We encourage every woman who is haunted by the memory of her abortion, or who believes that it has affected her physical or mental health to seek the help that is freely available. Speak to your doctor, perhaps referring to material from this book. Equally we urge medical professionals and counsellors to provide women considering abortion with accurate information about the medical and psychological risks it carries in its train.

References

Abbreviations
AJOG   American Journal of Obstetrics and Gynecology
BMJ   British Medical Journal
BJOG   British Journal of Obstetrics and Gynaecology
CMAJ   Canadian Medical Association Journal
IFPP   International Family Planning Perspectives
JAMA   Journal of the American Medical Association
JOGC   Journal of Obstetrics and Gynaecology Canada
NEJM   New England Journal of Medicine

1. Abortion Recovery International (ARIN). "About Us: Principles of Care." *Abortion Recovery International: Restoring Lives and Relationships after Abortion.* 2013. http://www.abortionrecovery.org/aboutus/principlesofcare/tabid/247/Default.aspx.
2. Abraham C. "Simple Test, Complex Questions." *Globe and Mail*, Feb 7, 2009. http://www.theglobeandmail.com/news/national/simple-test-complex-questions/article1148236/?page=all.
3. Acharya PS and Gluckman SJ. "Bacteremia Following Placement of Intracervical Laminaria Tents." *Clinical Infectious Diseases* 29, no. 3 (1999): 695-7.
4. Achilles SL and Reeves MF. "Prevention of Infection After Induced Abortion: Release Date October 2010 SFP Guideline 2012." *Contraception* 83, no. 4 (2012): 295-309.
5. Adams KM and Nelson JL. "An Investigative Frontier in Autoimmunity and Transplantation." *JAMA* 291, no. 9 (March 2004): 1127-31.
6. Adhikari N, Ghimire A and Ansari I. "Sex Preference in Urban Nepal." *Journal of the Institute of Medicine (Online)* 30, no. 2 (August 2008): 1-22.
7. Adler NE, David HP, Major BN, Roth S, Russo N and Wyatt G. "Psychological Responses After Abortion." *Science* 248, no. 4951 (6 April, 1990): 41-4.
8. Akerlof GA, Yellen JL and Katz ML. "An Analysis of Out-of-Wedlock Childbearing in the United States." *Quarterly Journal of Economics* 111, no. 2 (1996): 277-317.
9. Alexander GR. "Appendix B: Prematurity at Birth: Determinants, Consequences, and Geographic Variation." In *Preterm Birth: Causes, Consequences and Prevention.* Eds. Behrman RE and Butler AS. Washington, DC: National Academies Press (US), 2007.
10. Alio AP, Salihu HM, Nana PN, et al. "Association between Intimate Partner Violence and Induced Abortion in Cameroon." *International Journal of Gynecology & Obstetrics* 112, no. 2 (February 2011): 83-7.
11. Amaro H, Fried LE, Cabral H and Zuckerman B. "Violence During Pregnancy and Substance Use." *American Journal of Public Health* 80, no. 5 (May 1990): 575-9.

12. American Association of Pro-life Obstetricians & Gynecologists. "AAPLOG Response to the APA Task Force Report." (September 2008). www.aaplog.org/complications-of-induced-abortion/induced-abortion-and-mental-health/aaplog-response-to-the-apa-task-force-report/.

13. American Cancer Society (ACS). *Breast Cancer Facts and Figures 2011-2012.* Atlanta, GA: ACS, Inc., Table 1.

14. American Medical Association (AMA), Council on Ethical and Judicial Affairs. *Code of Medical Ethics: Current Opinions with Annotations.* Chicago: AMA Press, 2007.

15. American Medical Association (AMA). "Patient Physician Relationship Topics: Informed Consent." 2011. http://www.ama-assn.org/ama/pub/physician-resources/legal-topics/patient-physician-relationship-topics/informed-consent.page.

16. American Psychological Association (APA), Task Force on Mental Health and Abortion. *Report of the Task Force on Mental Health and Abortion.* Washington, DC: Author, 2008.http://www.apa.org/pi/wpo/mental-health-abortion-report.pdf.

17. Ananth CV, Smulian JC and Vintzileos AM. "The Association of Placenta Previa with History of Cesarean Delivery and Abortion: A Meta-Analysis." *AJOG* 177, no. 5 (November 1997): 1071-8.

18. Ando T and Davies TF. "Postpartum Autoimmune Thyroid Disease: The Potential Role of Fetal Microchimerism."*Journal of Clinical Endocrinology & Metabolism* 88, no. 7 (2003): 2965-71.

19. Andrieu N, Duffy SW, Rohan TE, et al. "Familial Risk, Abortion and Their Interactive Effect on the Risk of Breast Cancer— A Combined Analysis of Six Case-Control Studies."*British Journal of Cancer* 72, no. 3 (September 1995): 744-51.

20. Antsaklis A and Anastasakis E. "Selective Reduction in Twins and Multiple Pregnancies." *Journal of Perinatal Medicine* 39, no. 1 (January 2011): 15-21.

21. Anum EA, Brown HL and Strauss JF. "Health Disparities In Risk For Cervical Insufficiency." *Human Reproduction* 25, no. 11 (November 2010): 2894-900.

22. Appleby L. "Suicide During Pregnancy and In the First Postnatal Year."*BMJ* 302, no. 6769 (19 January 1991): 137–40.

23. Aronoff D, Hao Y, Chung J, et al."Misoprostol Impairs Reproductive Tract's Innate Response to C. Sordellii." *Journal of Immunology* 180, no. 12 (2008): 8222-30.

24. Ashok P, Templeton A, Wagaarachchi P and Fleet G. "Factors Affecting the Outcome of Early Medical Abortion: A Review of 4132 Consecutive Cases."*BJOG* 109, no. 11 (2002): 1281-89.

25. Attané I. "The Demographic Impact of a Female Deficit in China, 2000-2050." *Population and Development Review* 32, no. 4 (2006): 755-6.

26. Auger N, Daniel M and Moore S. "Sex Ratio Patterns According to Asian Ethnicity in Québec, 1981-2004." *European Journal of Epidemiology* 24, no. 1 (2009): 17-24.

27. AUL Action: The Legislative Action Arm of Americans United for Life. *Investigating the Confirmation Testimony of Elena Kagan before the US Senate Judiciary Committee and the Negative Impact of her Amendment of the 1997 Policy Statement of the American College of Obstetricians and Gynecologists (ACOG) on the Federal Administration of Justice and the U.S. Supreme Court.* Washington, DC: AUL Action, July 15, 2010. http://www.aul.org/featured-images/Kagan-Ethics-Report.pdf.

28.   Autry AM, Hayes EC, Jacobson GF, et al. "A Comparison of Medical Induction and Dilation and Evacuation for Second-Trimester Abortion." *AJOG* 187, no. 2 (2002): 393-7.

29.   Ayuk PT, Dudley S, McShane H, Rees M and Mackenzie IZ. "Efficacy of Follow Up and Contact Tracing of Women Who Test Positive for Genital Tract Chlamydia Trachomatis Prior to Pregnancy Termination." *Journal of Obstetrics and Gynaecology* 24, no. 6 (2004): 687-9.

30.   Barnett W, Freudenberg N and Willie R. "Partnership After Induced Abortion: A Prospective Controlled Study." *Archives of Sexual Behavior* 21, no. 5 (October 1992): 443-55.

31.   Bartz D and Golberg A. "Medication Abortion." *Clinical Obstetrics and Gynecology* 52, no. 2 (2009): 140-50.

32.   *Bautista v All Women's Health Services* (7 Jul. 2003; settled 24 Jan. 2005), Multnomah Co., 0307-07422 (Or Cir Ct).

33.   Beckwith FJ. "Absolute Autonomy and Physician-Assisted Suicide: Putting a Bad Idea Out of its Misery." Joseph Koterski SJ, ed. *Life and Learning VII. Seventh University Faculty for Life Conference*, 1997. Loyola College, Baltimore. Washington, DC: University Faculty for Life, 1998.

34.   Bégin I. "Mortality and Morbidity Coding in Canada and the World – Pitfalls and Shortcomings." Unpublished paper: Ottawa, 1999.

35.   Behrman RS, Butler AS and Alexander GR. *Preterm Birth: Causes, Consequences, and Prevention.* Washington, DC: National Academy Press, 2007.

36.   Beijing Center for Disease Control and Prevention. "China Says Breast Cancer on Rise in Beijing, Shanghai." *Reuters*, 30 October 2007. http://in.reuters.com/article/2007/10/30/us-china-cancer-idINPEK20120020071030.

37.   Benos DJ, Bashari E, Chaves JM, et al. "The Ups and Downs of Peer Review." *Advances in Physiological Education* 31, no. 2 (June 2007): 145-52.

38.   Berer M. "Global Perspectives - National Laws and Unsafe Abortion: The Parameters of Change." *Reproductive Health Matters* 12, Supplement 24 (November 2004): 1-8.

39.   Berg CJ, Atrash HK, Koonin LM and Tucker M. "Pregnancy-related mortality in the United States, 1987-1990." *Obstetrics & Gynecology* 88, no. 2 (August 1996): 161-7.

40.   Berg JW, Appelbaum PS, Lidz CW and Parker LS. *Informed Consent: Legal Theory and Clinical Practice.* Oxford: Oxford University Press, 2001.

41.   Berkowitz RL. "From Twin to Singleton." *BMJ* 313, no. 7054 (17 August, 1996): 373-4.

42.   Berkowitz RL, Lynch L, Stone J and Alvarez M. "The Current Status of Multi-Fetal Pregnancy Reduction." *AJOG* 174, no. 4 (April 1996): 1265-72.

43.   Better Outcomes Registry and Network Ontario. *The Ontario Perinatal Surveillance System Report 2008.* http://www.bornontario.ca/_documents/Publications/Annual%20Report%202008.pdf.

44. Bhattacharya S, Lowit A, Bhattacharya S, et al. "Reproductive Outcomes Following Induced Abortion: A National Register-Based Cohort Study in Scotland."*BMJ Open* 2, no. 3 (6 August 2012): e000911.

45. Bianchi DW, Farina A, Weber W, et al. "Significant Fetal-Maternal Hemorrhage After Termination of Pregnancy: Implications for Development of Fetal Cell Microchimerism."*AJOG* 184, no. 4 (2001): 703-6.

46. Bill C-510: *An Act to Amend the Criminal Code (Coercion)*. 40th Parliament, 3rd Session. (1st Reading, April 14th, 2010). http://www.parl.gc.ca/HousePublications/Publication.aspx?Language=E&Mode=1&DocId=4427296&File=24#1.

47. Bjartling C, Osser S and Persson K. "The Association Between Mycoplasma Genitalium and Pelvic Inflammatory Disease after Termination of Pregnancy."*BJOG: An International Journal of Obstetrics & Gynaecology* 117, no. 3 (2010): 361-4.

48. Black MC and Breiding MJ. "Adverse Health Conditions and Health Risk Behaviors Associated with Intimate Partner Violence—United States, 2005." *Morbidity and Mortality Weekly Report (MMWR)* 57, no. 5 (2008): 113-7.

49. Blackwell AL, Thomas PD, Wareham K and Emery SJ. "Health Gains from Screening for Infection of the Lower Genital Tract in Women Attending for Termination of Pregnancy."*The Lancet* 342, no. 8865 (1993): 206-10.

50. Bland K. "William Hunter Herridge Lecture: Contemporary Management of Pre-Invasive and Early Breast Cancer." *American Journal of Surgery* 201, no. 3 (2011): 278-89.

51. Bland KI and Copeland EM, eds. *The Breast: Comprehensive Management of Benign and Malignant Disorders*. Philadelphia: Saunders, 1991.

52. ———.*The Breast: Comprehensive Management of Benign and Malignant Disorders*, 2nd. 2 vols. Philadelphia: W.B. Saunders, 1998.

53. ———.*The Breast: Comprehensive Management of Benign and Malignant Disorders*, 3rd. 2 vols. St. Louis, MO: Saunders, 2004.

54. ———.*The Breast: Comprehensive Management of Benign and Malignant Disorders*, 4th. 2 vols. Philadelphia: Saunders Elsevier, 2009.

55. Blomain K. "You can't have a baby – a numbness beyond desperation." [Customer Review of An Empty Lap: One Couple's Journey to Parenthood, by Jill Smolowe]. 31 October, 1997. http://www.amazon.com/An-EMPTY-LAP-Couples-Parenthood/product-reviews/0671004360/ref=cm_cr_pr_top_link_2?ie=UTF8&pageNumber=2&showViewpoints=0&sortBy=bySubmissionDateDescending.

56. Blumberg SJ, Bramlett MD, Kogan MD, Schieve LA, Jones JR and Lu MC. "Changes in Prevalence of Parent Reported Autism Spectrum Disorder in School-Aged U.S. Children."*National Health Statistics Reports* 65 (20 March, 2013): 1-11.

57. Boden JM, Fergusson DM and Horwood LJ. "Experience of Sexual Abuse in Childhood and Abortion in Adolescence and Early Adulthood." *Child Abuse & Neglect* 33, no. 12 (December 2009): 870-6.

58. Boecker W, Weigel S, Handel W and Stute P. "The Normal Breast." In *Preneoplasia of the Breast: A New Conceptual Approach to Proliferative Breast Disease*. Ed. Boecker W. Munich: Elsevier, 2006: 2-27.

59. Boeke AJ, van Bergen JE, Morre SA and van Everdingen JJ. "The Risk of Pelvic Inflammatory Disease Associated with Urogenital Infection with Chlamydia Trachomatis." Literature Review. *Nederlands Tijdschrift voor Geneeskunde* 149, no. 15 (2005): 878-84.

60. Boivin J, Andersson L, Skoog-Svanberg A, Hjelmstedt A, Collins A and Bergh T. "Psychological Reactions During In Vitro Fertilization: Similar Response Pattern in Husbands and Wives." *Human Reproduction* 13, no. 11 (November 1998): 3262-7.

61. Bouyer J, Coste J, Shojael T, et al. "Risk Factors for Ectopic Pregnancy: A Comprehensive Analysis Based on a Large Case-Control, Population-Based Study in France." *American Journal of Epidemiology* 157, no. 3 (2003): 185-94.

62. Boy A and Salihu HM. "Intimate Partner Violence and Birth Outcomes: A Systematic Review." *International Journal of Fertility and Women's Medicine* 49, no. 4 (2004): 159-64.

63. Boyon C, Collinet P, Boulanger L, et al."Fetal Microchimerism: Benevolence or Malevolence for the Mother?"*European Journal of Obstetrics & Gynecology and Reproductive Biology* 158, no. 2 (2011): 148-52.

64. Brake E. "Fatherhood and Child Support: Do Men Have a Right to Choose?"*Journal of Applied Philosophy* 22, no. 1 (March 2005): 55-73.

65. Brasic JR. "Screening People with Disturbed Sleep for Depression." *Perception and Motor Skills* 103 (2006): 765-6.

66. Brauner C, Overvad K, Tjonneland A and Attermann J. "Induced Abortion and Breast Cancer Risk Among Parous Women: A Danish Cohort Study." *Acta Obstetricia et Gynecologica Scandinavica* 92, no. 6 (2013): 700-5.

67. Braun T, Brauer M, Fuchs I, et al. "Mirror Syndrome: A Systematic Review of Fetal Associated Conditions, Maternal Presentation and Perinatal Outcome."*Fetal Diagnosis Therapy* 27, no. 4 (2010): 191-203.

68. Bravin J. "Dr. Koop: Keep Kagan off High Court." *Wall Street Journal*, 19 July 2010.

69. Breast Cancer Prevention Institute. "Epidemiological Studies: Induced Abortion and Breast Cancer Risk." Fact Sheet. September 2012. www.bcpinstitute.org.

70. Breeze ACG, Lees CC, Kumar A, Missfelder-Lobos HH and Murdoch EM. "Palliative Care for Prenatally Diagnosed Lethal Fetal Abnormality." *Archives of Disease in Childhood: Fetal and Neonatal* 92, no. 1 (2007): F56-8.

71. Brewer C. "Prevention of Post-Abortion Infection."*The Lancet* 342, no. 8874 (1993): 802.

72. Brewster DH, Stockton DL, Dobbie R, Bull D and Beral V. "Risk of Breast Cancer after Miscarriage or Induced Abortion: A Scottish Record Linkage Case-Control Study." *Journal of Epidemiology and Community Health* 59, no. 4 (2005): 283-7.

73. Brind J, Chinchilli VM, Severs WB and Summy-Long J. "Induced Abortion as An Independent Risk Factor for Breast Cancer: A Comprehensive Review and Meta-Analysis." *Journal of Epidemiology and Community Health* 50, no. 5 (1996): 481-96.

74. ———."Reply to Letter Re: Relation Between Induced Abortion and Breast Cancer." *Journal of Epidemiology and Community Health* 52, no. 3 (1998): 209-11.

75. ———. "Early Reproductive Events and Breast Cancer: A Minority Report."Paper presented at the National Cancer Institute Workshop, "Early Reproductive Events and Breast Cancer." Bethesda, MD: February 24–26, 2003.

76. ———."Induced Abortion as An Independent Risk Factor for Breast Cancer: A Critical Review of Recent Studies Based on Prospective Data." *Journal of American Physicians and Surgeons* 10, no. 4 (2005): 105-10.

77. Britt DW and Evans MI. "Sometimes Doing the Right Thing Sucks: Frame Combinations and Multi-Fetal Pregnancy Reduction Difficulty." *Social Science & Medicine* 65, no. 11 (December 2007): 2342-56.

78. Broen A, Moum T, Bödtker AS and Ekeberg O. "Reasons for Induced Abortion and Their Relation to Women's Emotional Distress: A Prospective, Two-Year Follow-up Study."*General Hospital Psychiatry* 27, no. 1 (January-February 2005): 36-43.

79. Bromage DI. "Prenatal Diagnosis and Selective Abortion: A Result of a Cultural Turn?"*Med Humanities* 32, no. 1 (June 2006): 38-42.

80. Bronson P. "It's Easier to Get an Abortion Than an Aspirin." *Cincinnati Enquirer*, September 27, 2005.

81. Brown HC, Jewkes R, Levin J, Dickson-Tetteh K and Rees H. "Management of Incomplete Abortion in South African Public Hospitals."*BJOG: An International Journal of Obstetrics and Gynaecology* 110, no. 4 (April 2003): 371-7.

82. Browning, EB. "First Book." *Aurora Leigh*. London: J. Miller, 1864. Reprinted: Chicago: Academy Chicago Printers (Cassandra Editions), 1979. 1-36. http://digital.library.upenn.edu/women/barrett/aurora/aurora.html.

83. Brynner R and Stephens T. *Dark Remedy: The Impact of Thalidomide and Its Revival as a Vital Medicine*. Cambridge, MA: Perseus, 2001.

84. Buchmann E, Kunene B and Pattinson R. "Legalized Pregnancy Termination and Septic Abortion Mortality in South Africa." *International Journal of Gynaecology and Obstetrics* 101, no. 2 (May 2008): 191-2.

85. Bu L, Voigt L, Yu Z, Malone K and Daling J. "Risk of Breast Cancer Associated with Induced Abortion in a Population at Low Risk of Breast Cancer." *American Journal of Epidemiology* 141, no. S85 (1995) (abstract 337).

86. Buor D and Bream K. "An Analysis of the Determinants of Maternal Mortality in Sub-Saharan Africa."*Journal of Women's Health* 13, no. 8 (October 2004): 926-38.

87. Burd L, Severud R, Kerbeshian J and Klug MG. "Prenatal and Perinatal Risk Factors for Autism." *Journal of Perinatal Medicine* 27, no. 6(1992): 441-50.

88. Bygdeman M and Swahn ML."Progesterone Receptor Blockage: Effect on Uterine Contractility and Early Pregnancy."*Contraception* 32, no. 1 (1985): 45-51.

89. Calhoun BC, Napolitano P, Terry M, Bussey C and Hoeldtke NJ. "Perinatal Hospice: Comprehensive Care for the Family of the Fetus with a Lethal Condition." *Journal of Reproductive Medicine* 48, no. 11 (May 2003): 343-8.

90. Calhoun BC, Shadigian E and Rooney B. "Cost Consequences of Induced Abortion as an Attributable Risk for Preterm Birth and Impact on Informed Consent."*Journal of Reproductive Medicine* 52, no. 10 (2007): 929-37.

91. Campanario JM and Acedo E. "Rejecting Highly Cited Papers: The Views of Scientists Who Encounter Resistance to Their Discoveries from Other Scientists." *Journal of the American Society for Information Science and Technology* 58, no. 5 (2007): 734-43.

92. Campbell JC. "Health Consequences of Intimate Partner Violence." *The Lancet* 359, no. 9314 (13 April 2002): 1331-6.

93. Campbell O, Gipson R, Issa EH, et al. "National Maternal Mortality Ratio in Egypt Halved Between 1992-93 and 2000."*Bulletin of the World Health Organization* 83, no. 6 (2005): 462-71.

94. Campion B. "An Argument for Continuing a Pregnancy Where the Fetus is Discovered to be Anencephalic." In *Life and Learning IX: Proceedings of Ninth Annual Meeting*. University Faculty for Life in Trinity International University, 1999. Ed. Koterski JW. Washington, DC: University Faculty for Life, 2000.

95. Canadian Association for Community Living. "A Family's Heartbreaking Plight Sheds Light on Deeper Issues." Press Release, 2009.

96. Canadian Institute for Health Information (CIHI). "Quick Stats: Induced Abortions Performed in Canada in 2009."*Canadian Institute for Health Information.* http://www.cihi.ca/cihi-ext-portal/pdf/internet/ta_09_alldatatables20111028_en.

97. Canadian Medical Association. *CMA Code of Ethics (Update 2004)*, 2011. http://policybase.cma.ca/PolicyPDF/PD04-06.pdf.

98. Carroll JC. "Maternal Age-Based Prenatal Screening for Chromosomal Disorders – Attitudes of Women and Health Care Providers Towards Changes." *Canadian Family Physician* 59, no. 1 (2013): e30-47.

99. Carroll P. "The Breast Cancer Epidemic: Modeling and Forecasts Based on Abortion and Other Risk Factors." *Journal of American Physicians and Surgeons* 12, no. 3 (2007): 72-8.

100. *Carter v Benjamin et al.* (Apr. 2000; settled Oct. 2003), Philadelphia, No. 3890 (Pa Ct Com Pl).

101. Caruso S, Di Mari L, Cacciatore A, Mammana G, Agnello C and Cianci A. "Antibiotic Prophylaxis with Prulifloxacin in Women Undergoing Induced Abortion: A Randomized Controlled Trial."Translated from Italian. *Minerva Ginecologica* 60, no. 1 (February 2008): 1-5.

102. Cassidy E. "Multifetal Pregnancy Reduction (MFPR): The Psychology of Desperation and The Ethics of Justification." In *Life and Learning IX: Proceedings of Ninth Annual Meeting, University Faculty for Life in Trinity International University 1999*. Ed. Koterski, JW. Washington, DC: University Faculty for Life, 2000: 331-46.

103. — — — ."Psychological Decision-Making Models: An Extension of Miller's Abortion Decision Models to Miscarriage and Genetic Abortion in Light of the Human Genome Project. [Unpublished Conference Paper]. University Faculty for Life, June 1997.

104. Castadot RG. "Pregnancy Termination: Techniques, Risks, and Complications and Their Management." *Fertility and Sterility* 45, no. 1 (January 1986): 5-17.

105. Centers for Disease Control and Prevention. "Pelvic Inflammatory Disease (PID): CDC Fact Sheet."2011. http://www.cdc.gov/std/pid/stdfact-pid.htm.

106. Central Bureau of Statistics [Kenya], Ministry of Health [Kenya], and ORC Macro. *Demographic and Health Survey 2003*. Calverton, Maryland: Author, 2004.

107. Chamlin MB, Myer AJ, Sanders BA and Cochran JK. "Abortion as Crime Control: A Cautionary Tale." *Criminal Justice Policy Review* 19, no. 2 (2008): 135-52.

108. Charles VE, Polis CB, Sridhara SK and Blum RW. "Abortion and Long-Term Mental Health Outcomes: A Systematic Review of the Evidence."*Contraception* 78, no. 6 (December 2008): 436-50.

109. Charon R. "Narrative Medicine: Attention, Representation, Affiliation." *Narrative* 13, no. 3(October 2005): 261-70.

110. Chatterjee P. "Sex Ratio Imbalance Worsens in Vietnam." *The Lancet* 374, no. 9699 (24 October 2009): 1410.

111. Chen S, Li J and Van den Hoek A. "Universal Screening or Prophylactic Treatment for Chlamydia Trachomatis infection Among Women Seeking Induced Abortions: Which Strategy is More Cost-Effective?" *Sexually Transmitted Diseases* 34, no. 4 (2007): 230-6.

112. Chen SM, van den Hoek A, Shao CG, et al. "Prevalence of and Risk Factors for STIs Among Women Seeking Induced Abortions in Two Urban Family Planning Clinics in Shandong Province, People's Republic of China." *Sexually Transmitted Infections* 78, no. 3 (2002): e1-3.

113. Cherlin AJ. "American Marriage in the Early Twenty-First Century." *Marriage and Child Wellbeing* 15, no. 2 (October 2005): 33-55.

114. Chervenak FA, McCullough LB and Wapner R. "Three Ethically Justified Indications for Selective Termination in Multifetal Pregnancy: A Practical and Comprehensive Management Strategy." *Journal of Assisted Reproduction and Genetics* 12, no. 8 (September 1995): 531-6.

115. Che Y, Zhou W, Gao E and Olsen J. "Induced Abortion and Prematurity in a Subsequent Pregnancy: A Study from Shanghai."*Journal of Obstetrics and Gynaecology* 21, no. 3 (2001): 270-3.

116. Child TJ, Thomas J, Rees M, and MacKenzie IZ. "A Comparative Study of Surgical and Medical Procedures: 932 Pregnancy Terminations up to 63 days Gestation." *Human Reproduction* 16, no. 1 (January 2001): 67-71.

117. Chopra M, Daviaud E, Pattinson R, Fonn S and Lawn JE. "Saving the Lives of South Africa's Mothers, Babies, and Children: Can the Health System Deliver?"*The Lancet* 374, no. 9692 (August 2009): 835-46.

118. Choudhury, S et al. Molecular Profiling of Human Mammary Gland Links Breast Cancer Risk to a $p27^+$ Cell Population with Progenitor Characteristics. Cell Stem Cell 2013 July; 13, 117-130.

119. Chung CS, Smith RG, Steinhoff PG and Mi MP. "Induced Abortion and Ectopic Pregnancy in Subsequent Pregnancies."*American Journal of Epidemiology* 115, no. 6 (1982): 879-87.

120. Cinq-Mars C, Wright J, Cyr M and McDuff P. "Sexual At-Risk Behaviors of Sexually Abused Adolescent Girls." *Journal of Child Sexual Abuse* 12, no. 2 (2003): 1-18.

121. Clavel-Chapelon F and Gerber M. "Reproductive Factors and Breast Cancer Risk: Do They Differ According to Age at Diagnosis?" *Breast Cancer Research and Treatment* 72, no. 2 (March 2002): 107-15.
122. Cobia DC, Robinson K and Edwards L. "Intimate Partner Violence and Women's Sexual Health: Implications for Couples Therapists." *The Family Journal: Counseling and Therapy for Couples and Families* 16, no. 3 (2008): 249-53.
123. Cocchi G, Gualdi S, Bower C, et al. "International Trends of Down Syndrome 1993-2004: Births in Relation to Maternal Age and Terminations of Pregnancies."*Birth Defects Research. Part A, Clinical and Molecular Teratology* 88, no. 6 (June 2010): 474-9.
124. Coggins M and Bullock LFC. "The Wavering Line in the Sand: The Effects of Domestic Violence and Sexual Coercion." *Issues in Mental Health Nursing* 24, no.6/7 (2003): 723-38.
125. Cohen J. "How to Avoid Multiple Pregnancies in Assisted Reproduction." *Human Reproduction* 13, Supplement 3 (June 1998): 197-218.
126. Coleman PK. "Abortion and Mental Health: Quantitative Synthesis and Analysis of Research Published 1995-2009."*British Journal of Psychiatry* 199, no. 3 (2011): 180-6.
127. ———.Author's reply. *British Journal of Psychiatry* 200, no. 1 (2012): 79-80.
128. ———."Induced Abortion and Increased Risk of Substance Abuse: A Review of the Evidence."*Current Women's Health Reviews* 1, no. 1 (2005): 21-34.
129. Coleman PK, Maxey CD, Spence M and Nixon CL. "Predictors and Correlates of Abortion in the Fragile Families and Well-Being Study: Paternal Behavior, Substance Abuse and Partner Violence." *International Journal of Mental Health and Addiction* 7, no. 3 (2009): 405-22.
130. Coleman PK, Reardon DC and Calhoun BC. "Reproductive History Patterns and Long-Term Mortality Rates: A Danish, Population-Based Record Linkage Study."*European Journal of Public Health* 23, no. 4 (August 2013): 569-74.
131. Coleman PK, Rue VM and Coyle CT. "Induced Abortion and Intimate Relationship Quality in the Chicago Health and Social Life Survey." *Public Health* 123, no. 4 (2009): 331-8.
132. Coleman PK, Rue VM, Coyle CT and Maxey CD. "Induced Abortion and Child-Directed Aggression among Mothers of Maltreated Children." *Internet Journal of Pediatrics and Neonatology* 6, no. 2 (2007).
133. Coker AL. "Does Physical Intimate Partner Violence Affect Sexual Health? A Systematic Review." *Trauma, Violence, & Abuse* 8, no. 2 (2007): 149-77.
134. Collaborative Group on Hormonal Factors in Breast Cancer. "Breast Cancer and Abortion: Collaborative Reanalysis of Data from 53 Epidemiological Studies, Including 83,000 Women with Breast Cancer from 16 countries." *The Lancet* 363, no. 9414 (2004): 1007-16.
135. College of Physicians and Surgeons of Ontario. *CPSO Policy Statement: Consent to Medical Treatment*. Policy 4-05, 2006.
136. Collett TS. "Abortion Malpractice: Exploring the Safety of Legal Abortion." In *Life and Learning* V: *Fifth University Faculty for Life Conference*. Ed. Koterski JW. Milwaukee: Marquette University, June 1995: 243-74.

137. Collier R. "Prenatal DNA Test Raises Both Hopes and Worries." *CMAJ* 180, no. 7 (31 March, 2008): 705-8.
138. Collins FS and Mahoney MJ. "Hydrocephalus and Abnormal Digits after Failed First-Trimester Prostaglandin Abortion Attempt."*Journal of Pediatrics* 102, no. 4 (April 1983): 620-1.
139. Council of Europe. "Romania, Table 2: births, deaths, and legal abortions." *Recent Demographic Developments in Europe: Demographic Yearbook 2003* (2004). http://www.coe.int/t/e/social_cohesion/population/RTAB2.xls.
140. Cozzarelli C, Sumer N and Major B. "Mental Models of Attachment and Coping with Abortion." *Journal of Personality and Social Psychology* 74, no. 2 (February 1998): 453-67.
141. Crane JMG, Van den Hof MC, Dodds L, Armson A and Liston R. "Maternal Complications with Placenta Previa." *American Journal of Perinatology* 17, no. 2 (2000): 101-5.
142. Crawford C. "The Genetics Genie."*Abilities Magazine*. 2002-2003. Roeher Institute.
143. Creinin MD. "Randomized Comparison of Efficacy, Acceptability and Cost of Medical versus Surgical Abortion." *Contraception* 62, no. 3 (2000): 117-24.
144. Crowley T, Low N, Turner A, Harvey I, Bidgood K and Horner P. "Antibiotic Prophylaxis to Prevent Post-Abortal Upper Genital Tract Infection in Women with Bacterial Vaginosis: Randomised Controlled Trial."*BJOG* 108, no. 4 (2001): 396-402.
145. Crutcher M. *Lime 5: Exploited by Choice*. Denton, Texas: Life Dynamics, 1996.
146. Cunningham FG, Leveno KJ, Bloom SL, Hauth JC, Rouse DJ and Spong CY, eds. *Williams Obstetrics*. 23rd edition. New York: McGraw-Hill, 2010.
147. Dabash R and Rhoudi-Fahimi F. *Abortion in the Middle East and North Africa*. Washington, DC: Population Reference Bureau, 2008.
148. Dahl E, Beutel M, Brosig B, Grüssner S, Stöbel-Richter Y, Tinneberg HR and Brähler E. "Social Sex Selection and the Balance of the Sexes: Empirical Evidence from Germany, the UK, and the US." *Journal of Assisted Reproduction and Genetics* 23, no. 7-8 (2006): 311-18.
149. Dahl E. "Procreative Liberty: The Case for Preconception Sex Selection." *Reproductive BioMedicine Online* 7, no. 4 (October-November 2003): 380-4.
150. Daif JL, Levie M, Chudnoff S, Kaiser B and Shahabi S. "Group a Streptococcus Causing Necrotizing Fasciitis and Toxic Shock Syndrome After Medical Termination of Pregnancy."*Obstetrics and Gynecology* 113, no. 2 (2009): 504-6.
151. Daling JR, Brinton LA, Voigt LF, et al. "Risk of Breast Cancer Among White Women Following Induced Abortion." *American Journal of Epidemiology* 144, no. 4 (1996): 373-80.
152. Daling JR, Malone KE, Voigt LF, White E, and Weiss NS. "Risk of Breast Cancer Among Young Women: Relationship to Induced Abortions." *Journal of the National Cancer Institute Cancer Spectrum* 86, no. 21 (1994): 1584-92.
153. Dalton VK, Saunders NA, Harris LH, Williams JA and Lebovic DI. "Intrauterine Adhesions after Manual Vacuum Aspiration for Early Pregnancy Failure." *Fertility and Sterility* 85, no. 6 (2006): 1823.e1-e3.

154. Das Gupta M, Chung W and Shuzhuo L. "Evidence for an Incipient Decline in Numbers of Missing Girls in China and India." *Population and Development Review* 35, no. 2 (2009): 401-16.

155. Dayan L. "Pelvic Inflammatory Disease."*Australian Family Physician* 35, no. 11 (2006): 858-62.

156. Dean G, Cardenas L, Darney P and Goldberg A. "Acceptability of Manual versus Electric Aspiration for First Trimester Abortion: A Randomized Trial." *Contraception* 67, no.3 (March 2003): 201-6.

157. Decarli A, La Vecchia C, Negri E and Franceschi S. "Age at Any Birth and Breast Cancer in Italy." *International Journal of Cancer* 67, no. 2 (17 July, 1996): 187-9.

158. De Crespigny L and Savulescu J "Is Paternalism Alive and Well in Obstetric Ultrasound?: Helping Couples Choose Their Children." *Ultrasound in Obstetrics & Gynecology* 20, no. 3 (2002): 213-16.

159. Del Campo C. "Abortion Denied: Outcome of Mothers and Babies." *CMAJ* 130 (15 February, 1984): 361-6.

160. deVeber Institute for Bioethics and Social Research. "Interviews and Surveys of Canadian and American Women Regarding Their Experience of Induced Abortion." Unpublished. Toronto: deVeber Institute, 2011.

161. ———."Survey of Canadian Physicians on Women's Health after Induced Abortion". Unpublished Paper. Toronto: deVeber Institute, 1997.

162. Devries KM, Kishor S, Johnson H, et al. "Intimate Partner Violence During Pregnancy: Analysis of Prevalence Data from 19 Countries." *Reproductive Health Matters* 18, no. 36 (November 2010): 158-70.

163. Dhaliwal LK, Gupta KR and Gopalan S. "Induced Abortion and Subsequent Pregnancy Outcome." *Journal of Family Welfare* 49, no. 1 (June 2003): 50-5.

164. Diedrich J and Steinauer J. "Complications of Surgical Abortion." *Clinical Obstetrics and Gynecology* 52, no. 2 (2009): 205-12.

165. Disability Rights Education and Defense Fund, Generations Ahead, National Women's Health Network, Reproductive Health Technologies Project and World Institute on Disability. "The Prenatally and Postnatally Diagnosed Conditions Awareness Act." Fact Sheet. October 16, 2008. http://dredf.org/InfoSheetBrownbackKennedy.pdf.

166. Dixon DP. "Informed Consent or Institutionalized Eugenics? How the Medical Profession Encourages Abortion of Fetuses with Down Syndrome." *Issues in Law & Medicine* 24, no. 1 (2008): 3-59.

167. Dolle JM, Daling JR, White E, et al. "Risk Factors for Triple-Negative Breast Cancer in Women Under the Age of 45 Years." *Cancer Epidemiology, Biomarkers and Prevention* 18, no. 4 (2009): 1157-66.

168. Donohue III JJ and Levitt SD. "The Impact of Legalized Abortion on Crime." *Quarterly Journal of Economics* 116, no. 2(2001): 379-420.

169. ———."Measurement Error, Legalized Abortion, and the Decline in Crime: A Response to Foote and Goetz." *Quarterly Journal of Economics* 123, no. 1 (2008): 425-440.

170. Dubner SJ. "The Probability That a Real-Estate Agent is Cheating You (And Other Riddles of Modern Life): Inside the Curious Mind of the Heralded Young Economist Steven Levitt." *New York Times Magazine,* August 3, 2003. In *Freakonomics: A Rogue Economist Explores the Hidden Side of Everything.* New York: William Morrow, 2006.

171. Duchan E and Patel DR. "Epidemiology of Autism Spectrum Disorders." *Pediatric Clinics of North America* 59, no. 1(February 2012): 27-43.

172. Dunn S, Wise MR, Johnson LM, et al. "Chapter 10: Reproductive and Gynaecological Health." In Bierman AS, ed. *Project for an Ontario Women's Health Evidence-Based Report (POWER),* Volume 2. POWER: Toronto, 2011. http://powerstudy.ca/wp-content/uploads/downloads/2012/10/Chapter10-ReproductiveandGynaecologicalHealth.pdf.

173. Dytrych Z, Matejcek Z, Schüller V, David HP and Friedman HL. "Children Born to Women Denied Abortion." *Family Planning Perspectives* 7, no. 4 (July-August 1975): 165-71.

174. Eaton WW, Mortensen PB, Thomsen PH and Frydenberg M. "Obstetric Complications and Risk for Severe Psychopathology in Childhood." *Journal of Autism and Developmental Disorders* 31, no. 3 (2001): 279-85.

175. Ebenstein A and Leung S. "Son Preference and Access to Social Insurance: Evidence from China's Rural Pension Program." *Population and Development Review* 36, no. 1 (March 2010): 47-70.

176. Elam-Evans LD, Strauss LT, Herndon J, et al. "Abortion Surveillance: United States, 2000." *MMWR Surveillance Summaries* 55, no. SS12 (28 November, 2003). *Centres for Disease Control and Prevention:* www.cdc.gov/mmwr/preview/mmwrhtml/ss5212al.htm.

177. Elliott JP. "Multifetal Reduction of Triplets to Twins Improves Perinatal Outcome." *AJOG* 171, no. 1 (July 1994): 278.

178. Ely GE and Otis MD. "An Examination of Intimate Partner Violence and Psychological Stressors in Adult Abortion Patients." *Journal of Interpersonal Violence* 26, no. 16 (November 2011): 3248-66.

179. Erdmans MP and Black T. "What They Tell You to Forget: From Childhood Sexual Abuse to Adolescent Motherhood." *Qualitative Health Research* 18, no. 1 (2008): 77-89.

180. Erlandsson G, Montgomery SM, Cnattingius S and Ekbom A. "Abortions and Breast Cancer: Record Based Case-Control Study." *International Journal of Cancer* 103, no. 5 (2003): 676-9.

181. Evans MI and Britt DW. "Fetal Reduction." *Seminars in Perinatology* 29, no. 5 (October 2005): 321-9.

182. Evans MI, Goldberg JD, Horenstein J, et al. "Selective Termination for Structural, Chromosomal, and Mendelian Anomalies: International Experience." *AJOG* 181, no. 4 (October 1999): 893-7.

183. Evans MI, Quintero RA and Fletcher JC. "Ethical Issues Surrounding Multifetal Pregnancy Reduction and Selective Termination." *Clinical Perinatology* 23, no. 3 (September 1996): 437-51.

184. Faden RR and Beauchamp TL. *A History and Theory of Informed Consent.* Oxford: Oxford University Press, 1986.
185. Fairweather D. "Autoimmune Disease: Mechanisms."*Encyclopedia of Life Sciences.* Chicester, UK: John Wiley & Sons, Ltd., 2007: 1-7. www.els.net.
186. Faiz AS and Ananth CV. "Etiology and Risk Factors for Placenta Previa: An Overview and Meta-Analysis of Observational Studies." *Journal of Maternal–Fetal & Neonatal Medicine* 13, no. 3 (March 2003): 175-90.
187. Fanslow J, Silva M, Whitehead A and Robinson E. "Pregnancy Outcomes and Intimate Partner Violence in New Zealand." *Australian and New Zealand Journal of Obstetrics and Gynaecology* 48, no. 4 (August 2008): 391-7.
188. Fawcus SR, van Coeverden de Groot HA and Isaacs S. "A 50-Year Audit of Maternal Mortality in the Peninsula Maternal and Neonatal Service, Cape Town (1953-2002)."*BJOG: An International Journal of Obstetrics & Gynaecology* 112, no. 9 (September 2005): 1257-63.
189. Ferlay J, Héry C, Autier P and Sankaranarayanan R. "Chapter 1: Global Burden of Breast Cancer." In *Breast Cancer Epidemiology.* Ed. Li CI. New York: Springer, 2010: 1-19.
190. Fergusson DM, Horwood LJ and Boden JM. "Abortion and Mental Health Disorders: Evidence from a 30-Year Longitudinal Study." *British Journal of Psychiatry* 193 (2008): 444–51.
191. — — — .Letter to the *British Journal of Psychiatry Online,* 5 October 2011.
192. Ferguson JE, Burkett BJ, Pinkerton JV, et al."Intra-amniotic 15(s)-15-Methyl Prostaglandin F2 Alpha and Termination of Middle and Late Second-Trimester Pregnancy for Genetic Indications: A Contemporary Approach."*AJOG* 169, no. 2:1 (1993): 332-40.
193. Fernandez H, Fadheela A, Chauveaud-Lambling A, Frydman R and Gervaise A. "Fertility After Treatment of Asherman's Syndrome Stage 3 and 4." *Journal of Minimally Invasive Gynecology* 13, no. 5 (2006): 398-402.
194. Fernandez H and Gervaise A. "Ectopic Pregnancies After Infertility Treatment: Modern Diagnosis and Therapeutic Strategy."*Human Reproduction Update* 10, no. 6 (2004): 503-13.
195. Ferris LE, McMain-Klein M, Colodny N, Fellows GF and Lamont J. "Factors Associated with Immediate Abortion Complications." *CMAJ* 154, no. 11 (June 1996): 1677-85.
196. Fischer M, Bhatnagar J, Guarner J, et al. "Fatal Toxic Shock Syndrome Associated with Clostridium Sordellii after Medical Abortion." *NEJM* 353, no. 22 (1 December, 2005): 2352-60.
197. Fjerstad M, Trussell J, Sivin I, Lichtenberg ES and Cullins V. "Rates of Serious Infection after Changes in Regimens for Medical Abortion."*NEJM* 361, no. 2 (2009): 145-51.
198. Flett GMM and Templeton A. "Surgical Abortion: Best Practice & Research."*Clinical Obstetrics and Gynaecology* 16, no. 2 (2002): 247-61.
199. Foote CL and Goetz CF. "The Impact of Legalized Abortion on Crime: Comment." *Quarterly Journal of Economics* 123, no. 1 (2008): 407-23.

200. Forssman H and Thuwe I. "Continued Follow-Up Study of 120 Persons Born After Refusal of Application for Therapeutic Abortion." *Acta Psychiatrica Scandinavica* 64, no. 2 (1981): 142-9.

201. Frejka T, Jones GW and Sardon JP. "East Asian Childbearing Patterns and Policy Developments." *Population and Development Review* 36, no. 3 (2010): 579-606.

202. Galloway G. "Was Maurice Vellacott Right About Abortion?" *Globe and Mail*, 8 January 2010.

203. Garcia-Moreno C, Jansen HAFM, Ellsberg M, Heise L and Watts C. *WHO Multi-country Study on Women's Health and Domestic Violence Against Women: Initial Results on Prevalence, Health Outcomes and Women's Responses.* Geneva: World Health Organization, 2005.

204. Garel M, Stark C, Blondel B, Lefebvre G, Vauthier-Brouzes D and Zorn JR. "Psychological Reactions after Multifetal Pregnancy Reduction: A 2-Year Follow-Up Study." *Human Reproduction* 12, no. 3 (March 1997): 617-22.

205. Garg S and Nath A. "Female Feticide in India: Issues and Concerns." *Journal of Postgraduate Medicine* 54, no. 4 (2008): 276-9.

206. Garner BA and Black HC, eds. "Duress". *Black's Law Dictionary.* 9th edition. Saint Paul: West Group, 2009.

207. Gary MM and Harrison D. "Analysis of Severe Adverse Events Related to the Use of Mifepristone as an Abortifacient."*Annals of Pharmacotherapy* 40, no. 2 (February 2006): 191-7.

208. Gebrehiwot Y and Liabsuetrakul T. "Trends of Abortion Complications in a Transition of Abortion Law Revisions in Ethiopia."*Journal of Public Health* 31, no. 1 (March 2009): 81-7.

209. Gemzell-Danielsson K, and Lalitkumar S. "Second Trimester Medical Abortion with Mifepristone – Misoprostol and Misoprostol Alone: A Review of Methods and Management."*Reproductive Health Matters* 16, no. 31 (2008): 162-72.

210. Gentles I. "Good News for the Fetus: Two Fallacies in the Abortion Debate." *Policy Review* 40 (Spring 1987): 50-4.

211. George SM. "Millions of Missing Girls: From Fetal Sexing to High Technology Sex Selection in India." *Prenatal Diagnosis* 26, no. 7 (July 2006): 604-9.

212. Germain M, Krohn MA and Daling JR. "Reproductive History and The Risk of Neonatal Sepsis."*Pediatric and Perinatal Epidemiology* 9, no. 1 (1995): 48-58.

213. Gersho-Cohen J, Berger SM and Klickstein HS. "Roentgenography of Breast Cancer Moderating Concept of 'Biologic Predeterminism.'" *Cancer* 16, no. 8 (August 1963): 961-4.

214. Gilbert KR. "Taking a Narrative Approach to Grief Research: Finding Meaning in Stories."*Death Studies* 26, no. 3 (2002): 223-39.

215. Gilchrist AC, Hannaford PC, Frank P and Kay CR. "Termination of Pregnancy and Psychiatric Morbidity. *British Journal of Psychiatry* 167, no. 2 (August 1995): 243-8.

216. Gissler M, Berg C, Bouvier-Colle MH and Buekens P. "Methods for Identifying Pregnancy-Associated Deaths: Population-Based Data from Finland, 1987-2000."*Paediatric and Perinatal Epidemiology* 18, no. 6 (2004): 448-55.

217. Gissler M, Berg C, and Bouvier-Colle M. "Injury Deaths, Suicides, and Homicides Associated with Pregnancy, Finland 1987-2000." *European Journal of Public Health* 15, no. 5 (2004): 459-63.
218. Gissler M, Hemminki E and Lonnqvist J. "Suicides After Pregnancy in Finland, 1987-94: Register Linkage Study."*BMJ* 313, no. 7070 (December 1996): 1431-4.
219. Gissler M, Kauppila R, Merilainen J, Toukomaa H and Hemminki E. "Pregnancy-Associated Deaths in Finland 1987-1994—Definition Problems and Benefits of Record Linkage." *Acta Obstetricia et Gynecologica Scandinavica* 76, no. 7 (August 1997): 651-7.
220. Gleicher N, Campbell DP, Chan CL, et al. "The Desire for Multiple Births in Couples with Infertility Problems Contradicts Present Practice Patterns." *Human Reproduction* 10, no. 5 (May 1995): 1079-84.
221. Gnoth C, Maxrath B, Skonieczny T, Friol K, Godehardt E and Tigges J. "Final ART Success Rates: A 10 Years Survey." *Human Reproduction* 26, no. 8 (2011): 2239-46.
222. Goldacre MJ, Kurina LM, Seagroatt V and Yeates D. "Abortion and Breast Cancer: A Case Control Record Linkage Study." *Journal Epidemiology and Community Health* 55, no. 5 (2001): 336-7.
223. Gonzalez CH, Marques-Dias MJ, Kim CA, et al. "Congenital Abnormalities in Brazilian Children Associated with Misoprostol Misuse in First Trimester of Pregnancy."*The Lancet* 351, no. 9116 (30 May, 1998): 1624-7.
224. Gonzalez CH, Vargas FR, Perez AB, et al. "Limb Deficiency with or without Mobius Sequence in Seven Brazilian Children Associated with Misoprostol Use in the First Trimester of Pregnancy."*American Journal of Medical Genetics* 47, no. 1 (1993): 59-64.
225. Gonzalez R, Requejo JH, Nien JK, Merialdi M, Bustreo F and Betran AP. "Tackling Health Inequities in Chile: Maternal, Newborn, Infant, and Child Mortality Between 1990 and 2004." *American Journal of Public Health* 99, no. 7 (July 2009): 1220-6.
226. *Gonzales v. Carhart et al.* 127 S. Ct. 1610 (2007).
227. *Gonzales v Planned Parenthood Federation of America, Inc.*, 550 U.S. 124 (2007).
228. Gorrette N, Nabukera S and Salihu HM. "The Abortion Paradox in Uganda: Fertility Regulator or Cause of Maternal Mortality."*Journal of Obstetrics and Gynaecology* 25, no. 8 (November 2005): 776-80.
229. Government of Uganda. *UNGASS Country Progress Report Uganda: January 2008-December 2009*. UNAIDS: March 2010.http://data.unaids.org/pub/Report/2010/uganda_2010_country_progress_report_en.pdf.
230. Green JM, Hewison J, Bekker HL, Bryant LD and Cuckle HS. "Psychosocial Aspects of Genetic Screening of Pregnant Women and Newborns: A Systematic Review." *Health Technology Assessment* 8, no. 33. Southampton, UK: National Coordinating Centre for Health Technology Assessment, August 2004: iii, ix-x, 1-109.
231. Green JM. "Obstetricians' Views on Prenatal Diagnosis and Termination of Pregnancy: 1980 Compared with 1993."*BJOG* 102, no. 3 (1995): 228-32.
232. Grimes D. "Medical Abortion in Early Pregnancy: A Review of the Evidence."*Obstetrics & Gynecology* 89, no. 5, part 1 (May 1997): 790-6.

233. Grossman D, Blachard K and Blumenthal P. "Complications After Second Trimester Surgical and Medical Abortion." *Reproductive Health Matters* 16, no. 31 (2008): 173-82.

234. Groutz A, Yovel I, Amit A, Yaron Y, Azem F and Lessing JB. "Pregnancy Outcome after Multifetal Pregnancy Reduction to Twins Compared with Spontaneously Conceived Twins." *Human Reproduction* 11, no. 6 (June 1996): 1134-6.

235. Haldre K, Rahu K, Karro H and Rahu M. "Previous History of Surgically Induced Abortion and Complications of the Third Stage of Labour in Subsequent Normal Vaginal Deliveries." *Journal of Maternal-Fetal and Neonatal Medicine* 21, no. 12 (December 2008): 884-8.

236. Hall JG. "Arthrogryposis Associated with Unsuccessful Attempts at Termination of Pregnancy." *American Journal of Medical Genetics* 63, no. 1 (3 May, 1996): 293-300.

237. Hamama L, Rauch SA, Sperlich M, Defever E and Seng JS. "Previous Experience of Spontaneous or Elective Abortion and Risk for Posttraumatic Stress and Depression During Subsequent Pregnancy." *Depression and Anxiety* 27, no. 8 (August 2010): 699-707.

238. Hamelin C, Saloman C, Sitta R, Gueguen A, Cyr D and Lert F. "Childhood Sexual Abuse and Adult Sexual Health Among Indigenous Kanak Women and Non-Kanak Women of New Caledonia." *Child Abuse & Neglect* 34, no. 9 (September 2010): 677-88.

239. Hammond C. "Recent Advances in Second-Trimester Abortion: An Evidence-Based Review." *AJOG* 200, no. 4 (2009): 347-56.

240. Hamoda H, Flett GMM, Ashok PW and Templeton A. "Surgical Abortion Using Manual Vacuum Aspiration Under Local Anaesthesia: A Pilot Study of Feasibility and Women's Acceptability." *Journal of Family Planning and Reproductive Health Care* 31, no. 3 (July 2005): 185-8.

241. Hanstede MF, van Hof DB, van Groningen K and de Graaf IM. "Severe Complication after Termination of a Second Trimester Cervical Pregnancy." *Fertility and Sterility* 90, no. 5 (November 2008): e5-7.

242. Hardy G, Benjamin A and Abenhaim HA. "Effect of Induced Abortions on Early Preterm Births and Adverse Perinatal Outcomes." *JOGC* 35, no. 2 (February 2013): 138-43.

243. Harris J, Lippman ME, Morrow M and Osborne CK. *Diseases of the Breast*. 2nd ed. Baltimore, MD: Lippincott, Williams & Wilkins, 2000.

244. Hartge P. "Abortion, Breast Cancer, and Epidemiology." Editorial. *NEJM* 336, no. 2 (1997): 127-8.

245. Hassan MAM and Killick SR. "Is Previous Aberrant Reproductive Outcome Predictive of Subsequently Reduced Fecundity?" *Human Reproduction* 20, no. 3 (2005): 657-64.

246. Hathaway JE, Willis G, Zimmer B and Silverman JG. "Impact of Partner Abuse on Women's Reproductive Lives." *Journal of the American Medical Women's Association* 60, no. 1 (Winter 2005): 42-5.

247. Hatten KW. "Former Abortion Clinic Worker Breaks Silence, Speaks Out for Life." *LifeSiteNews*, 21 July 2011. http://www.lifesitenews.com/news/former-abortion-clinic-worker-speaks-out-for-life.

248. Hausknecht R. "Mifepristone and Misoprostol for Early Medical Abortion: 18 Months Experience in the United States."*Contraception* 67, no. 6 (June 2003): 463-5.

249. Hay C and Evans MM. "Has Roe v. Wade Reduced U.S. Crime Rates? Examining the Link Between Mothers' Pregnancy Intentions and Children's Later Involvement in Law-Violating Behaviour." *Journal of Research in Crime and Delinquency* 43, no. 1 (2006): 36-66.

250. Hayes JL and Fox MC. "Cervical Dilation in Second-Trimester Abortion."*Clinical Obstetrics and Gynecology* 52, no. 2 (2009): 171-8.

251. Health Grades Inc. "Prevalence and Incidence of Autoimmune Diseases."*Right Diagnosis*. (2013). http://www.rightdiagnosis.com/a/ai/prevalence.htm.

252. Heaman M, Kingston D, Chalmers B, Sauve R, Lee L and Young D. "Risk Factors for Preterm Birth and Small-for-Gestational Age Births Among Canadian Women."*Paediatric and Perinatal Epidemiology* 27, no. 1 (2013): 54-61.

253. Heisterberg L and Kringelbach M. "Early Complications after Induced First-Trimester Abortion." *Acta Obstetricia et Gynecologica Scandanavica* 66, no. 3 (1987): 201-4.

254. Hemminki E, Klemetti R, Sevon T and Gissler M. "Induced Abortions Previous to IVF: An Epidemiologic Register-Based Study from Finland." *Human Reproduction* 23, no. 6 (June 2008): 1320-3.

255. Henderson KD, Sullivan-Halley J, Reynolds P, et al. "Incomplete Pregnancy is Not Associated with Breast Cancer Risk: The California Teachers Study." *Contraception* 77, no. 6 (2008): 391-6.

256. Henshaw RC, Naji SA, Russell IT and Templeton AA. "A Comparison of Medical Abortion (Using Mifepristone and Gemeprost) with Surgical Vacuum Aspiration: Efficacy and Early Medical Sequelae."*Human Reproduction* 9, no. 11 (1994): 2167–72.

257. Henshaw SK and Van Vort J. "Abortion Services in the United States, 1991 and 1992." *Family Planning Perspectives* 26, no. 3 (May-June 1994): 100-6, 112.

258. Hern WM. "Selective Termination for Fetal Anomaly/Genetic Disorder in Twin Pregnancy at 32+ Menstrual Weeks." *Fetal Diagnostic Therapy* 19 (2004): 292-5.

259. Hesketh T, Li L and Zhu WX. "The Consequences of Son Preference and Sex-Selective Abortion in China and Other Asian Countries." *CMAJ* 183, no. 12 (6 September, 2011): 1374-7.

260. Hess RF. "Healing After Abortion: A Search for Forgiveness." *Journal of Christian Nursing* 26, no. 3 (September 2009): 154-8.

261. Hillis SD, Joesoef R, Marchbanks PA, et al. "Delayed Care of Pelvic Inflammatory Disease as a Risk Factor for Impaired Fertility."*AJOG* 168, no. 5 (1993): 1503-9.

262. Himpens E, van den Broeck C, Oostra A, Calders P and Vanhaesebrouck P. "Prevalence, Type, Distribution and Severity of Cerebral Palsy in Relation to Gestational Age: A Meta-Analytic Review."*Developmental Medicine and Child Neurology* 50, no. 5 (March 2008): 334-40.

263. Hirek M. "Népesedéspolitikánknéhánykérdése." *A KülönbUtódokért* 26, no. 10 (1973).

264. Hoeldtke NJ and Calhoun BC. "Perinatal Hospice." *AJOG*185, no. 3 (September 2001): 525-9.

265. Hogan MC, Foreman KJ, Naghavi M, et al. "Maternal Mortality for 181 countries 1980-2008: A Systematic Analysis of Progress toward Millennium Development Goal 5." *The Lancet* 375, no. 9726 (April 2010): 1609-23.

266. Hogan MC, Lopez AD, Lozano R, et al. *Building Momentum: Global Progress Toward Reducing Maternal and Child Mortality.* Seattle: Institute for Health Metrics and Evaluation, 2010.

267. Holmes LB. "Possible Fetal Effects of Cervical Dilation and Uterine Curettage During the First Trimester of Pregnancy."*Journal of Pediatrics* 126, no. 1 (January 1995): 131-4.

268. Holmes OW. "Address to Annual Meeting, Massachusetts Medical Society, 30 May 1860." In *Currents and Counter-Currents in Medical with Other Addresses and Essays.* Boston, Mass: Ticknor and Fields, 1861.

269. Holt VL, Daling JR, Voigt LF, et al. "Induced Abortion and the Risk of Subsequent Ectopic Pregnancy."*American Journal of Public Health* 79, no. 9 (1989): 1234-8.

270. Horon IL and Cheng D. "Enhanced Surveillance for Pregnancy-Associated Mortality: Maryland, 1993-1998." *JAMA* 285, no. 11 (21 March, 2001): 1455-9.

271. Horon IL. "Underreporting of Maternal Deaths on Death Certificates and the Magnitude of the Problem of Maternal Mortality."*American Journal of Public Health* 95, no. 3 (March 2005): 478-82.

272. "Hospital Pays $8.7m Settlement: Premature Baby was Abandoned with Dead Foetuses."*The National Post*, 31 July 1999: p. A1.

273. Howe HL, Senie RT, Bzduch H and Herzfeld P. "Early abortion and Breast Cancer Risk Among Women Under Age 40." *International Journal of Epidemiology* 18, no. 2 (1989): 300-4.

274. Hsieh CC, Wuu J, Lambe M, Trichopoulous D, Adami HO and Ekbom A. "Delivery of Premature Newborns and Maternal Breast Cancer Risk." *The Lancet* 353, no. 9160 (10 April, 1999): 1239.

275. Human Genome Management Information. "About the Human Genome Project." 2011. http://www.ornl.gov/sci/techresources/Human_Genome/project/about.shtml.

276. *Humes v Clinton* 792 P. (2d) 1032 (Kan. 1990).

277. Hung TH, Hsieh CC, Hsu JJ, Chiu TH, Lo LM and Hsieh TT. "Risk Factors for Placenta Previa in an Asian Population." *International Journal of Gynecology and Obstetrics* 97, no. 1 (April 2007): 26-30.

278. Hvistendahl M. *Unnatural Selection: Choosing Boys Over Girls, and the Consequences of a World Full of Men.* New York: Public Affairs, 2011.

279. ———. "The Women Shortage: How Sex Selection of Babies has Led to a Huge Surplus of Men and Why That's Bad for All of Us." Interview by Brian Bethune. *Macleans* (14 June 2011).http://www2.macleans.ca/2011/06/14/how-sex-selection-of-babies-has-led-to-a-huge-surplus-of-men-and-why-that's-bad-for-all-of-us/.

280. Indiana General Assembly. "Chapter 2: Requirements for Performance of Abortion; Criminal Penalties." *Indiana Code*. Title 16. Article 34.http://www.in.gov/legislative/ic/code/title16/ar34/.

281. Infante-Rivard C and Gauthier R. "Induced Abortion as a Risk Factor for Subsequent Fetal Loss." *Epidemiology* 7, no. 5 (September 1996): 540-2.

282. Institute of Medicine. "Preterm Birth: Causes, Consequences and Prevention." 13 July, 2006. www.iom.edu/Reports/2006/Preterm-Birth-Causes-Consequences-and-Prevention.aspx.

283. Institute Mensch, Ethik & Wissenschaft (IMEW). http://www.imew.de/index.php?id=513.

284. International Federation of Gynecology and Obstetrics (FIGO). "Resolution on 'Sex-Selection for Non-Medical Purposes'." London: March 2005. http://www.figo.org/projects/sex_selection.

285. Jabeen S, Haque M, Islam JU, Hossain MZ, Begum A and Kashem MA. "Breast Cancer and Some Epidemiological Risk Factors: A Hospital Based Study." *Journal of Dhaka Medical College* 22, no. 1 (2013): 61-6.

286. Jackson-Lee S. "Partial Birth Abortion Ban Act of 1997." *Congressional Record* 1997: H8654. http://www.c-spanarchives.org/congress/?q=node/77531&id=6761323.

287. Jacob S, Bloebaum L, Shah G and Varner MW. "Maternal Mortality in Utah." *Obstetrics & Gynecology* 91, no. 2 (February 1998): 187-91.

288. Jacobsson B, Hagberg G, Hagberg B, Ladfors L, Niklasson A and Hagberg H. "Cerebral Palsy in Preterm Infants: A Population-Based Case-Control Study of Antenatal and Intrapartal Risk Factors." *Acta Paediatrica* 91, vol. 8 (2002): 946-51.

289. Jacot FR, Poulin C, Bilodeau AP, et al. "A Five-Year Experience With Second-Trimester Induced Abortions: No Increase In Complication Rate As Compared to The First Trimester." *AJOG* 168, no. 2 (February 1993): 633-7.

290. Jain JK, Dutton C, Harwood B, et al. "A Prospective Randomized, Double-Blinded, Placebo-Controlled Trial Comparing Mifepristone and Vaginal Misoprostol to Vaginal Misoprostol Alone for Elective Termination of Early Pregnancy." *Human Reproduction* 17, no. 6 (2002): 1477-82.

291. Jain JK, Mechstroth KR, Park M, et al. "A Comparison of Tamoxifen and Misoprostol to Misoprostol Alone for Early Pregnancy Termination." *Contraception* 60, no. 6 (1999): 353-6.

292. Janssen PA, Holt VL, Sugg NK, Emanuel I, Critchlow CM and Henderson AD. "Intimate Partner Violence and Adverse Pregnancy Outcomes: A Population-Based Study." *AJOG* 188, no. 5 (2003): 1341-7.

293. Jasnosz KM, Shakir AM and Perper JA. "Fatal Clostridium Perfringens and Escherichia Coli Sepsis Following Urea-Instillation Abortion." *American Journal of Forensic Medicine and Pathology* 14, no. 2 (1993): 151-4.

294. Jefferson T, Alderson P, Wager E and Davidoff F. "Effects of Editorial Peer Review: A Systematic Review." *JAMA* 287, no. 21 (5 June, 2002): 2784-6.

295. Jejeebhoy SJ. "Associations between Wife-Beating and Fetal and Infant Death: Impressions from a Survey in Rural India." *Studies in Family Planning* 29, no. 3 (September 1998): 300-8.

296. Jensen JT, Astley SJ, Morgan E and Nichols MD. "Outcomes of Suction Curettage and Mifepristone Abortion in the United States." *Contraception* 59, no. 3 (1999): 153-9.

297. Jewkes RK, Fawcus S, Rees H, Lombard CJ and Katzenellenbogen J. "Methodological Issues in the South African Incomplete Abortion Study." *Studies in Family Planning* 28, no. 3 (September 1997): 228-34.

298. Jewkes RK, Gumede T, Westaway MS, Dickson K, Brown H and Rees H. "Why are Women Still Aborting Outside Designated Facilities in Metropolitan South Africa?" *BJOG: An International Journal of Obstetrics & Gynaecology* 112, no. 9 (September 2005): 1236-42.

299. Jewkes RK, Rees H, Dickson K, Brown H and Levin J. "The Impact of Age on the Epidemiology of Incomplete Abortions in South Africa after Legislative Change." *BJOG: An International Journal of Obstetrics & Gynaecology* 112, no. 3 (March 2005): 355-9.

300. Jewkes RK and Rees H. "Dramatic Decline in Abortion Mortality Due to the Choice on Termination of Pregnancy Act." *South African Medical Journal* 95, no. 4 (April 2005): 250.

301. Jha P, Kesler MA, Kumar R, et al. "Trends in Selective Abortions of Girls in India: Analysis of Nationally Representative Birth Histories from 1990 to 2005 and Census Data from 1991 to 2011." *The Lancet* 377, no. 9781 (4 June, 2011): 1921-8.

302. Jiang AR, Gao CM, Ding JH, Li SP, Liu YT, Cao HX, Wu JZ, Qian Y and Tajima K. "Abortions and Breast Cancer Risk in Premenopausal and Postmenopausal Women in Jiangsu Province of China." *Asian Pacific Journal of Cancer Prevention* 13 (2012): 33-5.

303. Johnson KL and Bianchi DW. "Fetal Cells in Maternal Tissue Following Pregnancy: What are the Consequences?" *Human Reproduction Update* 10, no. 6 (2004): 497-502.

304. Johnson LG, Mueller BA and Daling JR. "The Relationship of Placenta Previa and History of Induced Abortion." *International Journal of Gynecology and Obstetrics* 81, no. 2 (May 2003): 191-8.

305. Johnston HB, Gallo MF and Benson J. "Reducing the Costs to Health Systems of Unsafe Abortions: A Comparison of Four Strategies." *Journal of Family Planning and Reproductive Health Care* 33, no. 4 (2007): 250-7.

306. Jones RK and Henshaw K. "Mifepristone for Early Medical Abortion: Experiences in France, Great Britain, and Sweden." *Perspectives on Sexual and Reproductive Health* 34, no. 3 (2002): 154-60.

307. Jones RK, Kost K, Singh S, Henshaw SK and Finer LB. "Trends in Abortion in the United States." *Clinical Obstetrics and Gynecology* 52, no. 2 (2009): 119-29.

308. Jones RK, Moore AM and Frohwirth L. "Perceptions of Male Knowledge and Support Among U.S. Women Obtaining Abortions." *Women's Health Issues* 21, no. 2 (2011): 117-23.

309. Joseph KS, Kinniburgh B, Hutcheon JA, Mehrabadi A, Basso M, Davies C and Lee L. "Determinants of Increases in Stillbirth Rates from 2000 to 2010." *CMAJ* 185, no. 8 (14 May, 2013): E345-51.

310. Joyce T. "Did Legalized Abortion Lower Crime?" *Journal of Human Resources* 39, no. 1 (2004): 1-28.
311. Kaali SG, Szigetvari IA and Bartfai GS. "The Frequency and Management of Uterine Perforations During First-Trimester Abortions." *AJOG* 161, no. 2 (August 1989): 406-8.
312. Kahane LH, Paton D and Simmons R. "The Abortion-Crime Link: Evidence from England and Wales." *Economica* 75, no. 297 (February 2008): 1-21.
313. Kamath R, Mahajan KS, Ashok L and Sanai TS. "A Study on Risk Factors of Breast Cancer Among Patients Attending the Tertiary Care Hospital, in Udupi District." *Indian Journal Community Medicine* 38, no. 2 (2013): 95-9.
314. Karaer A, Avsar FA and Batioglu S. "Risk Factors for Ectopic Pregnancy: A Case-Control Study." *Australian and New Zealand Journal of Obstetrics and Gynaecology* 46, no. 6 (2006): 521-7.
315. Katz Rothman B. *The Tentative Pregnancy: Prenatal Diagnosis and the Future of Motherhood*. New York, NY: Viking, 1996.
316. Kaur R and Garg S. "Addressing Domestic Violence Against Women: An Unfinished Agenda." *Indian Journal of Community Medicine* 33, no. 2 (2008): 73-6.
317. Kaye DK, Mirembe M, Bantebya G, Johansson A and Ekstrom AM. "Domestic Violence as a Risk Factor for Unwanted Pregnancy and Induced Abortion in Mulago Hospital, Kampala, Uganda." *Tropical Medicine and International Health* 11, no. 1 (January 2006): 90-101.
318. Keeling J, Birch L and Green P. "Pregnancy Counselling Clinic: A Questionnaire Survey of Intimate Partner Abuse." *Journal of Family Planning and Reproductive Health Care* 30, no. 3 (July 2004): 165-8.
319. Kelly SE. "Choosing Not to Choose: Reproductive Responses of Parents of Children with Genetic Conditions or Impairments." *Sociology of Health and Illness* 31, no. 1 (2009): 81-97.
320. Kersting A, Dorsch M, Kreulich C, et al. "Trauma and Grief 2-7 Years After Termination of Pregnancy Because of Fetal Abnormalities." *Journal of Psychosomatic Obstetrics & Gynaecology* 26, no. 1 (2005): 9-14.
321. Kersting A, Kroker K, Steinhard J, et al. "Complicated Grief After Traumatic Loss: A 14-Month Follow Up Study." *European Archives of Psychiatry and Clinical Neuroscience* 257, no. 8 (December 2007): 437-43.
322. Kessler DA. *A Question of Intent: A Great American Battle with a Deadly Industry*. New York: Public Affairs, 2001.
323. Khachatryan L, Scharpf R and Kaan S. "Influence of Diabetes Mellitus Type 2 and Prolonged Estrogen Exposure Among Women in Armenia." *Health Care for Women International* 32, no. 11 (2011): 953-71.
324. Khadr Z. "Monitoring Socioeconomic Inequity in Maternal Health Indicators in Egypt: 1995-2005." *International Journal for Equity in Health* 8, no. 38 (November 2009): 8.
325. Khan KS, Wojdyla D, Say L, Gulmezoglu AM and Paul FA. "WHO Analysis of Causes of Maternal Death: A Systematic Review." *The Lancet* 367, no. 9516 (April 2006): 1066-74.

326. Khoshnood B, De Vigan C, Vodovar V, Breart G, Goffinet F and Blondel B. "Advances in Medical Technology and Creation of Disparities: The Case of Down Syndrome." *American Journal of Public Health* 96, no. 12 (December 2006): 2139-44.

327. Khoshnood B, Greenlees R, Loane M, Dolk H, EUROCAT Project Management Committee and EUROCAT Working Group. "Paper 2: EUROCAT Public Health Indicators for Congenital Anomalies in Europe." *Birth Defects Research. Part A, Clinical and Molecular Teratology* 91, Supplement 1 (March 2011): S16-22.

328. Kiely KC. "Everett Koop Urges Senators to Block Kagan." *USA Today,* 19 July 2010.

329. Kippen R, Evans A and Gray E. "Parental Preference for Sons and Daughters in a Western Industrial Setting: Evidence and Implications." *Journal of Biosocial Science* 39, no. 4 (2007): 583-97.

330. Kleiner GJ and Greston WM, eds. *Suicide in Pregnancy.* Boston: John Wright, 1984.

331. Kluger-Bell K. *Unspeakable Losses: Understanding the Experience of Pregnancy Loss, Miscarriage, and Abortion.* New York: W.W. Norton, 1998.

332. Kochanek KD, Kirmeyer SE, Martin JA, Strobino DM and Guyer B. "Annual Summary of Vital Statistics: 2009." *Pediatrics* 129, no. 2 (February 2012): 338-48.

333. Koch E, Thorp J, Bravo M, Gatica S, Romero CX, Aguilera H and Ahlers I. "Women's Education Level, Maternal Health Facilities, Abortion Legislation and Maternal Deaths: A Natural Experiment in Chile from 1957 to 2007." *PLoS ONE* 7, no. 5 (May 2012): e36613: 1-16.

334. Korenromp MJ, Page-Christiaens GC, van den Bout J, et al. "A Prospective Study on Parental Coping 4 Months After Termination of Pregnancy for Fetal Anomalies." *Prenatal Diagnosis* 27, no. 8 (2007): 709-16.

335. Kramer A. "Stages of Change: Surviving Intimate Partner Violence During and After Pregnancy." *Journal of Perinatal & Neonatal Nursing* 21, no. 4 (October/December 2007): 285-95.

336. Krieger N. "Exposure, Susceptibility, and Breast Cancer Risk: A Hypothesis Regarding Exogenous Carcinogens, Breast Tissue Development, and Social Gradients, Including Black/White Differences, in Breast Cancer Incidence." *Breast Cancer Research and Treatment* 13, no. 3 (1990): 205-23.

337. Krohn MA, Germain M, Mühlemann K and Hickok D. "Prior Pregnancy Outcome and the Risk of Intraamniotic Infection in the Following Pregnancy." *AJOG* 178, no. 2 (1998): 381-5.

338. Kulier R, Gulmezoglu AM, Hofmeyr GJ, Cheng LN and Campana A. "Medical Methods for First Trimester Abortion." *Cochrane Database of Systematic Reviews* 1, no. 9 (November 2011): CD002855.

339. Kunz J and Keller PJ. "HCG, HPL, Oestradiol, Progesterone and AFP in Serum in Patients with Threatened Abortion." *BJOG* 83, no. 8 (August 1976): 640-4.

340. Kusum K. "Sex Selection." In *Ethical Aspects of Human Reproduction.* Paris: John Libbey Eurotext, 1995.

341. Laffront I and Edelmann RJ. "Psychological Aspects of In Vitro Fertilization: A Gender Comparison." *Journal of Psychosomatic Obstetrics & Gynecology* 15, no. 2 (June 1994): 85-92.

342. Laing AE, Demenais FM, Williams R, Kissling G, Chen VW and Bonney GE. "Breast Cancer Risk Factors in African-American Women: The Howard University Tumor Registry Experience." *Journal of the National Medical Association* 85, no. 2 (1993): 931-9.
343. Laing AE, Demenais FM, Williams R, Kissling G, Chen VW and Bonney GE. "Reproductive and Lifestyle Factors for Breast Cancer in African-American Women." *Genetic Epidemiology* 11 (1994): A300.
344. Laliberte J. "Still No Mifepristone for Canada: Is it Safe?" *National Review of Medicine* 2, no. 16 (30 September, 2005): 1.
345. Lalonde AB, Okong P, Mugasa A and Perron L. "The FIGO Save the Mothers Initiative: The Uganda-Canada Collaboration." *International Journal of Gynaecology and Obstetrics* 80, no. 2 (February 2003): 204-12.
346. Lambe M. "Chapter 6: Reproductive Factors." In *Breast Cancer Epidemiology*. Ed. Li C. New York: Springer, 2010: 119-29.
347. Lambe M, Hsieh C, Chan H, Ekbom A, Trichopoulos D and Adami H. "Parity, Age at First and Last Birth, and Risk of Breast Cancer: A Population Study in Sweden." *Breast Cancer Research and Treatment* 38, no. 3 (January 1996): 305-11.
348. Lamichhane P, Harken T, Puri M, et al. "Sex-Selective Abortion in Nepal: A Qualitative Study of Health Workers' Perspectives." *Women's Health Issues* 21, Supplement 3 (May-June 2011): S37-41.
349. Lanfranchi A. "The Federal Government and Academic Texts as Barriers to Informed Consent." *Journal of American Physicians and Surgeons* 13, no. 1 (2008): 12-15.
350. Lasmar RB, Barrozo PR, Parente RC, et al. "Hysteroscopic Evaluation in Patients with Infertility." Translated from Portuguese. *Revista Brasileira de Ginecologia e Obstetricia* 32, no. 8 (August 2010): 393-7.
351. Lawson KL and Pierson RA. "Maternal Decisions Regarding Prenatal Diagnosis: Rational Choices or Sensible Decisions?" *JOGC* 29, no. 3 (2007): 240-6.
352. Lawton BA, Rose SB, Bromhead C, Gaitanos LA, MacDonald EJ and Lund KA. "High Prevalence of Mycoplasma Genitalium in Women Presenting for Termination of Pregnancy." *Contraception* 77, no. 4 (2008): 294-8.
353. Lecarpentier J, Noguès C, Mouret-Fourme E, et al. "Variation in Breast Cancer Risk Associated with Factors Related to Pregnancies According to Truncating Mutation Location, in the French National BRCA1 and BRCA2 Mutations Carrier Cohort (GENEPSO)." *Breast Cancer Research* 14, no. 4 (3 July, 2012): R99. http://breast-cancer-research.com/content/14/4/R99.
354. Lee JR, Ku SY, Jee BC, Suh CS, Kim KC and Kim SH. "Pregnancy Outcomes of Different Methods for Multifetal Pregnancy Reduction: A Comparative Study." *Journal of Korean Medical Science* 23, no. 1 (February 2008): 111-16.
355. Lee-Rife SM. "Women's Empowerment and Reproductive Experiences over the Lifecourse." *Social Science & Medicine* 71, no. 3 (August 2010): 634-42.
356. Leibner EC. "Delayed Presentation of Uterine Perforation." *Annals of Emergency Medicine* 26, no. 5 (November 1995): 643-6.
357. Leigh A and Wolfers J. "Abortion and Crime." *AQ: Australian Quarterly* 72, no. 4 (2000): 28-30, 40.

358. Leiva R. "Illegal Abortion and Safety: The Case of El Salvador." Letter in Response to "Transparency in the Delivery of Lawful Abortion Services," by Rebecca J. Cook. *CMAJ* 180, no. 3 (3 February 2009).http://www.cmaj.ca/content/180/3/272/reply#cmaj_el_53631?sid=e3298cf7-d9ea-4e90-9711-ec808ccf37ae.
359. Le MG, Bachelot A, Doyon F, Krama A and Hill C. "Oral Contraceptive Use and Breast or Cervical Cancer: Preliminary Results of a French Case-Control Study." *Hormones and Sexual Factors in Human Cancer Aetiology.* Eds. Wolff JP and Scott JS. Amsterdam: Elsevier, 1984: 139-47.
360. Leone T, Matthews Z and Zuanna GD. "Impact and Determinants of Sex Preference in Nepal." *IFPP* 29, no. 2 (June 2003): 69-75.
361. Leung TW, Leung WC, Chan PL and Ho PC. "A Comparison of the Prevalence of Domestic Violence between Patients Seeking Termination of Pregnancy and Other General Gynecology Patients." *International Journal of Gynecology and Obstetrics* 77, no. 1 (April 2002): 47-54.
362. Leuthner S and Jones EL. "Fetal Concerns Program: A Model for Perinatal Palliative Care." *American Journal of Maternal/Child Nursing* 32, no. 5 (2007): 272-8.
363. Levallois P and Rioux JE. "Prophylactic Antibiotics for Suction Curettage Abortion: Results of a Clinical Controlled Trial."*AJOG* 158, no. 1 (1988): 100-5.
364. Levitt SD and Dubner SJ. *Freakonomics: A Rogue Economist Explores the Hidden Side of Everything.* New York: William Morrow, 2006.
365. Li C, ed. *Breast Cancer Epidemiology.* New York: Springer, 2010.
366. Limperopoulos C, Bassan H, Sullivan NR, et al. "Positive Screening for Autism in Ex-Preterm Infants: Prevalence and Risk Factors." *Pediatrics* 121, no. 4 (April 2008): 758-65.
367. Lindahl V, Pearson JL and Colpe L. "Prevalence of Suicidality during Pregnancy and the Postpartum." *Archives of Women's Mental Health* 8, no. 2 (June 2005): 77–87.
368. Lindefors-Harris BM, Eklund G, Adami HO and Meirik O. "Response Bias in a Case-Control Study: Analysis Utilizing Comparative Data Concerning Legal Abortions and Two Independent Swedish Studies." *American Journal of Epidemiology* 134, no. 9 (1991): 1003-8.
369. Linos E, Spanos D, Rosner BA, et al. "Effects of Reproductive and Demographic Changes on Breast Cancer Incidence in China: A Modeling Analysis." *Journal of the National Cancer Institute* 100, no. 19(2008): 1352-60.
370. Lippman A. "Prenatal Genetic Testing and Screening: Constructing Needs and Reinforcing Inequalities." *American Journal of Law and Medicine* 17, nos. 1-2 (1991): 15-50.
371. Lipsky S, Holt VL, Easterling TR and Critchlow CW. "Police-Reported Intimate Partner Violence during Pregnancy: Who is at Risk?" *Violence and Victims* 20, no. 1 (February 2005): 69-86.
372. Lipworth L, Katsouyanni K, Ekbom A, Michels KB and Trichopoulos D. "Abortion and the Risk of Breast Cancer: A Case-Control Study in Greece." *International Journal of Cancer* 61, no. 2 (1995): 181-4.

373. Li S. "Imbalanced Sex Ratio at Birth and Comprehensive Intervention in China." *Hyderabad, India: 4th Asia Pacific Conference on Reproductive and Sexual Health Rights.* October 29-31, 2007.
374. Liu S, Joseph KS, Kramer MS, et al. "Fetal and Infant Health Study Group of the Canadian Perinatal Surveillance System: Relationship of Prenatal Diagnosis and Pregnancy Termination to Overall Infant Mortality in Canada." *JAMA* 287, no. 12 (March 2002): 1561-7.
375. Lloyd ME. "Gender Factors in Reviewer Recommendation for Manuscript Publication." *Journal of Applied Behavior Analysis* 23, no. 4 (1990): 539-43.
376. Lončar M, Medved V, Jovanovic N and Hotujac L. "Psychological Consequences of Rape on Women in 1991-1995 War in Croatia and Bosnia and Herzegovina." *Croatian Medical Journal* 47, no. 1 (2006): 67-75.
377. Lott JR and Whitley J. "Abortion and Crime: Unwanted Children and Out-of-Wedlock Births." *Economic Inquiry* 45, no. 2 (2007): 304-324.
378. Lowry RB. "Congenital Anomalies Surveillance in Canada." *Canadian Journal of Public Health* 99, no. 6 (November-December 2008): 483-5.
379. Lucaci L and Szucsik IA. "Statistical Study on the Incidence and Prevalence of Breast Cancer, In Arad County, Between the Years 1999-2009." *Arad Medical Journal* 13, no. 4 (November 2010): 5-10.
380. Lukse MP and Vacc NA. "Grief, Depression, and Coping in Women Undergoing Infertility Treatment." *Obstetrics & Gynecology* 93, no. 2 (February 1999): 245-51.
381. Luporsi E. "Breast Cancer and Alcohol." PhD dissertation. University of Paris-Sud, 1988.
382. Luttjeboer FY, Verhoeve HR, van Dessel HJ, van der Veen F, Mol BWJ and Coppus SFPJ. "The Value of Medical History Taking as Risk Indicator for Tuboperitoneal Pathology: A Systematic Review." *International Journal of Obstetrics and Gynaecology* 116, no. 5 (2009): 612-25.
383. Lyall K, Pauls DL, Spiegelman D, Ascherio A and Santangelo SL. "Pregnancy Complications and Obstetric Suboptimality in Association With Autism Spectrum Disorders in Children of the Nurses' Health Study II." *Autism Research* 5, no. 1 (February 2012): 21-30.
384. Macklin R. "The Ethics of Sex Selection and Family Balancing." *Seminars in Reproductive Medicine* 28, no. 4 (July 2010): 315-21.
385. Macones GA, Schemmer G, Pritts E, Weinblatt V, and Wapner RJ. "Multifetal Reduction of Triplets to Twins Improves Perinatal Outcome." *AJOG* 169, no. 4 (October 1993): 982-6.
386. Maconochie N, Doyle P, Prior S and Simmons R. "Risk Factors for First Trimester Miscarriage – Results from a UK Population-Based Case-Control Study." *BJOG* 114, no. 2 (February 2007): 170-86.
387. Major B, Cozzarelli C, Cooper ML, Zubek J, Richards C, Wilhite M and Gramzow RH. "Psychological Responses of Women After First-Trimester Abortion." *Archives of General Psychiatry* 57, no. 8 (2000): 777-84.

388. March CM. "Asherman's Syndrome." *Seminars in Reproductive Medicine* 29, no. 2 (March 2011): 83-94.

389. Marques-Dias MJ, Gonzalez CH and Rosemberg S. "Möbius Sequence in Children Exposed in Utero to Misprostol: Neuropathological Study of Three Cases."*Birth Defects Research. Part A, Clinical and Molecular Teratology* 67, no. 12 (December 2003): 1002-7.

390. Martinson BC, Anderson MS and deVries R. "Scientists Behaving Badly." *Nature* 435 (9 June, 2005): 737-8.

391. Matejcek Z, Dytrych Z and Schüller V. "Children from Unwanted Pregnancies."*Acta Psychiatrica Scandinavica* 57 (1978): 67-90.

392. Maternal Mortality Estimation Inter-Agency Group. *Trends in Maternal Mortality: 1990 to 2010: WHO, UNICEF, UNFPA and the World Bank Estimate.* Geneva: World Health Organization, 2012.

393. Mauelshagen A, Sadler LC, Roberts H, Harilall M and Farquhar CM. "Audit of Short Term Outcomes of Surgical and Medical Second Trimester Termination of Pregnancy."*Reproductive Health* 30, no. 6:16 (2009): 1-6.

394. Mayo Clinic. "Complicated Grief."*Mayo Clinic* (11 September 2011). http://www.mayoclinic.com/health/complicated-grief/DS01023.

395. Mbele AM, Snyman L and Pattinson RC. "Impact of the Choice on Termination of Pregnancy Act on Maternal Morbidity and Mortality in the West of Pretoria." *South African Medical Journal (SAMJ)* 96, no. 11 (November 2006): 1196-8.

396. Mbonye AK. "Abortion in Uganda: Magnitude and Implications." *African Journal of Reproductive Health* 4, no. 2 (October 2000): 104-8.

397. Mbonye AK, Mutabazi MG, Asimwe JB, et al. "Declining Maternal Mortality Ratio in Uganda: Priority Interventions to Achieve the Millennium Development Goal." *International Journal of Gynaecology and Obstetrics* 98, no. 3 (July 2007): 287-8.

398. McCoyd JL. "'I'm Not a Saint': Burden Assessment as an Unrecognized Factor in Prenatal Decision Making."*Qualitative Health Research* 18, no. 11 (November 2008): 1489-1500.

399. McFarlane J, Campbell JC, Sharps P and Watson K. "Abuse During Pregnancy and Femicide: Urgent Implications for Women's Health." *Obstetrics & Gynecology* 100, no. 1 (2002): 27-36.

400. McFarlane J, Malecha A, Watson K, et al. "Intimate Partner Sexual Assault Against Women: Frequency, Health Consequences, and Treatment Outcomes." *Obstetrics & Gynecology* 105, no. 1 (January 2005): 99-108.

401. McKenna T and O'Brien K. "Case Report: Group B Streptococcal Bacteremia and Sacroiliitis after Mid-Trimester Dilation and Evacuation."*Journal of Perinatology* 29, no. 9 (2009): 643-5.

402. McKinney M, Downey J and Timor-Tritsch I. "The Psychological Effects of Multi-Fetal Pregnancy Reduction." *Fertility and Sterility* 64, no. 1 (July 1995): 51-61.

403. McKinney MK, Tuber SB and Downey JI. "Multifetal Pregnancy Reduction: Psychodynamic Implications." *Psychiatry* 59, no. 4 (Winter 1996): 393-407.

404.   Mead PB, Hager WD, and Faro S, eds. *Protocols for Infectious Diseases in Obstetrics and Gynecology.* 2nd ed. Malden, MA: Blackwell Science, 2000.

405.   Meckstroth KR and Mishra K. "Analgesia/Pain Management in First Trimester Surgical Abortion." *Clinical Obstetrics and Gynecology* 52, no. 2 (June 2009): 160-70.

406.   Medical Practitioners Board of Victoria. *Report on Late Term Terminations of Pregnancy April 1988.* Victoria, Australia: Acute Health Division, Department of Human Services, 1998. http://www.dhs.vic.gov.au/ahs/archive/report/report7.htm.

407.   Meirik O, Adami HO and Eklund G. "Letter Re: Relation Between Induced Abortion and Breast Cancer." *Journal of Epidemiology and Community Health* 52, no. 3 (1998): 209-11.

408.   Meites E, Zane S and Gould C. "Letter to the New England Journal of Medicine." *NEJM* 363, no. 14 (30 September, 2010): 1382-3.

409.   Melbye M, Wohlfahrt J, Andersen A-MN, Westergaard T and Andersen PK. "Preterm Delivery and Risk of Breast Cancer." *British Journal of Cancer* 80, no. 3/4 (1999): 609-13.

410.   Melbye M, Wohlfahrt J, Olsen JH, et al. "Induced Abortion and the Risk of Breast Cancer." *NEJM* 336 (1997): 81-5.

411.   Mendieta W, Bohemer L and Cabrera RJ. "Nicaragua and Abortions." Letter to the Editor. *Washington Times*, 20 December 2007. http://www.washingtontimes.com/news/2007/dec/20/letters-to-the-editor-97819183/?page=all.

412.   Merli MG and Hertog S. "Masculine Sex Ratios, Population Age Structure and the Potential Spread of HIV in China." *Demographic Research* 22, no. 3 (2010): 63-94.

413.   Miech RP. "Pathophysiology of Mifepristone-Induced Septic Shock Due to Chlostridium Sordelli." *Annals of Pharmacology* 39, no. 9 (September 2005): 1483-8.

414.   — — — . "The Role of Fetal Microchimerism in Autoimmune Disease." *International Journal of Clinical and Experimental Medicine* 3, no. 2 (2010): 162-8.

415.   Miller E, Jordan B, Levenson R and Silverman JG. "Reproductive Coercion: Connecting the Dots between Partner Violence and Unintended Pregnancy." *Contraception* 81, no. 6 (2010): 457-9.

416.   Miller G. "Neurological Disorders: The Mystery of the Missing Smile." *Science* 316, no. 5826 (2007): 826-7.

417.   Miller WB. "An Empirical Study of the Psychological Antecedents and Consequences of Induced Abortion." *Journal of Social Issues* 48, no. 3 (Fall 1992): 67-93.

418.   Milliez JM. "Sex Selection for Non-Medical Purposes." *Reproductive BioMedicine Online* 14, no. S1 (2007): pp. 114-7.

419.   Mittal S and Misra SL. "Uterine Perforation Following Medical Termination of Pregnancy by Vacuum Aspiration." *International Journal of Gynaecology and Obstetrics* 23, no. 1 (February 1985): 45-50.

420.   Mogilevkina I, Markote S, Avakyan Y, Mrochek L, Liljestrand J and Hellberg D. "Induced Abortions and Childbirths: Trends in Estonia, Latvia, Lithuania, Russia, Belarussia and the Ukraine During 1970 to 1994." *Acta Obstetricia et Gynecologica Scandanavica* 75, no. 10 (November 1996): 908-11.

421. Molin A. "Risk Of Damage to the Cervix by Dilatation for First-Trimester Induced Abortion by Suction Aspiration." *Gynecologic and Obstetric Investigation* 35, no. 3 (1993): 152-4.
422. Moodley J and Akinsooto VS. "Unsafe Abortions in a Developing Country: Has Liberalisation of Laws on Abortions Made a Difference?" *African Journal of Reproductive Health* 7, no. 2 (August 2003): 34-8.
423. Moore AM, Frohwirth L and Miller E. "Male Reproductive Control of Women Who Have Experienced Intimate Partner Violence in the United States." *Social Science and Medicine* 70, no. 11 (2010): 1737-44.
424. Moore RC. "Husband Mourns Outcome of Wife's Painful Decision."*American Medical News*(14 October, 1991): 24.
425. Moreno-Ruiz NL, Borgatta L, Yanow S, et al. "Alternatives to Mifepristone for Early Medical Abortion."*International Journal of Gynaecology and Obstetrics* 96, no. 3 (2005): 212-18.
426. Morgan CL, Evans M and Peters JR. "Suicides After Pregnancy: Mental Health May Deteriorate as a Direct Effect of Induced Abortion."*BMJ* 314, no. 7084 (March 1997): 902-3.
427. *Morgan v MacPhail*, 550 Pa. 202, 704 A (2d) 617 (1997).
428. Morgentaler Clinic. "The Procedure." 2008. http://www.morgentaler.ca/procedure.html.
429. Morris JK and Wald NJ. "Prevalence of Neural Tube Defect Pregnancies in England and Wales From 1964 to 2004." *Journal of Medical Screening* 14 (2007): 55-9.
430. Moster D, Lie RT and Markestad T. "Long-Term Medical and Social Consequences of Preterm Birth." *NEJM* 359, no. 3 (17 July, 2008): 262-73.
431. Mota N, Burnett M and Sareen J. "Associations Between Abortion, Mental Disorders and Suicidal Behaviour in a Nationally Representative Sample." *Canadian Journal of Psychiatry* 55, no. 5 (April 2010): 239-47.
432. Mrozec A. "Canada's Lost Daughters." *Western Standard*(June 2006): 33-9.
433. Munk-Olsen T, et al. "Induced First-Trimester Abortion and Risk of Mental Disorder."*NEJM* 364, no. 4 (27 January, 2011): 332-9.
434. Myers KA and Farquhar DR. "Improving the Accuracy of Death Certification." *CMAJ* 158, no. 10 (May 1998): 1317-23.
435. Naieni KH, Ardalan A, Mahmoodi M, Motevalian A, Yahyapoor Y and Yazdizadeh B. "Risk Factors of Breast Cancer in North of Iran: A Case-Control in Mazandaran Province." *Asian Pacific Journal of Cancer Prevention* 8, no. 3 (2007): 395-8.
436. Nakazibwe C. "Maternal Health Care Wins District Vote in Uganda." *Bulletin of the World Health Organization* 84, no. 11 (November 2006): 847-9.
437. National Breast Cancer Coalition. "Truth #30: I Can Influence What Happens in Washington D.C. About Breast Cancer." *National Breast Cancer Coalition.*2011. http://www.breastcancerdeadline2020.org/know/31-myths-and-truths/truth-30-i-can-influence-capitol-hill.html.
438. National Cancer Institute. "Breast Cancer Prevention." 20 September, 2011. http://www.cancer.gov/cancertopics/pdq/prevention/breast/Patient/page3.

439. ———. "Cancer prevalence." *SEER Cancer Statistics Review 1975-2005* (2008).
440. National Center for Health Statistics. *Health, United States, 2007.* Hyattsville, MD: With Chartbook on Trends in the Health of Americans, 2007. http://www.cdc.gov/nchs/data/hus/hus07.pdf.
441. National Collaborating Centre for Mental Health (NCCMH). *Induced Abortion and Mental Health: A Systematic Review of the Mental Health Outcomes of Induced Abortion, Including Their Prevalence and Associated Factors.* London: Academy of Medical Royal Colleges, December 2011.
442. National Committee on Confidential Enquiries into Maternal Deaths (NCCEMD). *Saving Mothers 2005-2007: Fourth Report on Confidential Enquiries into Maternal Deaths in South Africa -Expanded Executive Summary.* Pretoria, South Africa: National Department of Health, March 2007. http://www.doh.gov.za/docs/reports/2007/savingmothers.pdf.
443. National Institute of Health, The Autoimmune Diseases Coordinating Committee. *Progress in Autoimmune Diseases Research, Report to Congress* (March 2005). http://www.niaid.nih.gov/topics/autoimmune/documents/adccfinal.pdf.
444. *National Memorial for the Unborn.*2010.http://www.memorialfortheunborn.org/tabid/55/default.aspx.
445. National Statistics Department of Health. *Abortion Statistics, England and Wales: 2012.* London: HMSO, 2013.
446. Nesheim BI. "Induced Abortion by the Suction Method: An Analysis of Complication Rates."*Acta Obstetricia et Gynecologica Scandinavica* 63, no. 7 (1984): 591-5.
447. Newcomb PA, Storer BE, Longnecker MP, Mittendorf R, Greenberg ER, and Willett WC. "Pregnancy Termination in Relation to Risk of Breast Cancer." *JAMA* 275, no. 4 (1996): 283-7.
448. Ney PG, Fung T and Wickett AR. "Relationship Between Induced Abortion and Child Abuse and Neglect: Four Studies." *Pre- and Perinatal Psychology Journal* 8, no. 1 (October 1993): 43-63.
449. Nguyen N, Winikoff B, Clark S, et al. "Safety, Efficacy and Acceptability of Mifepristone-Misoprostol Medical Abortion in Vietnam."*IFPP* 25, no. 1 (1999): 10-14.
450. Nie JB. "Limits of State Intervention in Sex-Selective Abortion: The Case of China." *Culture, Health & Sexuality* 12, no. 2 (February 2010): 205-19.
451. Nielsen IK, Engdahl E and Larsen T. "[Pelvic Inflammation after Induced Abortion] Danish." *Ugeskr Laeger* 154, no. 40 (28 September 1992): 2743-6.
452. Niinimäki M, Pouta A, Bloigu A, et al. "Immediate Complications After Medical Compared with Surgical Termination of Pregnancy." *Obstetrics & Gynaecology* 114, no. 4 (October 2009): 795-804.
453. Nishiyama F. "The Epidemiology of Breast Cancer in Tokushima Prefecture." *Shikoku Ichi* 38 (1982): 333-43.
454. Nordvig L, Secher NJ and Andersen S. "Psykologiske Aspekter, Brugerholdninger Og-Forventninger I Forbindelse Med Ultralydskanning I Graviditeten." *Medicinsk Teknologivurdering* 6, no. 13 (2006).
455. Norris S. "Reproductive Infertility: Prevalence, Causes, Trends and Treatments." *Parliamentary Research Branch: In Brief* (2 January, 2001): 1-4.

456. Oddens BJ, den Tonkelaar I and Nieuwenhuyse H. "Psychosocial Experiences in Women Facing Fertility Problems: A Comparative Survey." *Human Reproduction* 14, no. 1 (January 1999): 255-61.

457. Ohio Revised Code. Title [47] XLVII Occupations – Professions. Chapter 4731: Physicians; Physicians; Limited Practitioners.

458. Oklahoma Statutes §63-1-738.3b.E.

459. Okong P, Byamugisha J, Mirembe F, Byaruhanga R and Bergstrom S. "Audit of Severe Maternal Morbidity in Uganda – Implications for Quality of Obstetric Care." *Acta Obstetricia et Gynecologica Scandinavica* 85, no. 7 (2006): 797-804.

460. Onsrud M, Sjøvejan S, Luhiriri R and Mukwege D. "Sexual Violence-Related Fistulas in the Democratic Republic of Congo." *International Journal of Gynecology and Obstetrics* 103, no. 3 (December 2008): 265-9.

461. OptionLine. "Get Help: Locate a Pregnancy Help Center Near You." *OptionLine*, 2012. http://www.optionline.org/get-help.

462. Orinda V, Kakande H, Kabarangira J, Nanda G and Mbonye AK. "A Sector-Wide Approach to Emergency Obstetric Care in Uganda." *International Journal of Gynecology and Obstetrics* 91, no. 3 (December 2005): 285-91.

463. Osser S and Persson K. "Postabortal Pelvic Infection Associated with Chlamydia Trachomatis and the Influence of Humoral Immunity." *AJOG* 150, no. 6 (November 1984): 699-703.

464. Østbye T, Wenghofer EF, Woodward CA, Gold G and Craighead J. "Health Services Utilization After Induced Abortions in Ontario: A Comparison Between Community Clinics and Hospitals." *American Journal of Medical Quality* 16, no. 3 (2001): 99-106.

465. Qvigstad E, Skaug K, Jerve F, Fylling P and Ulstrup JC. "Pelvic Inflammatory Disease Associated with Chlamydia Trachomatis Infection after Therapeutic Abortion: A Prospective Study." *British Journal of Venereal Diseases* 59, no. 3 (June 1983): 189-92.

466. Owolabi OT and Moodley J. "A Randomized Trial of Pain Relief in Termination of Pregnancy in South Africa." *Tropical Doctor* 35, no. 3 (July 2005): 136-9.

467. Ozeren M, Bilekli C, Aydemir V, et al. "Methotrexate and Misoprostol Used Alone or in Combination for Early Abortion." *Contraception* 59, no. 6 (June 1999): 389-94.

468. Ozmen V, Ozcinar B, Karanlik H, et al. "Breast Cancer Risk Factors in Turkish Women - A University Hospital Based Nested Case Control Study." *World Journal of Surgical Oncology* 7, no. 37 (2009): 37-44.

469. Palmer JR, Rosenberg L, Rao RS, et al. "Induced Abortion in Relation to Risk of Breast Cancer (United States)." *Cancer Causes and Control* 8, no. 6 (1997): 841-9.

470. Papiernik E. "The Role of Emergency Obstetric Care in Preventing Maternal Deaths: An Historical Perspective on European Figures Since 1751." *International Journal of Gynecology and Obstetrics* 50, no. Supplement 2 (October 1995): S73-7.

471. Parazzini F, Chatenoud L, Tozzi L, Di Cintio E, Benzi G and Fedele L. "Induced Abortion in the First Trimester of Pregnancy and Risk of Miscarriage." *BJOG* 105, no. 4 (April 1998): 418-21.

472.   Parkhurst JO, Penn-Kekana L, Blaauw D, et al. "Health Systems Factors Influencing Maternal Health Services: A Four-Country Comparison."*Health Policy* 73, no. 2 (August 2005): 127-38.
473.   Parsons LH and Harper MA. "Violent Maternal Deaths in North Carolina." *Obstetrics & Gynecology* 94, no. 6 (1999): 990-3.
474.   Pastuszak AL, Schüler L, Speck-Martins CE, et al. "Use of Misoprostol During Pregnancy and Möbius' Syndrome in Infants."*NEJM* 338 (1998): 1881-5.
475.   Patel CJ and Kooverjee T. "Abortion and Contraception: Attitudes of South African University Students."*Health Care for Women International* 30, no. 6 (June 2009): 550-68.
476.   Paul ME, Mitchell CM, Rogers AJ, Fox MC and Lackie EG. "Early Surgical Abortion: Efficacy and Safety."*AJOG* 187, no. 2 (2002): 407-11.
477.   Pearce DM. "The Feminization of Ghetto Poverty."*Society* 21, no. 1 (1983): 70-4.
478.   Penney GC, Thomson M, Norman J, et al. "A Randomised Comparison of Strategies for Reducing Infective Complications of Induced Abortion." *BJOG* 105, no. 6 (1998): 599-604.
479.   Penney G. "Treatment of Pain During Medical Abortion." *Contraception* 74, no. 1 (July 2006): 45-7.
480.   Pennings G. "Ethics of Sex Selection for Family Balancing." *Human Reproduction* 11, no. 11 (1996): 2339–45.
481.   Perry K. "Abortion Provider Loses Ruling." *Cincinnati Enquirer*, 9 December 2010, C1.
482.   Phillips SP. "Violence and Abortions: What's a Doctor to Do?" *CMAJ* 172, no. 5 (1 March, 2005): 653-4.
483.   Piane GM. "Evidence-Based Practices to Reduce Maternal Mortality: A Systematic Review."*Journal of Public Health* 31, no. 1 (March 2009): 26-31.
484.   Pilkington E. "Sex Selection and the Rise of Generation XY: A New Book Explores Western Involvement in what has Become a Scourge of the Developing World: Sex Selection of Babies." *The Guardian*, 17 June, 2011.http://www.guardian.co.uk/world/2011/jun/17/sex-selection-rise-generation-xy?INTCMP=SRCH.
485.   Pioro M, Roxanne M and Nisker J. "Wrongful Birth Litigation and Prenatal Screening."*CMAJ* 179, no. 10 (4 November, 2008): 1027–30.
486.   Pizzo T, Knop F and Mengue S. "Prenatal Exposure to Misoprostol and Congenital Anomalies: Systematic Review and Meta-Analysis."*Reproductive Toxicology* 22, no. 4 (2006): 666-71.
487.   Polansky S. "Overcoming the Obstacles: A Collaborative Approach to Informed Consent in Prenatal Screening in Canada." *Health Law Journal* 14 (2006): 21-44.
488.   Ponnuru R. *The Party of Death: The Democrats, the Media, the Courts, and the Disregard for Human Life*. Washington, DC: Regnery Publishing, Inc., 2006.
489.   Pop-Eleches C. "The Impact of an Abortion Ban on Socioeconomic Outcomes of Children: Evidence from Romania." *Journal of Political Economy* 114, no. 4 (August 2006): 744-73.

490. Population Division of the United Nations Secretariat. *Abortion Policies: A Global Review*.3 vols. New York, NY: Population Division, Department of Economic and Social Affairs, United Nations Secretariat, 2002.http://www.un.org/esa/population/publications/abortion/index.htm.

491. Prada E, Mirembe F, Ahmed FH, Nalwadda R and Kiggundu C. *Abortion and Postabortion Care in Uganda: A Report from Health Care Professionals and Health Facilities*. New York: The Alan Guttmacher Institute, 2005.http://www.guttmacher.org/pubs/2005/05/28/or17.pdf.

492. Pregnancy and Infant Loss Awareness Network (PAIL Network). "Pregnancy and Infant Loss: About US." Pickering, ON: Author, 2012. www.pailnetwork.ca.

493. Pridmore BR and Chambers DG. "Uterine Perforation During Surgical Abortion: A Review of Diagnosis, Management and Prevention." *Aust N Z J Obstet Gynaecol* 39, no. 3 (August 1999): 349-53.

494. Pud Dand Amit A. "Anxiety as a Predictor of Pain Magnitude Following Termination of First-Trimester Pregnancy." *Pain Medicine* 6, no. 2 (March 2005): 143-8.

495. Puri S, Adams V, Ivey S and Nachtigall RD. "'There is Such a Thing as Too Many Daughters, but Not Too Many Sons': A Qualitative Study of Son Preference and Fetal Sex Selection among Indian Immigrants in the United States." *Social Science & Medicine* 72, no. 7 (April 2011): 1169-76.

496. Radestad A, Bui TH, Nygren KG, Koskimies A and Petersen K. "The Utilization Rate and Pregnancy Outcome of Multifetal Pregnancy Reduction in the Nordic Countries." *Acta Obstetricia et Gynecologica Scandanavica* 75, no. 7 (August 1996): 651-3.

497. Rahangdale L. "Infectious Complications of Pregnancy Termination." *Clinical Obstetrics and Gynecology* 52, no. 2 (2009): 198-204.

498. Raj A, Liu R, McCleary-Sills J and Silverman JG. "South Asian Victims of Intimate Partner Violence More Likely than Non-Victims to Report Sexual Health Concerns." *Journal of Immigrant Health* 7, no. 2 (April 2005): 85-91.

499. Rak JM, Maestroni L, Balandraud N, et al. "Transfer of the Shared Epitope Through Microchimerism in Women with Rheumatoid Arthritis."*Arthritis & Rheumatism* 60, no. 1 (2009): 73-80.

500. Raymond EG and Grimes DA. "The Comparative Safety of Legal Induced Abortion and Childbirth in the United States." *Obstetrics & Gynecology* 119, no. 2 (February 2012): 215-19.

501. Reardon DC and Coleman PK. "Short and Long Term Mortality Rates Associated with First Pregnancy Outcome: Population Register Based Study for Denmark 1980-2004." *Medical Science Monitor* 18, no. 9 (2012): PH71-6.

502. Reardon DC and Cougle JR. "Depression and Unintended Pregnancy in the National Longitudinal Survey of Youth: A Cohort Study."*BMJ* 324, no. 7330 (January 2002):151-2.

503. Reardon DC and Ney P. "Abortion and Subsequent Substance Abuse."*American Journal of Drug and Alcohol Abuse* 26, no. 1 (February 2000): 61-75.

504. Reardon DC, Ney PG, Scheurer FJ, Congle JR and Coleman PK. "Suicide Deaths Associated with Pregnancy Outcome: A Record Linkage Study of 172,279 Low Income American Women." *Archives of Women's Mental Health* 3, Supplement 2 (2001): 104.

505. Reardon DC. "Report Misses Association of Violence with Pregnancy" (Letter in response to "Violence as a Public Health Problem," by Jonathan Shepherd). *BMJ* 326, no. 7380(11 January 2003): 104.
506. Rees H, Katzenellenbogen J, Shabodien R, et al. "The Epidemiology of Incomplete Abortion in South Africa: National Incomplete Abortion Reference Group." *South African Medical Journal* 87, no. 4 (April 1997): 432-7.
507. *Reibl v. Hughes*, [1980] 2 S.C.R. 880.
508. Reinhard SC. "Burden Assessment Scale for Families of the Seriously Mentally Ill."*Evaluation and Program Planning* 17, no. 2 (1994): 261-9.
509. Reissman CK. "Strategic Uses of Narrative in the Presentation of Self and Illness: A Research Note." *Social Science & Medicine* 30, no. 11(1990): 1195–200.
510. Renker PR. "Keep a Blank Face. I Need to Tell You What Has been Happening to Me." *American Journal of Maternal Child Nursing* 27, no. 2 (March-April 2002): 109-16.
511. Renner RM, Jensen JT, Nichols MD and Edelman AB. "Pain Control in First-Trimester Surgical Abortion: A Systematic Review of Randomized Controlled Trials." *Contraception* 81, no. 5 (May 2010): 372-88.
512. Remennick LI. "Reproductive Patterns and Cancer Incidence in Women: A Population Based Correlation Study in the USSR." *International Journal of Epidemiology* 18, no.3 (989): 498-510.
513. Ring-Cassidy E and Gentles I, eds. *Women's Health after Abortion: The Medical and Psychological Evidence*. 2nd ed. Toronto: deVeber Institute for Bioethics and Social Research, 2003.
514. Robinson G, Stotland N and Nadelson. "RE: Abortion and Mental Health: Quantitative Synthesis and Analysis of Research Published 1995-2009." (Letter). *British Journal of Psychiatry*. 22 September, 2011. http://bjp.rcpsych.org/content/199/3/180.abstract/reply.
515. Robinson GE, Stotland NL, Russo NF, Lang JA and Occhiogrosso M. "Is There an 'Abortion Trauma Syndrome'? Critiquing the Evidence."*Harvard Review of Psychiatry* 17, no. 4 (2009): 268-90.
516. Rohan TE, McMichael AJ and Baghurst PA. "A Population-Based Case-Control Study of Diet and Breast Cancer in Australia." *American Journal of Epidemiology* 128, no. 3 (1988): 478-89.
517. Rookus MA and van Leeuwen FE. "Induced Abortion and Risk for Breast Cancer: Reporting (Recall) Bias in a Dutch Case-Control Study." *Journal of the National Cancer Institute* 88, no. 23 (1996): 1759-64.
518. Rooney B and Calhoun BC. "Induced Abortion and Risk of Later Preterm Births." *Journal of the American Physicians and Surgeons* 8, no. 2 (2003): 46-9.
519. Rooney B, Calhoun BC and Roche LE. "Does Induced Abortion Account for Racial Disparity in Preterm Births, and Violate the Nuremberg Code?" *Journal of American Physicians and Surgeons* 13, no. 4 (2008): 102-4.
520. Rose NR and Mackay IR, eds. *The Autoimmune Diseases*, 3rd ed. San Diego: Academic Press, 1998.

521. Rosenburg L. "Induced Abortion and Breast Cancer: More Scientific Data are Needed." *Journal of the National Cancer Institute* 86, no. 21 (2 November, 1994): 1569-70.

522. Rosenberg L, Palmer JR, Laufman DW, Strom BL, Schottenfeld D and Shapiro S. "Breast Cancer in Relation to the Occurrence and Time of Induced and Spontaneous Abortion." *American Journal of Epidemiology* 127, no. 5 (1988): 981-9.

523. Royal College of Obstetricians and Gynaecologists (RCOG). *The Care Of Women Requesting Induced Abortion: Evidence-Based Clinical Guideline* 7. London: RCOG Press, 2000; September 2004; November 2011. http://www.rcog.org.uk/files/rcog corp/Abortion%20guideline_web_1.pdf.

524. Ruiz-Rodríguez M, Wirtz VJ and Nigenda G. "Organizational Elements of Health Service Related to a Reduction in Maternal Mortality: The Cases of Chile and Colombia."*Health Policy* 90, no. 2/3 (November 2009): 149-55.

525. Russo J, Balogh GA and Russo IH. "Full-Term Pregnancy Induces A Specific Genomic Signature in the Human Breast." *Cancer Epidemiology, Biomarkers, & Prevention* 17, no. 1 (January 2008): 51-66.

526. Russo J, Hu YF, Yang X and Russo IH. "Chapter 1: Development, Cellular, and Molecular Basis of Human Breast Cancer."*Journal of the National Cancer Institute Monograph* 27 (2000): 17-37.

527. Russo J, Lynch H and Russo IH. "Mammary Gland Architecture as a Determining Factor in the Susceptibility of the Human Breast to Cancer." *The Breast Journal* 7, no. 5 (2001): 278-91.

528. Russo J, Rivera R and Russo IH. "Influence of Age and Parity on Development of the Human Breast." *Breast Cancer Research Treatment* 23 (1992): 211-18.

529. Russo J and Russo IH. "Susceptibility of the Mammary Gland to Carcinogenesis." *American Journal of Pathology* 100, no. 2 (1980): 497-512.

530. Sahni M, Verma N, Narula D, Varghese RM, Sreenivas V and Puliyel JM. "Missing Girls in India: Infanticide, Feticide and Made-to-Order Pregnancies? Insights from Hospital-Based Sex-Ratio-at-Birth over the Last Century." *PLoS ONE* 3, no. 5 (2008): e2224. http://www.plosone.org/article/fetchObject.action?uri=info%3Adoi%2F10.1371%2Fjournal.pone.0002224&representation=PDF.

531. Sarkar K and Miller FW. "Possible Roles and Determinants of Microchimerism in Autoimmune and Other Disorders."*Autoimmunity Reviews* 3, no. 6 (2004): 453-63.

532. Saunders C, ed. *The Management of Malignant Disease Series*. London: Edward Arnold, 1978.

533. Sawaya GF, Grady D, Kerlikowske K and Grimes DA. "Antibiotics at the Time of Induced Abortion: The Case for Universal Prophylaxis Based on a Meta-Analysis." *Obstetrics & Gynecology* 87, no. 5, part 2 (1996): 884-990.

534. Saxton M. "Disability Rights and Selective Abortion." In *Abortion Wars, A Half Century of Struggle: 1950 to 2000*. Ed., Rickie Solinger. Berkeley, CA: University of California Press, 1998.

535. Schenker JG. "Etiology of and Therapeutic Approach to Synechia Uteri." *European Journal of Obstetrics and Gynecology and Reproductive Biology* 65, no. 1 (March 1996): 109-13.

536. Schiff MA and Grossman DC. "Adverse Perinatal Outcomes and Risk of Postpartum Suicide Attempt in Washington State, 1987–2001." *Pediatrics* 118, no. 3 (September 2006): e669–75.

537. Schreiner-Engel P, Walther VN, Mindes J, Lynch L and Berkowitz RL. "First-Trimester Multi-Fetal Pregnancy Reduction: Acute and Persistent Psychologic Reactions." *AJOG* 172, no. 2 (Part 1) (February 1995): 541-7.

538. Schuberg K. "Abortion Ban Does Not Mean More Maternal Deaths, Chilean Study Finds." *CNSNews.com*, 1 March 2010.http://cnsnews.com/news/article/abortion-ban-does-not-mean-more-maternal-deaths-chilean-study-finds.

539. Schuller V and Stupkova E. "The Unwanted Child in the Family." *International Mental Health Research Newsletter* 14, no. 3 (Fall 1972): 2-16.

540. Seavilleklein V. "Challenging the Rhetoric of Choice in Prenatal Screening." Ph.D. Dissertation. Halifax, NS: Dalhousie University,2008.

541. Sedgh G, Henshaw SK, Singh S, Bankole A and Drescher J. "Legal Abortion Worldwide: Incidence and Recent Trends." *IFPP* 33, no. 3 (2007): 106-16.

542. Segi M, Fukushima I, Fujisaku S, et al. "An Epidemiological Study of Cancer in Japan." *GANN* 48 (1957): 1-43.

543. Sen A. "Does Increased Abortion Lead to Lower Crime? Evaluating the Relationship between Crime, Abortion, and Fertility." *B.E. Journal of Economic Analysis and Policy* 7, no. 1(September 2007): Article 48, 1-36.

544. ———."More Than 100 Million Women Are Missing." *New York Times*, 20 December 1990. http://www.nybooks.com/articles/archives/1990/dec/20/more-than-100-million-women-are-missing/.

545. Sentilhes L, Audibert F, Dommerques M, Descamps P, Frydman R and Mahieu-Caputo D. "Multifetal Pregnancy Reduction: Indications, Technical Aspects and Psychological Impact." *Presse Medicale* 37, no. 2 (part 2) (2008): 295-306.

546. Shah PS and Zao J. "Induced Termination of Pregnancy and Low Birthweight and Preterm Birth: A Systematic Review and Meta-Analyses."*BJOG: An International Journal of Obstetrics & Gynaecology* 116, no. 11 (May 2009): 1425-42.

547. Shalev J, Meizner I, Rabinerson D, et al. "Improving Pregnancy Outcome in Twin Gestations with One Malformed Fetus by Postponing Selective Feticide in the Third Trimester." *Fertility and Sterility* 72, no. 2 (1999): 257-60.

548. Shannon C, Brothers LP, Philip NM and Winikoff B. "Ectopic Pregnancy and Medical Abortion." *Obstetrics and Gynecology* 104, no. 1 (2004): 161-7.

549. Shaver J. *Gianna: Aborted…and Lived to Tell about It*. Colorado Springs, CO: Focus on the Family Publishing, 1995.

550. Shaw M."Airbrushing Away Diversity."Ottawa Citizen, 2 March, 2008. http://www.canada.com/ottawacitizen/news/story.html?id=7ef9c418-70c1-49cc-bbbf-cb1ae997b326.

551. Sheiner E, Shoham-Vardi I, Hallak M, Hershkowitz R, Katz M and Mazor M. "Placenta Previa: Obstetric Risk Factors and Pregnancy Outcome." *Journal of Maternal-Fetal Medicine* 10, no. 6 (December 2001): 414-19.

552. Shevell MI. "Eugenics by Another Name?" *Canadian Journal of Neurological Science* 34, no. 4 (November 2007): 494-5.

553. Skotko BG. "Prenatally Diagnosed Down Syndrome: Mothers Who Continued Their Pregnancies Evaluate their Health Care Providers." *AJOG* 192, no. 3 (2005): 670-7.
554. SickKids. "First in Canada: Baby has Heart Procedure While Inside her Mother's Womb and is Now Doing Fine." 2009. http://www.sickkids.ca/AboutSickKids/News-Room/Past-News/2009/first-in-canada.html.
555. Sik Yau Kan A, Caves N, Yuen Wai Wong S, Hung Yu Ng E and Chung Ho P. "A Double-Blind, Randomized Controlled Trial on the Use of a 50:50 Mixture of Nitrous Oxide/Oxygen in Pain Relief During Suction Evacuation for the First Trimester Pregnancy Termination." *Human Reproduction* 21, no. 10 (October 2006): 2606-11.
556. Sik Yau Kan A, Hung Yu Ng E and Chung Ho P. "The Role and Comparison of Two Techniques of Paracervical Block for Pain Relief During Suction Evacuation for First-Trimester Pregnancy Termination." *Contraception* 70, no. 2 (August 2004): 159-63.
557. Silverman JG, Decker MR, McCauley HL, et al. "Male Perpetration of Intimate Partner Violence and Involvement in Abortions and Abortion-Related Conflict." *American Journal of Public Health* 100, no. 8 (2010): 1415-17.
558. Singh RH, Ghanem KG, Burke AE, Nichols MD, Rogers K and Blumenthal PD. "Predictors and Perception of Pain in Women Undergoing First Trimester Surgical Abortion." *Contraception* 78, no. 2 (August 2008): 155-61.
559. Singh S. "Hospital Admissions Resulting from Unsafe Abortion: Estimates from 13 Developing Countries." *The Lancet* 368, no. 9550 (November 2006): 1887-92.
560. Singh S, Prada E, Mirembe F and Kiggundu C. "The Incidence of Induced Abortion in Uganda." *IFPP* 31, no. 4 (December 2005): 183-91.
561. Slater PE, Davies AM and Harlap S. "The Effect of Abortion Method on the Outcome of Subsequent Pregnancy." *Journal of Reproductive Medicine* 26, no. 3 (March 1981): 123-8.
562. Smith C, Bush J and Sutija VG. "Adverse Obstetric History and Ectopic Pregnancy." *Journal of Reproductive Medicine* 52, no. 9 (2007): 801-4.
563. Smith CD, Carlin EM, Heason J, Liu TY, Jushuf IA and Hammond RH. "Genital Infection and Termination of Pregnancy: Are Patients Still At Risk?" *The Journal of Family Planning and Reproductive Health Care* 27, no. 2 (April 2001): 81-4.
564. Somerville M. "Consultation sur le dépistage prenatal du syndrome de down menée par le comissaire à la santé et au bien-être" ("Consultation on Prenatal Screening for Down Syndrome Conducted by the Commissioner for Health and Well-Being"). [Written Submission]. *Commissaire à la santé et au bien-être*. Montréal : Ministère de la Santé et des Services Sociaux du Québec, 2008.
565. Sørensen JL, Thranov I, Hoff G, Dirach J and Damsgaard MT. "A Double-Blind Randomized Study of the Effect of Erythromycin in Preventing Pelvic Inflammatory Disease after First-Trimester Abortion." *BJOG* 99, no. 5 (May 1992): 434-8.
566. Sørenson SB, Wiebe DJ and Berk RA. "Legalized Abortion and the Homicide of Young Children: An Empirical Investigation." *Analyses of Social Issues and Public Policy* 2, no. 1 (December 2002): 239-56.
567. Souter I and Goodwin TM. "Decision-making in Multifetal Pregnancy Reduction for Triplets." *American Journal of Perinatology* 15, no. 1 (January 1998): 63-71.

568. South Carolina Legislature. "Section 44: Health; Chapter 41: Abortions; Article I: Abortions Generally; Section 44-41-10: Definitions." *South Carolina Code of Laws*. Unannotated Online Edition. http://www.scstatehouse.gov/code/title44.php.

569. South Dakota Task Force to Study Abortion. *Report of The South Dakota Task Force to Study Abortion*. Submitted to the Governor and Legislature of South Dakota, December 2005: 1-71. www.dakotavoice.com/Docs/South%20Dakota%20Abortion%20Task%20Force%20Report.pdf.

570. Speckhard A and Rue V. "Complicated Mourning: Dynamics of Impacted Post Abortion." *Pre- and Perinatal Psychology Journal* 8, no. 1 (October 1993): 5-32.

571. Statistics Canada. *Canadian Socio-economic Information Management System (CANSIM)*. Database. Government of Canada: Statistics Canada. http://www5.statcan.gc.ca/cansim/. "Table 75-001: Estimated Population of Canada, 1605 to Present."

572. — — — ."Table 051-005: Estimates of Population, Canada, Provinces and Territories, Quarterly (Persons). "*CANSIM*. Government of Canada. Accessed 26 September, 2012.http://www5.statcan.gc.ca/cansim/a26?lang=eng&retrLang=eng&id=0510005&tabMode=dataTable&srchLan=-1&p1=-1&p2=9.

573. — — — . "Table 106-9005: Induced Abortions in Hospitals and Clinics, by Area of Report and Type of Facility Performing the Abortion Canada, Provinces and Territories, Annual (Number)." Government of Canada: *CANSIM* database. Accessed June 2012.http://www5.statcan.gc.ca/cansim/a26?lang=eng&retrLang=eng&id=1069005&pattern=abortion&tabMode=dataTable&srchLan=-1&p1=1&p2=1.

574. Steinbock B. "Sex Selection: Not Obviously Wrong." *Hastings Center Report* 32, no. 1 (January-February 2002): 23-8.

575. Steinburg L. "A Social Neuroscience Perspective on Adolescent Risk-Taking." *Development Review* 28, no. 1 (March 2008). Study 1: 78-106.

576. Stevens A and Nelson JL. "Maternal and Fetal Microchimerism: Implications for Human Diseases." *NeoReviews* 3, no. 1 (1 January, 2002): e11-e19.

577. Stevens PE. "Marginalized Women's Access to Health Care: A Feminist Narrative Analysis."*ANS. Advances in Nursing Science* 16, vol. 2 (December 1993): 39-56.

578. Stone J, Belogolovkin V, Matho A, Berkowitz RL, Moshier E and Eddleman K. "Evolving Trends in 2000 Cases of Multifetal Pregnancy Reduction: A Single-Center Experience." *AJOG* 197, no. 4 (October 2007): 394.e1-4.

579. Stone J, Ferrara L, Kamrath J, et al. "Contemporary Outcomes with the Latest 1000 Cases of Multifetal Pregnancy Reduction (MPR)." *AJOG* 199, no. 4 (October 2008): 406.e1-4.

580. Strahan TW. "Studies Suggesting That Induced Abortion May Increase the Feminization of Poverty." *Studies in Pro-Life Feminism* 1, no. 3 (1995): 235-47.

581. Suliman S, Ericksen T, Labuschgne P, de Wit R, Stein DJ and Seedat S. "Comparison of Pain, Cortisol Levels, and Psychological Distress in Women Undergoing Surgical Termination of Pregnancy Under Local Anaesthesia versus Intravenous Sedation." *BMC Psychiatry* 7, no. 24 (June 2007): 24-32.

582. Sullins P. "Abortion and Family Formation: Circumstance or Culture?" In *Life and Learning XIII: Proceedings of Thirteenth University Faculty for Life Conference,2003*, ed. Joseph Koterski, S.J. Washington, D.C.: University Faculty for Life, 2004: 31-64.http://uffl.org/vol13/sullins03.pdf.

583. Summers AM, Langlois S, Wyatt P, Wilson RD and Society of Obstetricians and Gynaecologists of Canada. "Prenatal Screening for Fetal Aneuploidy." *JOGC* 29, no. 2 (February 2007): 146-79.

584. Sun Y, Che Y, Gao E, Olsen J and Zhou W. "Induced Abortion and Risk for Subsequent Miscarriage." *International Journal of Epidemiology* 32, no. 3 (June 2003): 449-54.

585. Suter SM. "Genetics and the Law: The Ethical, Legal and Social Implications of Genetic Technology and Biomedical Ethics: Sex Selection, Non-Directiveness and Equality." *University of Chicago Law School Round Table* 473, no. 34 (1996).

586. ———."Sex Selection, Nondirectiveness, and Equality." *University of Chicago Law School Roundtable* 3, no. 2 (1996): 473-89.

587. Sutkin G, Capelle SD, Schlievert PM and Creinin MD. "Toxic Shock Syndrome after Laminaria Insertion."*Obstetrics and Gynecology* 98, no. 5 (Part 2) (November 2001): 959-61.

588. Swingle HM, Colaizy TT, Zimmerman MB and Morriss FH. "Abortion and the Risk of Subsequent Preterm Birth: A Systematic Review with Meta-analyses." *The Journal of Reproductive Medicine* 54, no. 2 (February 2009): 95-108.

589. Sykes P. "Complications of Termination of Pregnancy: A Retrospective Study of Admissions to Christchurch Women's Hospital 1989 and 1990." *New Zealand Medical Journal* 106, no. 951 (March 10, 1993): 83-5.

590. Tabsh KM. "A Report of 131 Cases of Multifetal Pregnancy Reduction." *Obstetrics & Gynecology* 82, no. 1 (July 1993): 57-60.

591. Taft AJ and Watson LF. "Termination of Pregnancy: Associations with Partner Violence and Other Factors in a National Cohort of Young Australian Women." *Australian and New Zealand Journal of Public Health* 31, no. 2 (April 2007): 135-42.

592. Talamini R, Franceschi S, La Vecchia C, et al. "The Role of Reproductive and Menstrual Factors in Cancer of the Breast Before and After Menopause." *European Journal of Cancer* 32A, no. 2 (February 1996): 303-10.

593. Tang OS, Thong KJ, and Baird DT. "Second Trimester Medical Abortion with Mifepristone and Gemeprost: A Review of 956 Cases."*Contraception* 64, no. 1 (July 2001): 29-32.

594. Tang OS, Xu J, Cheng L, Lee SW and Ho PC. "Pilot Study on the Use of Sublingual Misoprostol with Mifepristone in Termination of First Trimester Pregnancy to 9 Weeks Gestation."*Human Reproduction* 17, no. 7 (July 2002): 1738-40.

595. Taylor BD and Haggerty CL. "Management of *Chlamydia Trachomatis* Genital Tract Infection: Screening and Treatment Challenges."*Infection and Drug Resistance* 4 (2011): 19-29.

596. Taylor VM, Kramer MD, Vaughan TL and Peacock S. "Placenta Previa in Relation to Induced and Spontaneous Abortion: A Population-Based Study." *Obstetrics and Gynecology* 82, no. 1 (July 1993): 88-91.

597. Tennessee Code. 39-15-202.
598. Tenore JL. "Ectopic Pregnancy." *American Family Physician* 61, no. 4 (February 2000): 1080-8.
599. Tharaux-Deneux C, Bouyer J, Job-Spira N, Coste J and Spira A. "Risk of Ectopic Pregnancy and Previous Induced Abortion." *American Journal of Public Health* 88, no. 3 (March 1998): 401-5.
600. Thiele AT and Leier B. "Towards an Ethical Policy for the Prevention of Fetal Sex Selection in Canada." *JOGC* 32, no. 1 (January 2010): 54-7.
601. Thonneau P, Fougeyrollas B, Ducot B, et al. "Complications of Abortion Performed Under Local Anesthesia." *European Journal of Obstetrics and Gynecology and Reproductive Biology* 81, no. 1 (October 1998): 59-63.
602. Thorn V. "Project Rachel: Faith in Action, A Ministry of Compassion and Caring." In *Post-Abortion Aftermath*, ed. Mannion M. Kansas City, MO: Sheed and Ward, 1994: 144-63.
603. Thorp JM, Hartmann KE and Shadigian E. "Long-Term Physical and Psychological Health Consequences of Induced Abortion: Review of the Evidence." *Obstetrical & Gynecological Survey* 58, no. 1 (January 2002): 67-79.
604. Torres-Sánchez L, López-Carrillo L, Espinoza H and Langer A. "Is Induced Abortion a Contributing Factor to Tubal Infertility in Mexico? Evidence from a Case-Control Study." *BJOG: International Journal of Obstetrics and Gynaecology* 111, no. 11 (November 2004): 1254-60.
605. Thorsén C, Aneblom G and Gemzell-Danielsson K. "Perceptions of Contraception, Non-Protection and Induced Abortion Among a Sample of Urban Swedish Teenage Girls: Focus Group Discussions." *European Journal of Contraception & Reproductive Health Care* 11, no. 4 (December 2006): 302-9.
606. Trott E, Ziegler W and Levey J. "Major Complications Associated with Termination of a Second Trimester Pregnancy: A Case Report." *Delaware Medical Journal* 67, no. 5 (May 1995): 294-6.
607. Tzonou A, Hsieh CC, Trichopoulos D, et al. "Induced Abortions, Miscarriages, and Tobacco Smoking as Risk Factors for Secondary Infertility." *Journal of Epidemiology and Community Health* 47, no. 1 (February 1993): 36-9.
608. Uganda Bureau of Statistics (UBOS) and Macro International Inc. *Uganda Demographic and Health Survey 2006*. Calverton, Maryland, USA: UBOS and Macro International Inc., 2007.
609. Unchoice Campaign. "Portraits of Coercion: America's Silent Epidemic." Elliot Institute: The UnChoice.com, 2006. http://theunchoice.com/pdf/FactSheets/PortraitsOfCoercion.pdf.
610. UNICEF Regional Office for CEECIS. "Country Profiles." *Transformative Monitoring for Enhanced Equity (TransMonEE) 2012 Database*. http://www.unicef-irc.org/databases/transmonee/2007/Country_profiles.xls.
611. ———. *Transformative Monitoring for Enhanced Equity (TransMonEE) 2012 Database*. http://www.transmonee.org/index.html.

612. UNICEF. *The State of the World's Children 2007: Women and Children – The Double Dividend of Gender Equality*. New York, NY: UNICEF, December 2006. http://www.unicef.org/sowc07/docs/sowc07.pdf.

613. –––. *The State of the World's Children 2009: Maternal and Newborn Health*. New York, NY: UNICEF, December 2008. http://www.unicef.org/sowc09/docs/SOWC09-FullReport-EN.pdf.

614. United Nations Population Division, Department of Economic and Social Affairs. "Abortion Policies: A Global Review." 2002. http://www.un.org/esa/population/publications/abortion/doc/italy.doc.

615. United Nations Population Fund (UNFPA). *Delivering on the Promise of Equality: UNFPA's Strategic Framework for Gender Mainstreaming and Women's Empowerment 2008-2011*. New York, NY: UNFPA, 2008. https://www.unfpa.org/webdav/site/global/shared/documents/publications/2007/gender_report_2007.pdf.

616. United Nations Statistics Division. "Table 12: Live Births by Gestational Age: 1990-1998." *United Nations Demographic Yearbook: Focusing on Natality (1999)*. New York, NY: UNSD. http://unstats.un.org/unsd/demographic/products/dyb/DYBNat/NatStatTab12.pdf.

617. United States Conference of Catholic Bishops (USCCB), Committee on Clergy, Consecrated Life, and Vocations. *Project Rachel Ministry: A Post-Abortion Resource Manual for Priests and Project Rachel Leaders*. Washington, DC: USCCB, 2009.

618. Unnithan-Kumar M. "Female Selective Abortion—Beyond 'Culture': Family Making and Gender Inequality in a Globalising India." *Culture, Health & Sexuality* 12, no. 2 (February 2010): 153-66.

619. Vatten LJ, Romundstad PR, Trichopoulos D and Skjaerven R. "Pregnancy Related Protection Against Breast Cancer Depends on Length of Gestation." *British Journal of Cancer* 87, no. 3 (July 2002): 289-90.

620. Verhoeve HR, Steures P, Flierman PA, van der Veen F and Mol BW. "History of Induced Abortion and the Risk of Tubal Pathology." *Reproductive BioMedicine Online* 16, no. 2 (February 2008): 304-7.

621. Verlinden I, Güngör N, Wouters K, Janssens J, Raus J and Michiels L. "Parity-Induced Changes in Global Gene Expression in the Human Mammary Gland." *European Journal of Cancer Prevention* 14, no. 2 (April 2005): 129-37.

622. Vietnamese Ministry of Health. *A Strategic Assessment of Policy, Programme and Research Issues Relating to Abortion in Vietnam: A Draft Report*. Hanoi, Vietnam: Author, 1997.

623. Vogel L. "Sex Selection Migrates to Canada." *CMAJ* 184, no. 3 (21 February, 2012): e163-4.

624. Vos T, Astbury J, Piers LS, et al. "Measuring the Impact of Intimate Partner Violence on the Health of Women in Victoria, Australia." *Bulletin of the World Health Organization* 84, no. 9 (September 2006): 739-44.

625. Wachbroit R and Wasserman D. "Patient Autonomy and Value-Neutrality in Nondirective Genetic Counseling." *Stanford Law & Policy Review* 6, no. 2 (Spring 1995): 103-11.

626. Wadhera S and Millar WJ. "Second Trimester Abortions: Trends and Medical Complications."*Health Reports* 6, no. 4 (1994): 441-54.
627. Wahlberg D. "Study: Breast Cancer Not Tied to Abortion." *Atlanta Journal Constitution*, 26 March, 2004.
628. *Wallace v Planned Parenthood, Southwest Ohio Region et al.* (2007). Hamilton Co., No. A0502691 (Ohio Ct Com Pl, Civ Div).
629. Ware M. *Peer Review: Benefits, Perspectives and Alternatives*(PRC Summary Papers).London, UK: Publishing Research Consortium (PRC). www.publishingresearch.net/documents/PRCsummary4Warefinal.pdf
630. White E, Daling JR, Norsted TL and Chu J. "Rising Incidence of Breast Cancer Among Young Women in Washington State." *Journal of the National Cancer Institute* 79, no. 2 (August 1987): 239-43.
631. Wiebe ER and Janssen P. "Universal Screening for Domestic Violence in Abortion." *Women's Health Issues* 11, no. 5 (September-October 2001): 436-41.
632. Wilkerson DS, Volpe AG, Dean RS and Titus JB. "Perinatal Complications as Predictors of Infantile Autism." *International Journal of Neuroscience* 112, no. 9 (September 2002): 1085-98.
633. Williams CM, Larson U and McCloskey LA. "Intimate Partner Violence and Women's Contraceptive Use." *Violence Against Women* 14, no. 12 (December 2008): 1382-96.
634. Williams GB and Brackley MH. "Intimate Partner Violence, Pregnancy and the Decision for Abortion." *Issues in Mental Health Nursing* 30, no. 4 (April 2009): 272-8.
635. Wilson BK and Haynie L. "Experiences of Women Who Seek Recovery Assistance Following an Elective Abortion: A Grounded Theory Approach." Doctor of Nursing Science (DNS)Dissertation, Louisiana State University Health Sciences Center School of Nursing,2004.
636. Wilson JT. "Mourning the Unborn Dead: American Uses of Japanese Buddhist Post-Abortion Rituals." PhD Dissertation [Unpublished], University of North Carolina at Chapel Hill, 2007.
637. Winikoff B, Sivin I, Coyaji K, et al. "Safety, Efficacy, and Acceptability of Medical Abortion in China, Cuba, and India: A Comparative Trial of Mifepristone-Misoprostol Versus Surgical Abortion."*AJOG* 176, no. 2 (February 1996): 431-7.
638. wiseGeek.com. "What is a Personal Affidavit?" Sparks, North Virginia: Conjecture Corporation, 2003-2013. www.wisegeek.com/what-is-a-personal-affidavit.htm.
639. Wong CYG, Ng EHY, Ngai SW and Ho PC. "A Randomized, Double Blind, Placebo-Controlled Study to Investigate the Use of Conscious Sedation in Conjunction with Paracervical Block for Reducing Pain In Termination of First Trimester Pregnancy by Suction Evacuation." *Human Reproduction* 17, no.5 (May 2002): 1222-5.
640. Woo J, Fine P and Goetzl L. "Abortion Disclosure and the Association with Domestic Violence." *Obstetrics and Gynecology* 105, no. 6 (June 2005): 1329-34.
641. World Bank."Promoting and Monitoring Gender Equality and Empowerment of Women." *Global Monitoring Report: Confronting the Challenges of Gender Equality and Fragile States.* Washington, DC: The World Bank, 2007: 105-38.

642. World Health Organization, Department of Reproductive Health and Research. *Unsafe Abortion: Global and Regional Estimates of Incidence of Unsafe Abortion and Associated Mortality in 2008*, 6th ed. Geneva: World Health Organization, 2011.

643. World Health Organization. *European Health for all Database* (HFA-DB). Copenhagen: Regional Office for Europe, January 2011.

644. ———. *Maternal Mortality in 2000: Estimates by UNICEF, WHO, & UNFPA*. Geneva: Department of Reproductive Health & Research. 2004.

645. ———. "Maternal Mortality Ratio (Per 100 000 Live Births)." *Health Statistics and Health Information Systems*. http://www.who.int/healthinfo/statistics/indmaternalmortality/en/index.html.

646. World Health Organization (WHO), Regional Office for Africa. *MPS: Making Pregnancy Safer: Implementing the MPS Initiative in Soroti District, Uganda*. Kampala, Uganda: WHO – Uganda, 2010. http://www.afro.who.int/en/downloads/cat_view/1501-english/969-countries/1015-uganda/1437-best-practise-reports.html.

647. Wright VC, Chang J, Jeng G and Macaluso M. "Assisted Reproductive Technology Surveillance - United States, 2003." *Division of Reproductive Health National Center for Chronic Disease Prevention and Health Promotion* 55, no. SS04 (26 May, 2006): 1-22. http://www.cdc.gov/mmwr/preview/mmwrhtml/ss5504a1.htm.

648. Xing P, Li J and Jin F. "A Case-Control Study of Reproductive Factors Associated with Subtypes of Breast Cancer in Northeast China." *Medical Oncology* 27, no. 3 (September 2010): 926-31.

649. Yamaguchi K and Kandel D. "Drug Use and Other Determinants of Premarital Pregnancy and Its Outcome: A Dynamic Analysis of Competing Life Events." *Journal of Marriage and the Family* 49 (May 1987): 257-70.

650. Yanhua C, Geater A, You J, et al. "Reproductive Variables and Risk of Breast Malignant and Benign Tumours in Yunnan Province, China." *Asian Pacific Journal of Cancer Prevention* 13, no. 5 (2012): 2179-84.

651. Yan Z, Lambert NC, Guthrie KA, et al. "Male Microchimerism in Women without Sons: Quantitative Assessment and Correlation with Pregnancy History." *American Journal of Medicine* 118, no. 8 (August 2005): 899-906.

652. Yassin KM. "Incidence and Socioeconomic Determinants of Abortion in Rural Upper Egypt." *Public Health* 114, no. 4 (July 2000): 269-72.

653. Yilmaz Z, Sahin FI, Bulakbasi, Yüregir OO, Tarim E and Yanik F. "Ethical Considerations Regarding Parental Decisions for Termination Following Prenatal Diagnosis of Sex Chromosome Abnormalities." *Genetic Counseling* 19, no. 3 (2008): 345-52.

654. Yimin C, Shouging L, Arzhu Q, et al. "Sexual Coercion Among Adolescent Women Seeking Abortion in China." *Journal of Adolescent Health* 31, no. 6 (December 2002): 482-6.

655. Yu D, Li TC, Xia E, Huang X, Liu Y and Peng X. "Factors Affecting Reproductive Outcome of Hysteroscopicadhesiolysis for Asherman's Syndrome." *Fertility and Sterility* 89, no. 3 (March 2008): 715-22.

656. Yu D, Wong YM, Cheong Y, Xia E and Li TC. "Asherman Syndrome – One Century Later." *Fertility and Sterility* 89, no. 4 (April 2008): 759-79.

657.   Zambri B. *Hope in Turmoil*. 3rd ed. Mississauga, 2013.
658.   Zaridze DG. 1988. Unpublished study. *In* Andrieu N, Duffy SW, Rohan TE, et al. "Familial Risk, Abortion and Their Interactive Effect on the Risk of Breast Cancer — A Combined Analysis of Six Case-Control Studies." *British Journal of Cancer* 72, no. 3 (September 1995): 744-51.
659.   Zeng Y, Xu M, Tan S and Yin L. "Analysis of the Risk Factors of Breast Cancer." Translated from the Chinese. *Nan Fang Yi Ke Da Xue Xue Bao* 30, no. 3 (2010): 622-3.
660.   Zhang RJ, Zhang XJ, Lu XJ, et al. "Study on the Correlation Between Induced Abortion and Reproductive Tract Infections." Translated from the Chinese. *Zhonghua Liu Xing Bing Xue Za Zhi* 32, no. 1 (January 2011): 29-32.
661.   Zhou C, Wang XL, Zhou XD and Hesketh T. "Son Preference and Sex-Selective Abortion in China: Informing Policy Options." *International Journal of Public Health* 57, no. 3 (June 2012): 459-65.
662.   Zhou XD, Li L, Yan Z and Hesketh T. "High Sex Ratio as a Correlate of Depression in Chinese Men." *Journal of Affective Disorders* 144, no. 1-2 (January 2013): 79-86.
663.   Zhou W, Gao E, Che Y and Olsen J. "Induced Abortion and Duration of Third Stage of Labour in a Subsequent Pregnancy." *Journal of Obstetrics and Gynaecology* 19, no. 4 (July 1999): 349-54.
664.   Zhou W, Nielsen GL, Møller M and Olsen J. "Short-Term Complications after Surgically Induced Abortion: A Register-Based Study of 56 117 Abortions."*Acta Obstetricia et Gynecologica Scandinavica* 81, no. 4 (April 2002): 331-6.
665.   Zhou W and Olsen J. "Are Complications After an Induced Abortion Associated with Reproductive Failures in a Subsequent Pregnancy?"*Acta Obstetricia et Gynecologica Scandinavica* 82, no. 2 (February 2003):177-81.
666.   Zhou W, Olsen J, Nielsen GL and Sabroe W. "Risk of Spontaneous Abortion Following Induced Abortion is Only Increased with Short Interpregnancy Interval." *Journal of Obstetrics and Gynaecology* 20, no. 1 (January 2000): 49-54.
667.   Zhu WX, Li L and Hesketh T. "China's Excess Males, Sex Selective Abortion, and One Child Policy: Analysis of Data from 2005 National Intercensus Survey." *BMJ* 338 (9 April 2009): b1211.
668.   Zlatnik FJ, Burmeister LF, Feddersen DA and Brown RC. "Radiological Appearance of the Upper Cervical Canal in Women with a History of Premature Delivery. II. Relationship to Clinical Presentation and to Tests of Cervical Compliance." *Journal of Reproductive Medicine* 34, no. 8 (August 1989): 525-30

Glossary

Abortion: the termination of pregnancy with the death of the embryo or fetus.
A **spontaneous** abortion is the unintended delivery and death of a child in utero with a gestational age younger than 24 weeks, known as a 'miscarriage.'
An **induced** abortion is the intentional termination of pregnancy and death of the child in utero either by surgical or medical means.
Medical abortions: abortions induced using a combination of medicines.
Surgical abortions: the most common form of induced abortions, using surgical instruments such as a curette or suction device (aspirator) depending on the stage of pregnancy.
Late term abortion: one performed at or after twenty weeks gestation; generally refers to the abortion of a baby that has reached the age of viability by means that ensure that the baby is dead at the time of birth.

adhesions: strands of scar tissue that are attached to internal organs.

affirmative duty of disclosure: the fiduciary duty of a physician to discuss with a patient both the positive and negative side effects and outcomes of a medical or surgical intervention or investigation.

amniocentesis: a procedure in which amniotic fluid is removed from the uterus of a pregnant mother for testing or treatment. A genetic amniocentesis analyzes the chromosomes within the fetal cells to determine whether there is an abnormality.

amniotic fluid: the fluid that surrounds and protects a fetus during pregnancy. This fluid contains fetal cells and various proteins produced by the fetus.

analgesia: medication that relieves pain.

Asherman's Syndrome: intra-uterine adhesions (scar tissue connecting the inner walls of the uterus), a complication of surgical curettage, as in a D&C or abortion. Also known as *synechia uteri*.

asymptomatic: a disease process that does not change the way a person feels.

Autism Spectrum Disorder (ASD): a condition of people who tend to have communication deficits, such as responding inappropriately in conversations, misreading nonverbal interactions, or having difficulty building friendships appropriate to their age. In addition, people with ASD may have developmental delays in other domains, be overly dependent on routines, highly sensitive to changes in their environment, or intensely focused on inappropriate items.

battery: any unlawful and unpermitted touching of another.

bodily integrity: having personal autonomy and/or self-determination over one's own body. A unique example of a Canadian law that promotes bodily integrity is the Ontario Health Care Consent Act that states that people have the right to consent to, or refuse, treatment, if they have mental capacity to understand and appreciate the consequences of the treatment decision that have been disclosed by their physician.

caesarean section: a surgical operation to deliver an infant.

Cerebral palsy (CP): a generally recognized term that describes a wide spectrum of disabilities related to brain damage occurring before, during or shortly after birth. The most common underlying pathologies are stroke or oxygen deprivation.

cervical incompetence: abnormal weakness of the cervix (the muscle that controls the aperture of the opening of the uterus) that can result in recurrent pregnancy loss. Also known as "cervical insufficiency".

child mortality: the death of a child under the age of 5 years (generally expressed as a rate or percentage).

coding: the international normative way of identifying diseases or symptoms (e.g. fever) by assigning a letter and number. Codes vary according to jurisdiction.

common law: the English law (both criminal and civil) that is based on custom, judicial precedent and statute. In some jurisdictions participants in "common-law" relationships have rights equal to those participants in formal legal relationships such as marriage.

comorbidity: a concomitant but unrelated disease process.

counter narrative: a narrative is a genre of discourse that attempts to make sense of an event or experience and signal this "sense" to others. Narratives order characters in space and connect past events to present states; they are the "real" stories of our lived lives. A counter narrative is a story that contests the claims or "sense" of another's story. Including counter narratives in research adds validity by introducing the ambiguities, inconsistencies and contradictions that arise as interviewees try to find ways to mitigate the interactive trouble of being misconstrued.

depression: is a common medical illness characterized by sadness, loss of interest or pleasure, feelings of guilt or low self-worth, disturbed sleep or appetite, feelings of tiredness, and poor concentration lasting for a period of 2 months or more.

diclofenac: generic name for an anti-inflammatory medication.

dilation: the opening (or dilating) of the cervix during childbirth, miscarriage, induced abortion, or gynecological procedure.

dilation and curettage (D&C): a surgical procedure in which the cervix is stretched open and the lining of the uterus is scraped off and removed.

dilation and evacuation (D&E): a surgical abortion performed by dilating the cervix and using a vacuum aspirator to suction out the fetus or "products of conception".

due care: the conduct that a reasonable man or woman will exercise in a particular situation, in looking out for the safety of others; also known as "due diligence".

dysmenorrhea: pain or discomfort during or just before a menstrual period.

ectopic pregnancy: a pregnancy that develops outside the uterus, most commonly in the fallopian tube, but sometimes in the ovary or, rarely, in the abdominal cavity or cervix; the condition creates a life-threatening situation that requires emergency treatment.

electric aspiration: a suction apparatus powered by electricity that is used in first trimester induced abortions to suction the fetal infant *in utero* and placenta out of the uterus. Short form: EVA.

embryo: a human offspring in the first 8 weeks after conception.

emergency obstetric care: timely medical/nursing or surgical care provided to women experiencing complications during pregnancy or delivery.

et al.: Latin abbreviation used in scientific notation meaning *and others*.

eugenics: Charles Darwin's cousin, Francis Galton, coined the term "eugenics" (Greek for "well-born") in 1883 to describe the process of improving or impairing "the racial qualities of future generations either physically or mentally." Eugenicists promoted sterilization, marriage laws and segregation of the mentally or physically handicapped for the purpose of creating a "superior" race.

feticide: the killing of fetus *in utero* or prior to full egression of the fetus from the birth canal.

fetus (also foetus): an unborn human more than 8 weeks after conception.

fibroids: benign whorls of uterine muscle within the uterine wall.

gendercide: intentional killing of human beings based on gender.

gestation: the period of time between conception and birth when a fetus is carried inside the womb/uterus. The gestational period for human beings is traditionally measured from the date of the onset of the last menstrual period to the time of birth—the average being 40 weeks.

gynecology: a branch of medicine dealing with medical or surgical problems related to the female reproductive organs.

hemorrhage: a copious loss of blood.

hysterectomy: surgical removal of the uterus.

hysteroscopicadhesiolysis: the cutting of adhesions within the uterus with the aid of a special light designed for visualizing the interior of the uterine cavity.

induced abortion: the deliberate termination of pregnancy, resulting in destruction of an embryo or fetus, by means of a surgical procedure, a pharmaceutical product, or other means.

infant mortality: the death of a child under the age of two.

infanticide: the intentional murder of infants.

infertility: the inability to conceive a child.

informed consent: a formal agreement of the patient to a specific course of action based on an adequate explanation about the nature of the proposed investigation or treatment and its anticipated outcome as well as the significant risks involved and alternatives available.

intrapartum: occurring during the time of labour or delivery.

intrauterine adhesions: scar tissue within the uterus secondary to trauma.

intra-uterine device (IUD): a small piece of plastic shaped like a "T" or "7" that is generally impregnated with progesterone or coated in copper that is placed inside the uterus to prevent conception, or the implantation of a fertilized ovum.

laparoscopy: a non-invasive surgical technique using a special flexible light attached to a camera that enables surgery to be done through "key-hole" incisions.

maternal injury: an injury to a mother related to pregnancy or delivery of a child.

maternal mortality: a death of a mother related to pregnancy or delivery of a child often expressed as a rate, or percentage.

maternal mortality ratio (MMR): the number of women who die during pregnancy and childbirth per 100,000 live births.

meta-analysis: a statistical method in which data from a number of similar experimental studies are combined and analyzed together in order to increase statistical power.

miscarriage: the spontaneous end of pregnancy and loss of a child generally in the first trimester; also known as spontaneous abortion.

morbidity: the state or condition of having a disease or symptom complex.

multiparous: having borne more than one child.

neonatal: pertaining to the four-week period following delivery regardless of gestational age at the time of delivery.

nulliparity: having never borne a child of more than 24 weeks gestation. Thus all abortions prior to 24 weeks are not counted in a woman's parity.

obstetrics: the division of medicine that focuses on the care of women during pregnancy, childbirth and the time immediately afterwards.

paracervical block (PCB): a local anaesthetic injected into the nerves around the cervix to diminish the pain caused by dilating the cervix.

parous or parity: a medical descriptor of a woman who has been pregnant and borne a child of a gestational age of 24 weeks or more, regardless of whether the child was alive or dead at the time of birth.

peer review: the evaluation of one's research by experts in the same field in order to maintain, enhance or validate the quality of one's work.

pelvic inflammatory disease (PID): an infection of the female reproductive organs by common sexually transmitted organisms (such as gonorrhea and chlamydia).

perinatal: pertaining to the period before and after delivery. The length of the period is dependent on jurisdiction and varies from starting at the twentieth week of gestation to the 28th week to ending at the first to sixth week after delivery.

peritonitis: a severe potentially life-threatening infection of the lining of the abdominal cavity, the membranes covering the intestines and abdominal organs.

placenta: a fetal maternal organ that connects the developing fetus to the uterine wall to allow nutrient uptake, waste elimination, and oxygen and carbon dioxide exchange via the mother's blood supply.

placenta previa: the natural growth of the placenta in the lower part of the uterus, near or partially or fully covering the internal opening of the cervix. The normal position for a placenta is in the upper portion of the uterus.

postpartum: the period of time following birth.

post-traumatic stress disorder (PTSD): a mental health condition characterized by nightmares, flashbacks and severe anxiety triggered by a terrifying event.

prenatal: the time period following conception and before birth.

preterm birth: the birth of a human baby under 37 weeks' gestation.

primigravida: a woman who is pregnant for the first time.

primiparous: an adjective used to denote a woman who has delivered a child of a gestational age greater than, or equal to, 24 weeks regardless of outcome.

psychotherapy: the treatment of mental disorders by psychological means.

qualitative research: a method of inquiry that seeks to understand human behavior and the reasons that govern such behavior by asking 'why' and 'how' questions of individuals using such techniques as focus groups or interviews.

quantitative research: the systematic empirical investigation of social phenomena via statistical, mathematical or computational techniques.

reporting bias: selective revealing or suppression of information by subjects involved in a study or the attribution of unexpected or undesirable experimental results to sampling or measurement errors by authors of a study.

sepsis: a systemic illness caused by microbial invasion of normally sterile parts of the body. Sepsis with organ damage has a mortality rate of 25 to 30 per cent and when accompanied by "shock" has a mortality rate of 40 to 70 per cent.

sequelae: secondary adverse results or complications of a disease, disorder, injury or medical or surgical intervention.

sex ratio at birth (SRB): the ratio of males to females at birth in a population.

sex-selective abortion: an abortion induced because the sex of the child *in utero* is not desired. This practice targets female children almost exclusively.

sexually transmitted disease (STD): an infection transmitted by bodily fluids during sexual activity.

sonography: a diagnostic imaging technique that uses ultrasound.

spontaneous abortion: the unintended delivery and death of a child *in utero* with a gestational age younger than 24 weeks, known as a 'miscarriage.' Eighty per cent of spontaneous abortions occur prior to eight weeks gestation due to a lethal chromosomal anomaly in the embryo.

sterilization: a medical term denoting a procedure that renders a fertile person infertile.

stillbirth: a baby of a gestational age greater than 23 weeks and five days that is born dead.

tort law: law that deals with legal actions between two individuals or organizations that do not involve the state (government) or a contract.

Trisomy 13: a genetic disorder in which there is an extra chromosome number 13, also known as Papau syndrome.

Trisomy 18: a genetic disorder in which there is an extra chromosome number 18, also known as Edwards syndrome.

Trisomy 21: a genetic disorder in which there is an extra chromosome number 21, also known as Down syndrome.

ultrasound: a diagnostic imaging modality that utilizes sound waves.

unsafe abortion: a procedure for terminating an unintended pregnancy carried out either by persons lacking the necessary skills or in an environment that does not conform to minimal medical standards, or both.

uterine perforation: a tear or rip in the uterine wall.

INDEX

Abortion
    chemical, 2, 102, 199, 211-2, 220
        See also medical or drug-induced.
    complications, 170-1, 177, 186-7, 207-8, 213, 218, 220, 301, 308, 327, 340, 345-6, 356, 358, 361
    physical, 89-252
    psychological, 253-365
    D&C (dilation and curettage), 92, 105, 190, 249
    D&E (dilation and extraction), 100, 188
    the experience of, 319-65
    failed, 30, 35-7, 95, 100-108, 213-4, 216, 219,
    failure rate, 101-2, 104, 212, 214-5, 220, 362
        See also Abortion, failed.
    first-trimester, 99, 103, 113, 119, 135, 147, 149, 150, 152, 172, 184, 188, 190, 192, 199, 212, 214, 218, 219, 249, 276, 309, 318
    hysterectomy, 92, 186-7, 288, 346
    hysterotomy, 92
    illegal, 6, 17, 20-1, 25-6, 30, 34-8, 62, 66-7, 70, 72-3, 122, 206, 267, 360
    incomplete. *See* Abortion, failed.
    induced, 1-3, 5, 8, 11-12, 19, 21-5, 28, 34-8, 40, 42, 51, 75, 85, 88-100, 102-3, 108-9, 111-113, 114-129, 131, 134-6, 138-9, 142, 151, 167-181, 183-92, 195, 199- 209, 211-220, 234-45, 252-5, 259, 261, 266, 269, 270, 274, 279, 281-2, 286, 289, 293-9, 302, 318, 320, 350, 352, 358-9, 361-4.
    See also Abortion, medical or drug-induced.
    late-term, 56, 104, 127, 164
    legalization of, 2, 8, 22, 28-31, 33-4, 35-7, 57-73, 122-3, 253, 257-70, 357, 363.
    Crime, abortion's impact on; Child Sexual Abuse (CSA).
    medical or drug-induced, 211-220.
        See also Abortion, induced.
    misinformation about, 139, 152-3, 161.
        See also Informed consent.

unsafe, 18-20, 30, 32, 35-28
politics of, 11, 37-8, 90, 100, 116, 136-7, 139-41, 201, 205, 207-8, 254, 271-2, 279
breast cancer, 90, 100, 116, 136-7, 139-41
maternal mortality, 37-8, 201, 205, 207-8
mental health, 254, 271-2, 279
reasons for, 46, 222, 259, 279, 285, 297, 306-7, 309
repeat, 170
second-trimester, 100, 103, 113, 147, 150, 188, 189, 191, 199, 215, 216, 217, 218
spontaneous (miscarriage), 107
surgical, 16, 89, 91-4, 95, 98-104, 106-8, 167-8, 172, 178-81, 183, 188, 193, 199, 211-17, 219-20, 236, 243, 248-50, 358, 361-2
therapeutic, 77, 171, 187, 307, 309
unsuccessful. *See* Abortion, failed.
Abortion clinics, providers, 89, 94, 97, 171, 172, 205, 207, 250, 302, 336-40, 346, 355, 358
follow up, 89, 302, 346, 355
Abuse, 3, 53, 252-3, 255, 257, 264-6, 270, 280, 286-7, 288-99, 327, 359-60, 363-4.
See also Intimate Partner Violence (IPV).
child abuse, 252-3, 257, 264-6, 270, 288-9, 292-3, 295, 363. *See also* Child Sexual Abuse (CSA).
verbal abuse, 327
Adoption, 64, 260, 268, 330
African-American women, 90, 128-9
breast cancer, 90, 128-9
Ambivalence, 233, 250, 291
American Medical Association (AMA), 76-8
American Psychological Association (APA), 1, 254, 279-80, 301, 303, 309-12, 318, 363-4
Amniocentesis, 6, 47, 3, 90, 146, 148-50, 226, 360
Anxiety, 5, 10, 12, 14, 154, 247, 250-2, 254-5, 266, 271, 274, 279, 280-1, 283, 289, 314, 316, 336, 346, 349-51, 354, 363
Asherman's Syndrome (intrauterine adhesions), 91, 179, 183, 185-6, 189, 193, 351. *See also* Endometrium.

Autism Spectrum Disorder (ASD), 3, 93, 235, 239, 240-5, 259, 362

Autoimmune disorders, autoimmune disease, 92, 195-200. *See* Microchimerism.

Battery, 79-80. *See also* Consent law.

Behavioural and social outcomes, 240
    crime, 2, 7-8, 48, 54-5, 57-73, 357

Bias, 49, 51, 52, 100, 101, 104, 125, 129-39, 152, 156, 174, 176, 205, 221, 241, 273, 274-5, 278-9, 312-18. *See also* Methodology.

Birth control, 62, 122, 138, 208, 298, 299
    See also Contraception.

Birth weight, 3, 93-4, 179, 189-90, 235-6, 239, 240-1, 243, 289-90, 362. *See also* Preterm.

Bleeding, 10, 18, 89, 98-100, 102, 106-8.
    See also Hemorrhage, Uterine bleeding.

Blindness, 93, 159, 235, 238, 362

Breast cancer. *See* Cancer.

Brind, Joel, 120, 131-3

Canada, Canadians, 7, 11, 13, 41, 51, 67, 71-2, 78-80, 82, 85, 86, 87, 92, 96-8, 100, 104, 105, 144, 146-8, 150, 152, 154, 160, 161, 174, 201-2, 204-8, 212, 216, 217, 223, 237, 243, 245, 250, 253, 265, 305, 307, 314-5, 320, 329, 349

Canadian Medical Association (CMA), 76-8, 307

Canadian Medical Certificates of Death, 207.
    See also Mortality, politics of abortion.

Cancer, 1, 2, 8, 75, 88, 89-90, 95, 96, 109-42, 176, 198, 216, 241-2, 346, 349, 351-3, 358-9, 363,
    of the breast, 1, 2, 8, 75, 88, 89-90, 95, 96, 109-42, 176, 241-2, 346, 349, 358-9, 363,
    of the cervix, 198, 346, 351-3

Centers for Disease Control (CDC), 61, 107, 144, 202, 205-7, 224, 240

Cerebral palsy, 3, 6, 40-2, 93, 105, 159, 235, 238-40, 243-5, 362

Cervix, cervical damage, cervical dilation, cervical incompetence, cervical insufficiency, cervical trauma, cervical lacerations, paracervical block, 2, 89, 91-2, 95-6, 100-1, 105-7, 112, 117-8, 150, 168-9, 179, 181, 183, 188-90, 193, 213, 215, 236, 243, 249-50, 346, 351, 361

Child abuse. *See* Abuse.

Childbirth, safety of, 93, 201-9, 362

Children, 1, 2, 3, 6, 7, 8, 40, 48, 52, 53, 56, 57, 61-6, 68, 72-3, 90, 91-4, 103-4, 106, 116, 119, 138, 144-6, 148, 153, 158-65, 218, 232-4, 235, 239-44, 253, 258-60, 264-70, 302, 317, 320-4, 327-9, 346, 349, 351-6, 357, 360, 362, 364. *See also* Premature; Child Sexual Abuse (CSA); Relationships; Families

unwanted, 7, 61-6, 68, 73

Chile, 5-6, 17, 19, 20-3, 39, 43, 357

Child Sexual Abuse (CSA), 264-6, 286, 288, 293, 295

China, 1, 6, 47-8, 53, 55, 104, 114-5, 121, 123, 138, 190, 212, 215, 357

One Child Policy, 6, 48, 123

Chlamydia trachomatis, 167, 169-72, 181

Choice, the illusion of, 3, 7, 52-3, 151-6, 228, 230, 255, 285, 286, 294-5, 299, 305, 332-3, 345, 354

Chorionic villi sampling (CVS), 90, 150, 360

Coding, 100, 187, 204, 207, 208,
of maternal mortality/morbidity, 204, 207, 208

Coercion, duress, pressure to abort, 10, 53, 86-7, 151, 222, 228, 230, 255, 286, 294-5, 299, 301, 303, 306-7, 319, 333-4, 354, 364. *See also* Pressure.

Coleman, Priscilla K, 254, 265-6, 269, 273, 275-82, 297

Complications. *See* Abortion.

consent, *See* Informed consent.

Contraception, 36, 62, 114, 136, 258-9, 261, 269, 292, 298, 321-2

Counselling, 12-15, 105, 143, 148, 150, 152, 157-9, 161, 279, 307-8, 314, 317, 324, 326, 327, 331

Crack-cocaine epidemic, 7, 57, 60, 71, 292

Crime, abortion's impact on, 2, 7-8, 54, 55, 57-73, 357

Daling, Janet, 124, 138

Denial and repression, 16, 234, 343-4

Denmark, Danish, 92-3, 98, 115-6, 121, 132-3, 145-6, 153, 202-3, 209, 254, 276-7, 282, 315

Depression, 5, 10, 12, 14, 55, 85, 89, 143, 163, 221, 250-2, 254-5, 266, 269, 271-83, 287-9, 297, 301-2, 303, 314-7, 340, 342, 346-7, 355-6, 359-60, 363-5

D&C (Dilation and curettage). *See* Abortion

D&E (Dilation and extraction). *See* Abortion

Domestic Violence. *See* Intimate Partner Violence.

'Dose-response' effect, 115, 121, 236

Down syndrome. *See* Trisomy 21.

Drugs. *See* Substance abuse, coercion.

Duress. *See* Informed consent.

Duty and breach of. *See* Informed consent.

Dysphoria. *See* Guilt.

Eating disorders, 271, 342

Echlin, Jean, palliative-care nurse, 1, 349-55

Ectopic pregnancy, 11, 22, 23, 91, 95, 96, 104, 167, 173, 174, 177-81, 187, 203, 204, 205, 208, 218, 220, 237, 361

Embodiment, 290

Embolism, 204, 207

Emergency Obstetric Care (EmOC), 6, 17, 19, 23, 25, 28, 39, 43, 357

Endometritis, 168, 171, 181

Endometrium, Asherman's Syndrome, 91, 179, 183-6, 189, 193, 351

England, *See* United Kingdom.

Epidemiology, 109-42

Epilepsy, 93, 235, 238, 362

European Society of Human Reproduction and Embryology, 237

Europe, 40-3, 51, 73, 122, 125, 127, 144, 145, 148, 171, 205, 227, 321

Families, fathers, husbands, parents, 3, 9-11, 13, 15-16, 50-4, 57, 64, 68, 86, 125, 143, 148-9, 150, 153, 156, 159-61, 164-5, 175, 204, 207, 221, 222, 228, 229, 232, 253, 257-70, 293, 298, 305, 307, 316, 320, 322, 324, 325, 328, 329, 334, 335, 349, 351-3, 355, 363, 365. *See also* Abuse, Men, Relationships, premarital, Adolescents, Marriage, Single-Parenthood, Children, One Child Policy.

Fertility, 22, 54, 61-4, 71-2, 138, 163, 175, 177, 178, 185, 250, 264, 291. *See also* Infertility, Subfecundity.

Fetus, 2, 48, 51, 82, 86, 93, 101, 103-5, 117-18, 144, 146-7, 149-50, 152, 154, 156, 159, 164, 188, 196, 199, 212-13, 219, 221-2, 225-8, 231-2, 234, 242, 251, 260, 289, 308-9, 340, 355, 361
    fetal abnormalities, anomalies and disabilities, 30, 91, 106, 143, 146, 149, 151, 153, 156, 162-4, 211, 226-8
    fetal deaths, 105, 131, 144, 225, 231, 289

Fever, 10, 186

Finland, 92, 99, 102,
    and breast cancer, 121
    and maternal mortality, 202-3, 209

Genetic anomalies, diseases, testing, 46, 51, 150, 156, 164

Gestational age, 100, 188, 214, 218, 227, 236-240, 288, 308, *See also* Prematurity.

Gonorrhea, 168-9. *See also* Pelvic inflammatory disease (PID)

Grief, 5, 9, 10-12, 15-6, 105, 162-3, 232, 234, 266, 279, 287, 327, 329-30, 339, 351, 355, 365

Guilt (dysphoria), 12, 14, 85, 105, 221, 222, 232, 233, 253, 257, 266, 283, 288, 330, 341, 343, 351, 363, 364

Guttmacher Institute, 202, 262

Healing, psychological, spiritual, 5, 9-16, 229, 302, 305, 316, 319, 330, 343-4, 347-8, 356, 365
    organizations, 13-15
    Abortion Recovery International (ARIN), 13
    Project Rachel, 13-15
    reconciliation, forgiveness, 5, 9, 13-5, 330, 343-4, 347, 350-2, 356, 365

Hemorrhage, 18, 27, 39, 89, 95-6, 98, 101, 106-7, 108, 187, 204, 207, 215, 220, 225

Hungary, Hungarian, 6, 17, 40, 42, 240, 357

Hysteroscopicadhesiolysis, 186. *See* Endometrium.

Hysterectomy. *See* Abortion.

Hysterotomy. *See* Abortion.

In vitro fertilization, 174-5, 221-5, 227, 229, 233-4

India, 1, 6-7, 47, 49-50, 51, 53, 55, 104, 116, 156, 179, 215, 285, 289, 297, 357

Infanticide, 48, 68
Infection, 10, 89, 95, 96, 98-9, 101, 103, 106-8, 150, 167-81, 186, 189, 204, 213, 217-8, 243, 288, 346, 356, 361, 362. *See also* Chlamydia trachomatis, Endometritis, Pelvic Inflammatory Disease, pelvis, uterine infection.
Infertility, 2, 91, 95, 96, 167-81, 183, 185-6, 193, 221, 223, 229, 232, 233, 288, 346, 361-2. *See also* Fertility.
Informed consent, 2, 8, 75-88, 142, 147, 151-8, 164-5, 175, 208, 221, 222, 228-30, 234, 245, 305, 307-10, 325
   duty, and breach of, 76, 80-2, 84, 87, 208
   ethical and legal codes, 76-9
   lawsuits, 8, 85
   and MFPR, 222, 228-30, 234
   negligence, 79, 80, 84
   and pain, degree of, 250,
   and prenatal testing, 151-8
   professional misconduct, 78-9
   right to, 2, 8, 76, 82-3, 87, 250, 357
Injury, physical, 8, 30, 35, 80 -81, 84, 85, 91, 112, 168, 184, 188, 255, 287, 289, 292. *See also* Negligence, Complications.
Intellectual impairment, 3, 241-2, 359
Intimate Partner Violence, 3, 255, 285-99, 364
Intrauterine adhesions. *See* Endometrium.
Isolation, alienation, 55, 287, 340, 343
Laparascopic sterilization, 184
Macrosomia, 290
Malpractice, 79, 207. *See also* Medical liability, Informed consent, professional misconduct.
Marriage, 7, 49, 54, 55, 61-3, 161, 222, 257-64, 268-9, 297, 316, 346, 351-2, 364
Maternal mortality. *See* Mortality.
Medical liability, 140, 152, 157
   See also Informed consent.
Men, 363.
   effects of abortion on, 285-6, 333-34, 349, 353
   powerlessness, disenfranchisement, 12
   legal rights, 85

paternal support, 268
pressure on women to abort, 63, 86, 151, 260, 268, 278, 295, 301, 303, 306, 316, 319, 324, 332, 353, 355
roles and responsibilities of, 258
trust, 287, 331, 346

Mental health, 3, 13, 29, 65, 254-55, 266, 269-83, 288, 309, 311-12, 328, 346, 363, 365. *See also* Anxiety, Coleman, Priscilla K, Depression, Grief, Guilt, Post-traumatic stress disorder (PTSD), Regret, Shame, Suicide.

Mental retardation. *See* Intellectual impairment.

Methodology, 100, 116, 134, 137, 201, 203, 209, 274, 282, 305, 362
biased, 52, 101, 156, 221, 274,
faulty, 91, 161, 201, 209,

Microchimerism, fetal, 195-200, 361

Mifepristone, 103-4, 211-20

Miscarriage. *See* Abortion, spontaneous.

Misoprostol, 103-4, 211-20

Morgantaler clinic, 250-1

Mortality, 6, 17-43, 92, 93, 164, 201-9, 217-8, 228, 235, 245, 281-2, 289, 291-2, 357, 362-3
adolescent, teenage, 265
infant, perinatal, 6, 17-43, 49, 93, 235, 245
maternal, 6, 17-34, 37-40, 42, 92, 164, 201-9, 217-8, 281-2, 289, 291-2, 357, 362-3. *See also* Hemorrhage, Suicide, Coding, United Kingdom, Scandinavia, Finland, Denmark, United States.
causes of, 18, 28, 39, 53, 181, 185, 196, 249, 292,
likelihood of, 100, 178, 190, 226, 240, 266, 275,
rate of, 3, 27, 33, 40-1, 62, 90-1, 95, 97-106, 108, 118, 147, 163,
risk of, 1-3, 8, 12, 30, 41, 65, 80, 84, 89, 91, 92-3, 99, 100, 104-7, 109-13, 115
biased statistics, 152, 204
reducing maternal mortality, 347
reporting system, 204, 206,
politicization of, 362

Moster, Dag, 238-9

Multi-fetal pregnancy reduction (MFPR), 221-234
Multiparity. *See* Pregnancy.
Nausea, 216, 217, 287, 288, 324, 362
Negligence, 79, 80, 84, *See also* Informed consent.
Neural tube defects, 150
   spina bifida, 145-7
Ney, Philip, 264-265
North America, 2, 16, 51, 79, 81, 100, 110, 116, 148, 159, 162, 201, 204, 205, 207-8, 223, 227-8, 240, 257, 340, 365
Nulliparity. *See* Pregnancy.
One Child Policy. *See* China.
Pain, 81, 94, 101, 167, 173, 216-7, 222, 247-9, 252, 283, 287-8, 305, 317, 325-6, 227-8, 342-3, 350, 352, 356
   pain perception, 250, 251
   severity of, 222, 251
   treatment of, 349, 353-4
   trivialization of, 252, 358
Pelvic Inflammatory Disease (PID), 91, 167-75, 178, 181, 288, 361-2
Perinatal palliative care, 91, 149, 158, 361
Planned Parenthood, 87-8, 102, 141, 172, 208, 336, 345, 355
Placenta, 92, 95, 96, 101, 103, 179, 183, 185, 190-3, 200, 361
   problems with, 101, 103, 185, 192, 200
   previa, 92, 95, 96, 179, 183, 190-3, 361
Population policy, 48, 322. *See also* China, One-Child Policy.
Post-traumatic Stress Disorder (PTSD), 143, 163, 184, 251-2, 287-9
Poverty, 8, 26, 29, 51, 58, 68, 253, 257, 267-9, 270, 308, 329, 357, 363
   feminization of, 253, 257, 257-9, 270, 363
Pregnancy, 9-13, 15-16, 18, 22, 28, 30, 46-8, 56, 62, 65, 86, 89-94, 100-101, 103, 105, 109-13, 116-19, 121-2, 125-8, 133, 135, 138, 141-4, 146, 148, 153-5, 157-9, 161-5, 167, 169-70, 174-7, 180-1, 184-6, 188-9, 190, 193, 195-200, 202-9, 212-4, 222-3, 226-34, 275-8, 281-2, 286-299, 306-10, 324, 326, 329-334, 336, 340, 345, 355, 358-60. *See also* Ectopic pregnancy.
   Early Pregnancy Factor, 198
   multiparity, 189

nulliparity, 89, 112, 126, 188
outside of marriage, 61-3, 258-260, 269
primiparity, 48
unwanted, 65, 266, 278, 292, 294, 298-9, 336, 360

Prematurity, premature births, preterm, low-weight births, 3, 40-1, 92-4, 111, 113, 128-9, 179, 180, 188-9, 190, 225, 231, 235-9, 238, 240-5, 290, 361, 362,
causes of, 18, 28, 39, 53, 181

Prenatal testing and genetic diagnosis, 2, 90-1, 143-65, 360-1
and eugenics, 91, 148, 158, 165
and disabilities rights movement, 152, 158-65

Pressure, 53, 86-7, 93, 136, 151, 153, 160, 259, 260, 268, 278, 295, 301, 303, 306-7, 316-17, 319-20, 324-5, 327, 333-6, 354, 360, 364. *See also* Coercion, Duress, Politics.

Preterm. *See* Prematurity.

Primiparity. *See* Pregnancy.

Prostaglandin, 102-3, 213

Psychiatric or mental illnesses or disturbances, 90-1, 156, 271-83, 329

Psychic or emotional numbing [affect], 317

Psychological impact, 257-83, 312-18, 340-7
harm, distress, 8, 85-8, 283, 363

Reardon, David, 347

Refused abortion, 253, 260, 324

Regret, 3, 154, 162, 301-2, 315, 317, 319, 329, 330-1, 338, 340-5, 355, 363. *See also* Guilt.

Relationships, impact of abortion on, 5, 10, 14-16. *See also* Families.
break-ups, dissolution, 161, 261-2, 346, 364
divorce, 161, 262-3, 346, 352
loss of sexual desire, libido, intimacy, sexual dysfunction, 316-7, 364
marriage, 49, 54-5, 61-3, 161, 222, 257-64, 268, 269, 297, 316-7, 346, 352, 364
parent-child, 65-6, 68, 73
premarital sexual, 62-3, 257, 259-60, 269

Relief, 301, 338, 339, 340-5, 347, 355

Religion, religious values, 10, 13-16, 45, 49, 137, 232, 259, 302, 305, 328, 345, 347, 354
Buddhist, 15

Catholic, 13-14, 345
Christianity, 13, 14-15, 347
Muslim, Islam, 328
Right-to-Know laws, 8, 75, 87. *See also* Informed consent.
Roe v. Wade, 59, 65, 68
Royal College of Obstetricians and Gynaecologists, 99, 106, 168, 184, 188, 358
RU-186. *See* Misopristone.
Sárkány, Jenö, 240
Saunders, Cicely, 350
Screening, 143-65, 240
Secrecy, 342, 344, 352, 353
Self-harm, self-destructive behaviour, 14, 301, 340, 346. *See also* Suicide.
Self-esteem, self-respect, 11, 316, 330, 331, 340, 342, 343, 346
Sex, as a risk factor, 240-1
Sexual dysfunction, 288, 316, 364
Sexually-transmitted disease (STD) or infection (STI), 54-5, 168, 181, 288
Sexual revolution, 63
Sex-selection, 6-7, 45-56
Shame, 14, 253, 266, 279, 287, 328, 337, 340, 343-5. *See also* Guilt.
Siblings, effect of abortion on, 10, 65, 267
Single-parenthood, 57, 63, 257-60, 268-9
Smoking, 90, 128, 140, 269, 317
Spina bifida. *See* Neural tube defects.
Spiritual impact, 5, 9-16, 302, 319, 329-30, 340, 343, 347-56
Subfecundity. *See* Infertility.
Substance abuse, 255, 266, 269, 271-83
Suicide, attempted suicide, 12, 163, 202-4, 209, 254-5, 271, 274, 278, 281-2, 283, 287, 292, 302, 314, 317, 326, 328, 340-1, 346, 355, 363. ,
See also Adolescents Mortality.
suicidal ideation, 287, 314, 317, 340, 346, 355,
Sweden, Swedish, 66, 121, 130, 156, 231, 238, 267
Third World, developing world, 7, 39-40, 212, 218-9, 320, 329
Trisomy 21, 91, 145-8, 150-3, 157, 161, 164
Trauma, 10, 92, 93, 163, 165, 168, 184, 185, 188-9, 227,

229, 232, 261, 288-9, 311, 330, 339, 355, 364, 365. *See also* Post-traumatic stress disorder (PTSD).

Ultrasonography (ultrasound), 7, 47, 49, 52, 82, 90, 147, 150, 153-4, 232, 324-5

United Kingdom, 8, 43, 68-70, 73, 121-2. *See also* Europe.
England, 69-70, 121-2, 145, 167, 212
Ireland, Northern Ireland, Irish Republic, Republic of Ireland, 6, 17, 40, 42-3, 69-70, 73, 121-2, 357
Scotland, 69-70, 121-2, 132, 237
Wales, 69-70, 121, 145, 212

United States (U.S.), America, Americans, 8, 13, 15, 41, 50-1, 55, 57-60, 62, 66-7, 69-70, 76-80, 82, 87, 90, 97, 99-100, 107, 114, 123, 124, 129, 141, 165, 168, 172, 177, 191, 196, 202, 204-8, 212, 215, 217, 218, 224, 225, 236-7, 243, 255, 258, 280, 287, 290, 292, 295, 310, 312, 320, 329-48, 358-9, 364. *See also* Crime, abortion's impact on; Centers for Disease Control (CDC); North America; American Psychological Association (APA); American Medical Association (AMA); African-Americans; American College of Obstetrics and Gynecology (ACOG), 140 and maternal mortality, 201, 202, 205-9, 217

Unwanted pregnancy, 62, 65-6, 266-7, 277-8, 292-3, 294, 298, 299, 336
and intimate partner violence, 292-3

Uterine
adhesions, 92, 190, 243
bleeding, 187, 190. *See also* Hemorrhage.
perforations, 2, 89, 91, 95, 96, 98, 100, 106, 168, 183, 184-5, 186, 189, 193, 217, 362
rupture, 186, 218, 362

Women's voices, narratives, 303-18, 319-65
at the end of life, 349-56

World Health Organization (WHO), 18-19, 28, 156, 204-6, 293-4
reporting guidelines of, 205-6

Wrongful birth, 147, 152

About the authors

ANGELA LANFRANCHI, MD, is a practising breast surgeon, Fellow of the American College of Surgeons, and Clinical Assistant Professor of Surgery at Robert Wood Johnson Medical School in New Jersey.

IAN GENTLES is a Fellow of the Royal Historical Society, and Professor of History at York University and Tyndale University College, Toronto, where he teaches a seminar on the history of human population. He is also the Research Director of the deVeber Institute for Bioethics and Social Research.

ELIZABETH RING-CASSIDY, Reg. Psych.(AB), MA(Psych)., is a Registered Psychologist, specializing in Development Psychology and Research. She is the Director of Student Services at Our Lady Seat of Wisdom Academy in Barry's Bay, Ontario and a Senior Research Associate at the deVeber Institute. Her areas of research include: child abuse, the psychological implications of abortion as well as assisted reproductive technologies.

To contact the deVeber Institute or the authors or to order *Complications: Abortion's Impact on Women*:

The deVeber Institute for Bioethics and Social Research

415 Oakdale Road Unit #215., Toronto, ON M3N 1W7

Telephone: 416-256-0555   Fax: 416-256-0611

Email: bioethics@deveber.org

Website: www.deveber.org